OCT Imaging in Glaucoma

Ki Ho Park • Tae-Woo Kim
Editors

OCT Imaging in Glaucoma

A guide for practitioners

Springer

Editors
Ki Ho Park
Department of Ophthalmology
Seoul National University Hospital
Seoul
Korea

Tae-Woo Kim
Department of Ophthalmology
Seoul National University Bundang
Hospital
Seongnam
Korea

ISBN 978-981-16-1180-3 ISBN 978-981-16-1178-0 (eBook)
https://doi.org/10.1007/978-981-16-1178-0

This Springer imprint is published by the registered company Springer Nature Singapore Pte Ltd.
The registered company address is: 152 Beach Road, #21-01/04 Gateway East, Singapore 189721, Singapore

Preface

Glaucoma is one of the leading causes of blindness. One cannot emphasize too much the importance of early detection of glaucoma to maintain patients' quality of life. The technology for imaging the optic nerve to detect glaucoma in its early stage and monitor the disease progression has been greatly advanced in recent decades. The use of optical coherence tomography (OCT), one of the top technologies, has expanded rapidly in our daily practice.

Nowadays, artificial intelligence combined with normative database of OCT helps us to interpret test results more accurately and conveniently. However, understanding the basic principles, algorithms, strengths, and weaknesses of OCT will enrich our knowledge and guide our decision-making with higher confidence in clinics. Further, the capacity of OCT to look into the deeper as well as microstructures of the optic nerve head and macula including their vasculature will significantly enhance our insight into the nature of glaucomatous neuronal damage.

We would like to thank all the authors from our department who contributed chapters herein. They are all experts on their respective subjects.

It is our hope that this book will be a rich source of information and guidance for practicing ophthalmologists, glaucoma specialists, and trainees.

Finally, we would like to extend great thanks and love to our families for their continuous support and encouragement, without which we could not have accomplished our goals.

Seoul, Korea

Ki Ho Park
Tae-Woo Kim

Contents

Principles of OCT Imaging

Kyoung Min Lee

Abstract

Optical coherence tomography (OCT) uses the interference between the light waves reflected by the reference and sample arms to obtain spatial information on tissue microstructure, which is used to construct an in-vivo cross-sectional image. OCT has become an essential part of daily practice in the field of ophthalmology and glaucoma over the past 30 years. This success was possible by tremendous advances of its technology toward better sensitivity and faster scan speed from Time-domain to Spectral-domain and Swept-source OCT. This chapter was written to describe the basic principles of OCT and how they enable its various applications, which are crucial to understand how such advances of OCT have been possible in the past, and why OCT still has boundless potential for future growth.

Keywords

Optical coherence tomography · Interferometer · Fourier transformation Spectral-domain OCT · Swept-source OCT

1 Introduction

Modern progress in medicine has largely been driven by the advent of tomographic imaging techniques such as X-ray computed tomography (CT), magnetic resonance imaging (MRI), and ultrasound imaging. These can generate a cross-sectional image of living tissue, thereby locating the diseased portion. Optical coherence tomography (OCT), meanwhile, can be described as the optical analog of ultrasound imaging (Huang et al. 1991; Fercher et al. 2003; Fercher 2010; Popescu et al. 2011; Drexler et al. 2014; Fujimoto and Swanson 2016; Aumann et al. 2019). In ultrasound imaging, a sound pulse is launched, the echoes of which are measured to create a cross-sectional image. In OCT, correspondingly, a light pulse is launched, but its reflections—in the aspect of its delays—cannot be measured directly because of its fast velocity; instead, the interference between the light waves reflected by the reference and sample arms, respectively, is measured to obtain spatial information on tissue microstructure. To understand this more deeply, let us start with light and its wave-like behavior.

K. M. Lee (✉)
Seoul National University Boramae Medical Center, Dongjak-gu, Seoul, Korea
e-mail: isletz00@snu.ac.kr

K. H. Park, T.-W. Kim (eds.), *OCT Imaging in Glaucoma*,
https://doi.org/10.1007/978-981-16-1178-0_1

2 Light

Light is an electromagnetic phenomenon. A particle that carries an electric charge (q_0) will generate an electric field (E) with different amounts of force (F_e) on a charge at different locations: $E/q_0 = F_e$. This in turn will generate an electromagnetic field that is well explained by Maxwell's equations (Brezinski 2006a) as follows:

1. Gauss' law for electric fields: $\nabla \bullet D = \rho$, which means that the net outward flow (D) through a closed surface is equal to the total charge (ρ) enclosed by that surface.
2. Gauss' law for a magnetic field: $\nabla \bullet B = 0$, which means that the divergence of the magnetic flux (B) is always zero and that there are no isolated magnetic changes.
3. Faraday's law: $\nabla \times E = -\partial B/\partial t$, which means that a magnetic field (B) change over time (t) produces an electric field (E).
4. Ampere's law: $\nabla \times H = J + \partial D/\partial t$, which means that a changing electric field (D) produces a magnetic field (H).

That is, a changing electric field produces a magnetic field, whereas a changing magnetic field produces an electric field. Since the two fields recreate each other indefinitely, a light can propagate in free space as an oscillating wave with the electric and magnetic fields located perpendicularly to each other (Fig. 1a). Each light, as an oscillating wave, has a frequency (f) and wavelength (λ): $c = f \times \lambda$. The energy transmitted by the light is proportional to the frequency: $E = h \times f$ (h =Planck's constant).

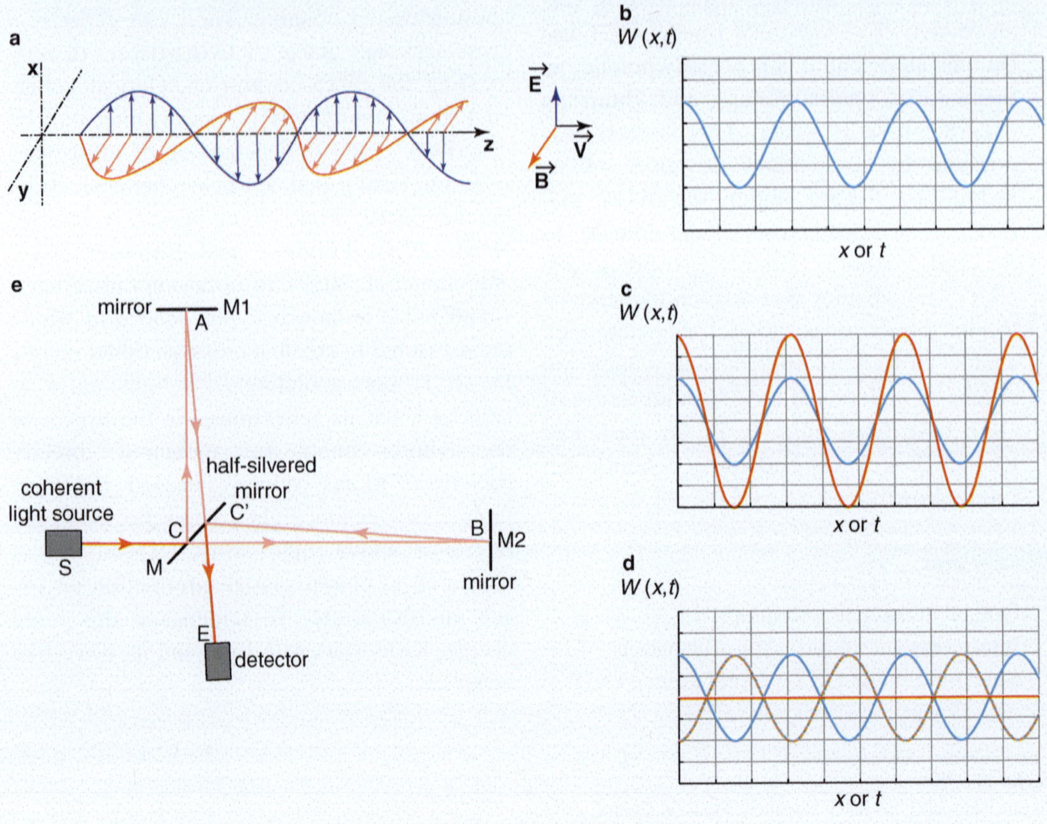

Fig. 1 Interference and Michelson interferometer. By mutual production, electric and magnetic waves can propagate eternally in space with a fixed oscillatory component: a frequency (**a**; figure taken from Wikipedia). The summation of two waves with the same frequency (**b**) can produce constructive (**c**) or destructive (**d**) interference according to a phase delay. The interference can be measured using the Michelson interferometer (**e**). The pattern of interference is determined by twice the length difference between M_1 and M_2 (round trip)

2.1 Interference

A point in a wave is determined by its spatial location (x) and time (t) (Fig. 1b).

$W_1(x,t) = A\cos(kx - \omega t)$, where A is the peak amplitude, $k = 2\pi/\lambda$ is the wavenumber, and $\omega = 2\pi f$ is the angular frequency of the wave. A second wave with a phase delay (φ) is $W_2(x,t) = A\cos(kx - \omega t + \varphi)$.

The summation of the two waves is as follows:

$$W_1 + W_2 = A\cos(kx - \omega t) + A\cos(kx - \omega t + \varphi) = 2A\cos\frac{\varphi}{2}\cos\left(kx - \omega t + \frac{\varphi}{2}\right)$$

This equation reveals that the new wave shares the same frequency and wavelength (both k and ω are unchanged). The amplitude of the new wave is determined by a factor of $2\cos\frac{\varphi}{2}$. When φ is an even multiple of π, $\left|\cos\frac{\varphi}{2}\right| = 1$, and so the amplitude is doubled, which phenomenon is known as constructive interference (Fig. 1c). When φ is an odd multiple of π, $\left|\cos\frac{\varphi}{2}\right| = 0$, and so the amplitude becomes zero, which phenomenon is known as destructive interference (Fig. 1d) (Brezinski 2006b).

More generally, if both the initial wave (W_1) and the summation of the initial and reflected waves ($W_1 + W_2$) are provided, the phase delay (φ) of W_2 can be calculated. The Michelson Interferometer is designed to measure this interference phenomenon (Fig. 1e). A beam splitter directs the course of light against two different mirrors (M_1 and M_2). Both mirrors reflect the lights: they share the same frequency and wavelength, but the lengths of their light paths are different (Fig. 1e). If the two mirrors reflect the lights equally, the length of difference alone determines the phase delay.

2.2 Coherence

To this point, calculations were based on light with a single frequency (monochromatic light). But real light sources are never monochromatic, even laser sources being quasi-monochromatic, for two reasons. First, light is produced by atomic transitions from a higher-energy state to a lower one, and the energy is directly related to the frequency: $E = h \times f$. The problem is that while the atoms are in the excited state, they are colliding, which results in the loss or gain of some energy. So, the energy and the frequency vary, they are not fixed, even from the beginning. Second, the atoms emitting light are moving in different directions, which fact, given that the interaction of light with a moving object results in a Doppler shift, induces a frequency shift (Brezinski 2006b).

Coherence is a measure of inter-wave correlation. Since a wave is dependent on spatial location (x) and time (t), coherence is measured in both the spatial and temporal aspects. Here, let us focus on temporal coherence. As the frequencies of different waves get closer and closer, the time during which the waves are in unison–the coherence time–will become longer and longer. On the other hand, the lights have a broader spectrum of frequencies, the lower the chances are that the waves will be in unison, and, correspondingly, the shorter the coherence time becomes. The coherence length is the distance that light travels during the coherence time; it signifies that the properties of the beam retain relatively constant characteristics only over that unit of length. Using the Michelson interferometer, the length difference can be detected only within the limit of the coherence length. Therefore, the coherence length is directly associated with the axial resolution, and that is why low-coherence light, which has broader spectral bandwidth, is preferred for Time-domain OCT.

2.3 Diffraction

Diffraction refers to various phenomena that occur when a wave encounters an obstacle or a slit, the aperture effectively becoming a secondary source of the propagating wave. Therefore, even a well-focused, aberration-free converging lens never focuses light to a single point but always has a trace of diffraction (Brezinski 2006b). Diffraction of a circular aperture produces the bright central irradiance surrounded by the series of concentric rings: the former is known as the Airy spot which contains 84% of the total irradiance, and the latter is known as the Airy pattern. Since the system can only resolve the structures to the width of the Airy function, the diffraction determines the resolution limit of the system. It is particularly important for the lateral resolution which is essentially dependent on the optics of the imaging device. A larger diameter lens and shorter wavelengths result in smaller Airy spot and therefore higher resolutions (Brezinski 2006b).

2.4 Tissue Interactions

When light is within materials rather than in a vacuum, it interacts with atoms and molecules, and this interaction is best described as the dipole moment: separation of opposite charges (Brezinski 2006c). Then, the electrical dipole oscillates and generates a second propagating electromagnetic wave with a different velocity. This velocity change in the light is known as refractive index: $n = c/v$.

The refractive index is frequency dependent: in a medium, different wavelengths will travel at different speeds, and this fact is called dispersion. Although dispersion can be used to decompose the light into its different frequency components as in Spectral-domain OCT, dispersion generally needs to be compensated for in OCT systems because dispersion makes the different wavelengths return at slightly different times.

When the impinging electromagnetic waves are near the resonance frequency, the electron absorbs the energy of a photon of a specific frequency and goes to a higher-energy state, a phenomenon known as absorption. More generally, atoms that are exposed to light absorb light energy and re-emit light in different directions with differing intensities, a phenomenon known as scattering. Keep in mind, meanwhile, that refractive index, dispersion, absorption, and scattering are related to each other in that they are all frequency (f) dependent.

3 Time-Domain OCT

The basic principle of Time-domain OCT is that of the Michelson interferometer's use of the light of a low-coherence source (Fig. 2a) (Huang et al. 1991; Fercher et al. 2003; Fercher 2010; Popescu et al. 2011; Drexler et al. 2014; Fujimoto and Swanson 2016; Aumann et al. 2019; Brezinski 2006d). By replacing one of the mirrors with a sample, one can measure the interference of back-scattered light from the sample and the reflected light from the reference mirror. The back-reflected lights from the two arms (reference and sample) are combined and interfere only if the optical path lengths match within the coherence length. Interference fringe bursts, roughly the amplitudes of the interference, are detected by the photodiode. For each sample point, the reference mirror is scanned in the depth (z) direction, and a complete depth profile is generated at the beam position: this is the A-scan (amplitude scan). For a cross-sectional image, the scan beam is moved laterally across the line, and repeats A-scans in the same way: this is the B-scan (named after "brightness scan" in ultrasonography) (Fig. 2b) (Fercher et al. 2003; Fercher 2010; Popescu et al. 2011; Drexler et al. 2014; Fujimoto and Swanson 2016; Aumann et al. 2019).

To compute the axial resolution, the wavelength profile of a light source must be considered, because it determines the coherence length.

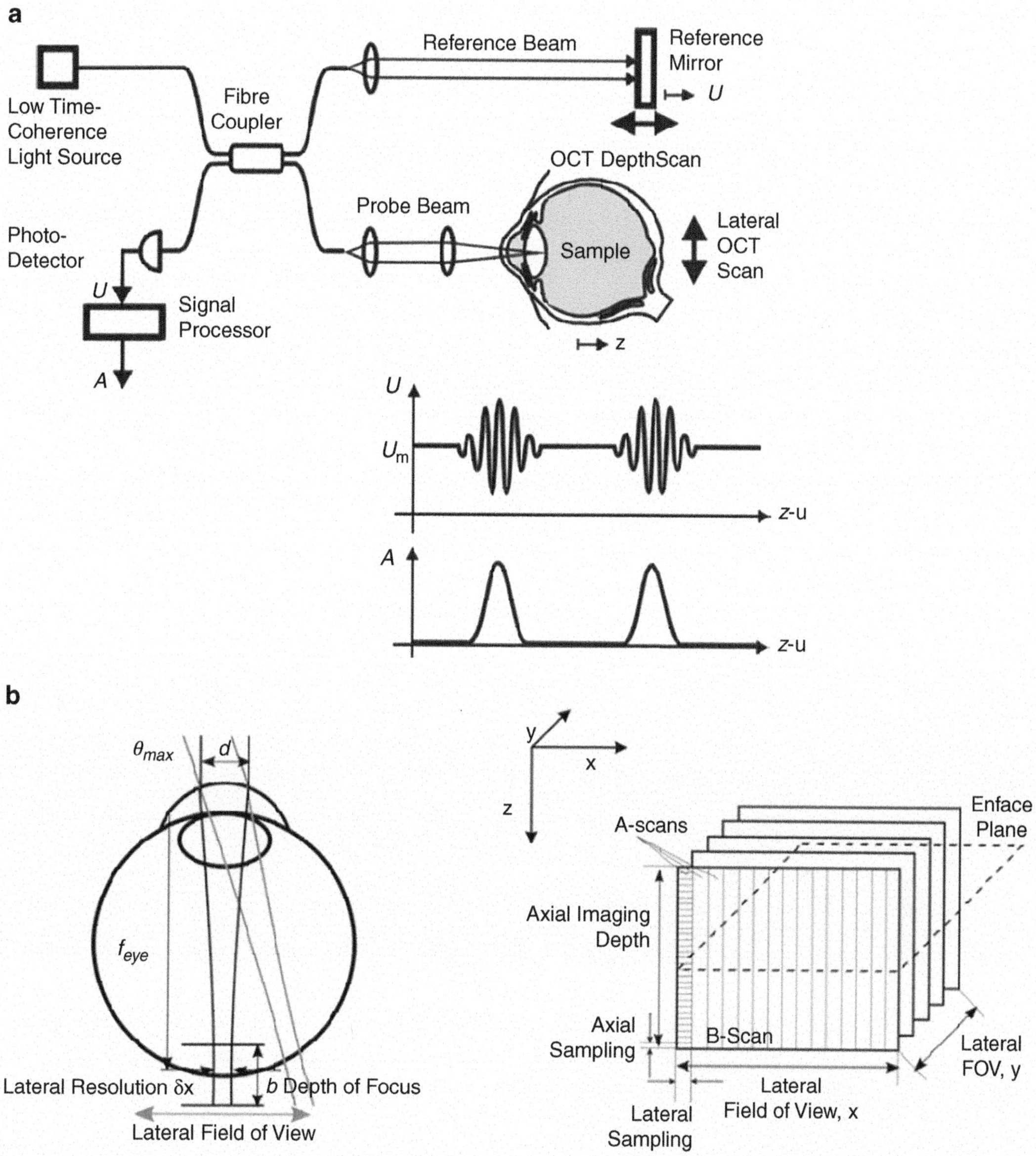

Fig. 2 Working principle of Time-domain OCT (TD-OCT). For the axial image, a light from the light source is split into the reference beam and the central beam. Back-reflected light from both arms is combined again and recorded by the detector. To record one depth profile of the sample (an A-scan), the reference arm needs to be scanned (**a**). This has to be repeated for each lateral scan position to construct a volume scan (**b**). Therefore, the lateral resolution of OCT depends on the focusing ability of the probing beam: which is to say, the optics of the system. Figures reprinted from (Aumann et al. 2019)

Let us assume a Gaussian spectrum of wavelengths, then the wavelength profile is determined by its wavelength (λ_0) and its spectral bandwidth ($\Delta\lambda$). Usually, the spectral bandwidth is described by the full width at half-maximum (FWHM): the width at the intensity level equal to half the maximum intensity. Then, the axial resolution (along the z axis) in free space equals the round-trip coherence length of the source light (Fercher 2010; Popescu et al. 2011; Drexler et al. 2014;

Fujimoto and Swanson 2016; Aumann et al. 2019; Brezinski 2006d):

$$\delta_z = \frac{2\ln 2}{\pi} \times \frac{\lambda_0^2}{\Delta\lambda}$$

This means, at the theoretical level at least, that a better axial resolution is dependent only on the light source: a shorter wavelength (λ_0) and broader spectral bandwidth ($\Delta\lambda$).

The lateral resolution is determined by the spot size of the probing beam, which is dependent on the optics of the imaging device (Fig. 2b; NA = numerical aperture of focusing lens) (Fercher 2010; Popescu et al. 2011; Drexler et al. 2014; Fujimoto and Swanson 2016; Aumann et al. 2019).

$$\delta_x = \frac{2\sqrt{\ln 2}}{\pi} \times \frac{\lambda_0}{\mathrm{NA}}$$

Tight focusing would increase the lateral resolution (via the increase of the NA) at the expense of focusing depth (the axial range). The confocal parameter, b, is twice the Rayleigh length (z_R):

$$b = 2 \times z_R = 2 \times \frac{\pi}{\lambda_0} \times \omega_0^2$$

Tight focusing will reduce the beam waist (ω_0: radial size of beam), and the axial range.

Time-domain OCT has several limitations. First, it requires movement of the reference arm corresponding to the z-axis location of the sample arm, which critically limits the scan speed. Second, only the light reflected from a thin tissue slice within the coherence length contributes to the OCT signal, while the detection system records, at each axial location over the full spectral bandwidth, the summated power reflected from all depth locations. To handle this glut of information, Fourier-domain OCT was introduced (Fercher 2010; Popescu et al. 2011; Drexler et al. 2014; Fujimoto and Swanson 2016; Aumann et al. 2019; de Boer et al. 2017a).

4 Fourier-Domain OCT

A Fourier series is an expansion of a periodic function in terms of an infinite sum of sines and cosines. Let us imagine two waves with different frequencies but the same amplitude and phase.

$W_1(x, t) = A \cos(k_1 x - \omega_1 t)$ and $W_2(x, t) = A \cos(k_2 x - \omega_2 t.)$

The summation of the two waves is as follows:

$$W_1 + W_2 = 2A\cos\left(\frac{k_1 - k_2}{2} \times x - \frac{w_1 - w_2}{2} \times t\right)\cos\left(\frac{k_1 + k_2}{2} \times x - \frac{w_1 + w_2}{2} \times t\right)$$

This equation clearly shows that the summated wave has two oscillating components: one with a rapidly varying part and the other with a slowly varying envelope (Fig. 3a) (Aumann et al. 2019; Brezinski 2006d). This means that the individual frequency components still exist, even after the summation of the waves. A Fourier series states that every singular frequency component can be traced back from the complex summated waves.

4.1 Fourier Transformation

Fourier transformation is a function that enables a perspective change from the time- or spatial domain to the frequency domain (Fig. 3b).

$$\hat{g}(f) = \int_{t_1}^{t_2} g(t) \times e^{-2\pi i f t}\, dt$$

To understand why this function acts as a Fourier transformation, it is required to understand the method of manipulating values on a two-dimensional plane using complex numbers: a point $(a, b) = a + bi$. This manipulation is particularly useful in the aspect of circular transformation since every point in the unit circle ($\cos\theta + i \bullet \sin\theta$) corresponds to $e^{i\theta}$ (Fig. 3c; Euler's equation). This means that one can transpose any function along the circle in the polar coordinate system by multiplying $e^{i\theta}$. During the Fourier transformation, $e^{-2\pi i}$ is multiplied in order to wrap a function $g(t)$ along the circle, and an integral is used to squeeze out its frequency pro-

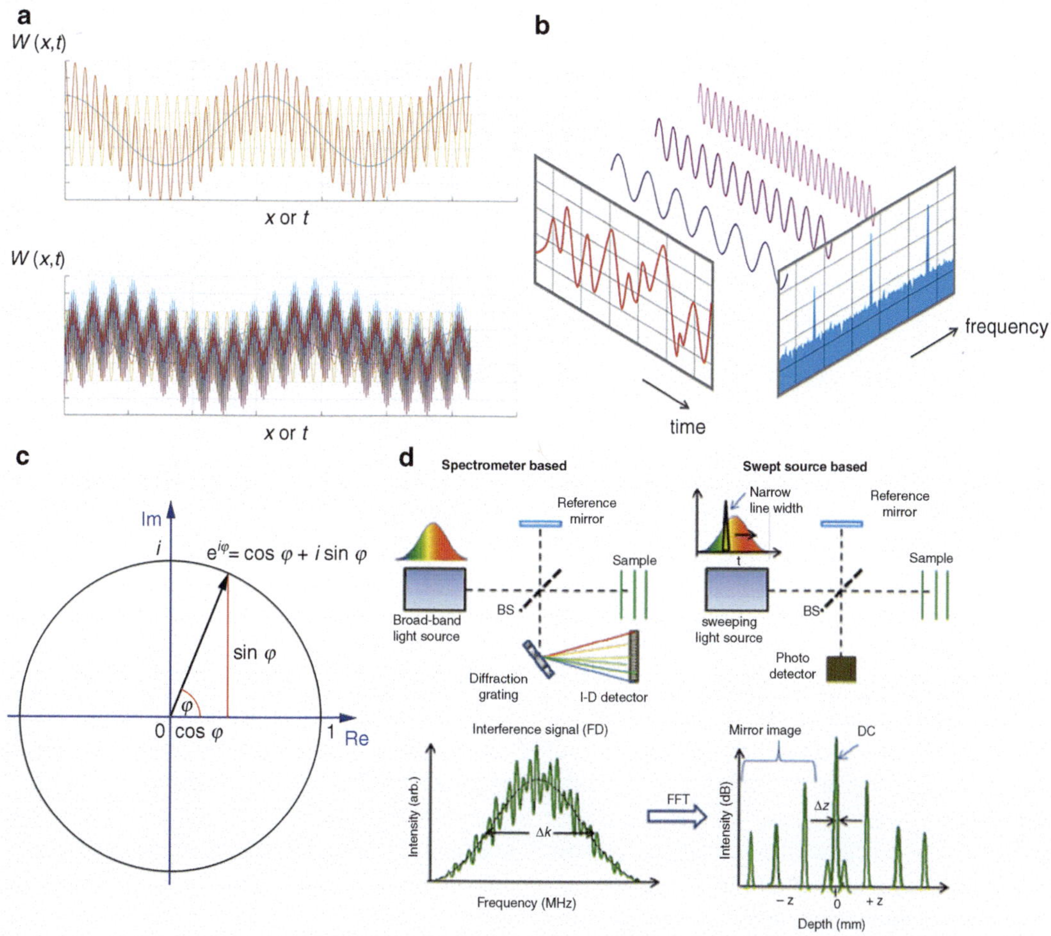

Fig. 3 Working principle of Fourier-domain OCT (FD-OCT). Despite the mixing of diverse frequencies, the summated waves (red waves) still bear the original individual components (**a**). With formulaic calculation, each component can be extracted from the mixed waves: Fourier-transformation (**b**; figure taken from Wikimedia). To understand how it works, waves should be described in the complex number system (**c**; figure taken from Wikipedia). In this polar coordinate system, any point in the waves is described by its real number portion and its imaginary number portion. Then, the waves can be translated into circular movement (phase information is translated into the angle from the x-axis, and the amplitude is translated into the distance from the reference point). Based on the Euler's equation, any point in the unit circle is $\cos\varphi + i \sin \varphi$, and can be translated as $e^{i\varphi}$ (**c**; figure taken from Wikipedia). Therefore, any wave can be transformed to rotate along the unit circle by simply multiplying $e^{i\varphi}$. The frequency profile is squeezed out during the integral process because the hills and valleys of complex waves are counterbalanced during the integration except for when the winding frequencies match exactly those of the individual frequency components. This means that although Fourier-domain OCT receives signals as summated waves, their individual frequency components can be back-calculated and isolated systematically. The total waves are obtained either by a spectrometer (a spectrometer-based OCT: Spectral-domain OCT) or by rapid sweeping of wavelengths from the source (Swept-source OCT). Both implementations record an interference spectrum that carries the depth information of the sample. Fast Fourier Transformation is then used to transform the interference signal into an A-scan (**d**; figures reprinted from (Aumann et al. 2019))

file. As the original function is transposed along the circle, the infinite length of function is winding along the circle over and over, and its hills and valleys are counterbalanced during the integral process except for when the winding frequencies match exactly with those of the individual waves of $g(t)$. At this moment, all the hills are arranged on the one side and the valleys on the other side, thereby the transformed function $\hat{g}(f)$ has spikes on those specific frequencies. After obtaining the frequency profiles from the mixed waves, the individual waves can be extracted and analyzed according to their frequencies (Fig. 3b).

The Fourier transform of the spectrum provides a back-reflection profile as a function of depth (Fig. 3d) (Fercher 2010; Popescu et al. 2011; Drexler et al. 2014; Fujimoto and Swanson 2016; Aumann et al. 2019). Depth information is obtained by the different interference profiles from the different path lengths in both arms: larger differences in the optical path length result in higher-frequency interference signals (Brezinski 2006d; de Boer et al. 2017a; Fercher et al. 1995; Leitgeb et al. 2000).

$$I(k) = G(k)\left(1 + 2\int_{z_0}^{\infty} a(z) \times \cos(2knz)\,dz + \iint_{z_0}^{\infty} a(z')\,a(z) \times e^{i \cdot 2kn(z-z')}\,dz\,dz'\right)$$

$I(k)$ is the total inference signal, $G(k)$ is the spectral intensity distribution of the light source, z_0 is the offset of the reference plane from the object surface, z is the axial location, $a(z)$ is the backscattering coefficient of the object signal with regard to the offset z_0, and n is the refractive index. The first term is the direct-current term, and the second term encodes the depth information z: as the light goes deeper, the frequency of oscillation gets higher. The third term describes the mutual interference of all elementary waves; in fact, it can be neglected, since the second term is much higher than the third term in a strongly scattered medium (Brezinski 2006d; de Boer et al. 2017a; Fercher et al. 1995; Leitgeb et al. 2000).

4.2 Spectral-Domain OCT

In this OCT mode's early development stage, it was called "spectral radar" (Ha Usler and Lindner 1998; Andretzky et al. 1999, 2000); this term probably best describes its mechanism. The photodiode detector is replaced by a spectrometer, which separates the different wavelength components spatially, and these lights are received by a charged-coupled device (CCD) (Fercher 2010; Popescu et al. 2011; Drexler et al. 2014; Fujimoto and Swanson 2016; Aumann et al. 2019; Brezinski 2006d; de Boer et al. 2017a; Fercher et al. 1995; Leitgeb et al. 2000). Therefore, only a narrow optical bandwidth corresponding to a long coherence length is measured by each detector element (de Boer et al. 2017a; Fercher et al. 1995; Leitgeb et al. 2000).

The strength of Spectral-domain OCT is speed. It does not require a moving reference arm, and the depth information is obtained all at once. High scan speed enables averaging, which reduces speckle noise (mutual interference of a set of coherent waves) and fluctuations in background noise. With n-times averaging, the signal-to-noise (SNR) ratio increases by $\sqrt{n}$ times. Therefore, Spectral-domain OCT provides higher sensitivity with better resolution than can Time-domain OCT (Leitgeb et al. 2003; Choma et al. 2003).

Spectral-domain OCT, however, has several weaknesses as well (Liu and Brezinski 2007). First, all Fourier-domain OCTs suffer diminished sensitivity with increases in imaging depth: this is the roll-off phenomenon. During Fourier transformation, a deeper axial location is encoded with a higher-frequency panel, but it is more difficult to capture a signal with a higher frequency. Further, in Spectral-domain OCT, the finite pixel size of the CCD array and the finite spectral resolution of the spectrometer limit the range of measurable frequency. Therefore, a deeper location beyond the obtainable CCD frequency range cannot be measured. Second, Spectral-domain OCT is limited by the capacity of the CCD, which has a limited spectral range. If a spectral range is too small, it cannot capture the full spectrum, and if it is too large, the pixel spacing is reduced, which results in a reduced measurement range without axial resolution improvement. Third, Fourier transform links z (depth) and k (frequency) spaces, whereas k (frequency) and λ (wavelength) have a nonlinear relationship: $k = 2\pi/\lambda$. Therefore, the signal is unevenly sampled in k space but evenly sampled in λ space, which results in broadening of the point spread function. Fourth, dispersion, which is also frequency dependent, has to be corrected by software. Fifth and finally, Spectral-domain OCT is more vulnerable to motion artifacts, due to the integration process of the CCD.

4.3 Swept-Source OCT

Many problems of Spectral-domain OCT are related to the use of the CCD rather than the photodiode detector. In Swept-source OCT, by contrast, the broadband light source is replaced by an optical source that rapidly sweeps a narrow linewidth over a broad range of wavelengths (Fercher 2010; Popescu et al. 2011; Drexler et al. 2014; Fujimoto and Swanson 2016; Aumann et al. 2019; Brezinski 2006d; de Boer et al. 2017a; Chinn et al. 1997). Therefore, only a narrow optical bandwidth corresponding to a long coherence length is measured sequentially in time by the single detector element (de Boer et al. 2017a; Chinn et al. 1997).

Swept-source OCT has the merit of using the photodiode detector rather than the CCD. But it is also subject to other innate weaknesses of Fourier-domain OCT (Liu and Brezinski 2007). Swept-source OCT, like Spectral-domain OCT, suffers the roll-off phenomenon, which is related to the instantaneous linewidth of the light source and the detection bandwidth of the analog-to-digital conversion (photodiode and digitizer) (de Boer et al. 2017a). Technologically, it is much easier to achieve a narrow instantaneous line width with a tunable light source than to manufacture a spectrometer covering a more-than-100 nm optical bandwidth with very high spectral resolution. Therefore, roll-off is easier to overcome in Swept-source OCT than in Spectral-domain OCT.

5 Further OCT Modifications

5.1 Enhanced Depth Imaging

OCT imaging of the deep layers of the optic nerve head complex is disturbed by (1) high scattering of the retinal pigment epithelium and (2) the roll-off phenomenon incurred with Fourier-domain OCT. These problems could be partially evaded by using the enhanced depth imaging (EDI) technique. By shifting the position of the reference mirror, the optimum imaging position is moved to the lower part of the sample, and the characteristic roll-off is reversed in depth: that is, deeper layers have smaller differences in optical path lengths, and thus are encoded in lower frequencies. Unfortunately, the EDI technique cannot handle the scattering obstacle (Aumann et al. 2019; Spaide et al. 2008; Mrejen and Spaide 2013).

5.2 OCT Angiography

Using the Doppler shift of the OCT signals, the flow in the vessels (mainly due to the flow of erythrocytes) can be visualized by OCT angiography (An and Wang 2008; Jia et al. 2012). This will be addressed in a separate chapter of this book.

5.3 Visible-Light OCT

Usually, OCT uses a light source in the near-infrared wavelength (800–1300 nm). By reducing the wavelength to visible light (450–700 nm), the axial resolution increases about 8 times and the lateral resolution increases about 1.6 times (Aumann et al. 2019; Nafar et al. 2016). Also, the spectral information can be used to determine the oxygen saturation levels of the vessels (Yi et al. 2015). This technique, however, needs careful correction for chromatic aberrations, and may potentially incur photo-chemical action, bleaching of the photopigments, and, thus too, subject discomfort. Inaccessibility below the intact retinal pigment epithelium (due to strong absorption) is a critical problem (Aumann et al. 2019).

5.4 OCT Elastography

Tissue elasticity, described by the Young modulus, can be measured by Brillouin scattering. But the wavelength shift is extremely small, and so a laser with a very narrow spectral band is required. Still, in the early developmental stage, OCT elastography doubtlessly will provide information on tissues' mechanical loadings someday (Aumann et al. 2019; Scarcelli and Yun 2012; Kirby et al. 2017).

5.5 Polarization-Sensitive OCT

When light is passed through tissue, the sample is capable of generating an altered state of back-reflected polarized light. Therefore, the polarization state of the back-scattered light gives additional information about the sample. The polarization of the light can be described with the Jones formalism (de Boer et al. 2017b): with calculation of a vector (to describe the direction of polarization) and a matrix (Jones matrix J; the polarization changing properties of a medium), the polarization state can be drawn. Polarization-sensitive OCT can be used for measuring tissue with high birefringence (Aumann et al. 2019; de Boer et al. 2017b). Currently, it incorporates swept-source technology, which enables better resolution (Yamanari et al. 2008; Braaf et al. 2014).

5.6 Adaptive Optics OCT

OCT system resolution is dependent on the light source for the axial direction and on the optical system for the lateral direction: currently about 3 μm in the axial direction, and about 9 μm in the lateral direction. The low resolution in the lateral direction is due to the fact that the diffraction-limited optical resolution is determined by the numerical aperture (NA), which can be maximized by pupil dilation. Optical aberration, however, increases rapidly with pupil diameter. In adaptive optics OCT, the optical aberrations are corrected using a deformable mirror. Consequently, the resolution of <3 μm in all dimensions can be achieved, which enables cellular imaging (Aumann et al. 2019; Kumar et al. 2013; Liu et al. 2017).

5.7 High-speed OCT

High scanning speed can reduce motion artifacts, increase A-scan density so as to improve digital lateral resolution, and increase the SNR ratio with averaging as in Fourier-domain OCT (Aumann et al. 2019). Currently, these goals are being achieved in two ways: (1) increasing the rate of sweep of the light source: Fourier Domain Mode Locked (FDML) Lasers with an MHz Sweep Rate (Huber et al. 2006; Klein et al. 2012), and (2) lateral parallelization of OCT data acquisition: Parallel OCT or Line-field Fourier-domain OCT, which illuminates tissue with either a line or over a full area, where each lateral pixel records the depth structure (Nakamura et al. 2007; Fechtig et al. 2015). For extension of this technology, Full-field Swept-source OCT has been developed. By replacing the line detector with a 2D image sensor, a complete 3D volume stack is constructed in just one sweep of the laser (Hillmann et al. 2016, 2017).

6 Conclusion

In the last paragraph of an epoch-making article (Huang et al. 1991) that coined the term "OCT," the authors stated that "Because OCT is an optical method, a variety of optical properties can be utilized to identify tissue structure and composition." In that paper, they presented only a prototype of Time-domain OCT but predicted the boundless development of future OCT in such manifestations as Spectral-domain OCT and Polarization-sensitive OCT. However, it took decades for their prediction to come true, because it required advances in the signal processing mechanism (including Fast Fourier transformation), higher speed of data transfer and conversion, and a sustainable light source of a specific spectrum as well. Notably, the light still has many and various useful properties to be discovered (or problematic ones to be coped with). Those useful properties will enable the development of new OCT iterations in the future.

References

An L, Wang RK. In vivo volumetric imaging of vascular perfusion within human retina and choroids with optical micro-angiography. Opt Express. 2008;16(15):11438–52.

Andretzky P, Lindner M, Herrmann J, et al. Optical coherence tomography by spectral radar: dynamic range estimation and in-vivo measurements of skin: SPIE; 1999.

Andretzky P, Knauer M, Kiesewetter F, Haeusler G. Optical coherence tomography by spectral radar: improvement of signal-to-noise ratio: SPIE; 2000.

Aumann S, Donner S, Fischer J, Müller F. Optical Coherence Tomography (OCT): principle and technical realization. In: Bille JF, editor. High resolution imaging in microscopy and ophthalmology: new frontiers in biomedical optics. Cham: Springer; 2019. p. 59–85.

Braaf B, Vermeer KA, de Groot M, Vienola KV, de Boer JF. Fiber-based polarization-sensitive OCT of the human retina with correction of system polarization distortions. Biomed Opt Express. 2014;5(8):2736–58.

Brezinski ME. Light and electromagnetic waves. In: Brezinski ME, editor. Optical coherence tomography. Burlington: Academic Press; 2006a. p. 31–55.

Brezinski ME. Interference, coherence, diffraction, and transfer functions. In: Brezinski ME, editor, Optical coherence Tomography. Burlington: Academic Press; 2006b. p. 71–94.

Brezinski ME. Light in matter. In: Brezinski ME, editor. Optical coherence tomography. Burlington: Academic Press; 2006c. p. 57–69.

Brezinski ME. Optical coherence tomography theory. In: Brezinski ME, editor. Optical coherence tomography. Burlington: Academic Press; 2006d. p. 97–145.

Chinn SR, Swanson EA, Fujimoto JG. Optical coherence tomography using a frequency-tunable optical source. Opt Lett. 1997;22(5):340–2.

Choma M, Sarunic M, Yang C, Izatt J. Sensitivity advantage of swept source and Fourier domain optical coherence tomography. Opt Express. 2003;11(18):2183–9.

de Boer JF, Leitgeb R, Wojtkowski M. Twenty-five years of optical coherence tomography: the paradigm shift in sensitivity and speed provided by Fourier domain OCT [Invited]. Biomed Opt Express. 2017a;8(7):3248–80.

de Boer JF, Hitzenberger CK, Yasuno Y. Polarization sensitive optical coherence tomography – a review [Invited]. Biomed Opt Express. 2017b;8(3):1838–73.

Drexler W, Liu M, Kumar A, Kamali T, Unterhuber A, Leitgeb R. Optical coherence tomography today: speed, contrast, and multimodality. J Biomed Optics. 2014;19(7):071412.

Fechtig DJ, Grajciar B, Schmoll T, et al. Line-field parallel swept source MHz OCT for structural and functional retinal imaging. Biomed Opt Express. 2015;6(3):716–35.

Fercher AF. Optical coherence tomography – development, principles, applications. Z Med Phys. 2010;20(4):251–76.

Fercher AF, Hitzenberger CK, Kamp G, El-Zaiat SY. Measurement of intraocular distances by backscattering spectral interferometry. Opt Commun. 1995;117(1):43–8.

Fercher AF, Drexler W, Hitzenberger CK, Lasser T. Optical coherence tomography – principles and applications. Rep Prog Phys. 2003;66(2):239–303.

Fujimoto J, Swanson E. The development, commercialization, and impact of optical coherence tomography. Invest Ophthalmol Vis Sci. 2016;57(9):Oct1–oct13.

Ha Usler G, Lindner MW. "Coherence radar" and "spectral radar"-new tools for dermatological diagnosis. J Biomed Opt. 1998;3(1):21–31.

Hillmann D, Spahr H, Pfäffle C, Sudkamp H, Franke G, Hüttmann G. In vivo optical imaging of physiological responses to photostimulation in human photoreceptors. Proc Natl Acad Sci. 2016;113(46):13138–43.

Hillmann D, Spahr H, Sudkamp H, et al. Off-axis reference beam for full-field swept-source OCT and holoscopy. Opt Express. 2017;25(22):27770–84.

Huang D, Swanson EA, Lin CP, et al. Optical coherence tomography. Science. 1991;254(5035):1178–81.

Huber R, Wojtkowski M, Fujimoto JG. Fourier Domain Mode Locking (FDML): a new laser operating regime and applications for optical coherence tomography. Opt Express. 2006;14(8):3225–37.

Jia Y, Morrison JC, Tokayer J, et al. Quantitative OCT angiography of optic nerve head blood flow. Biomed Opt Express. 2012;3(12):3127–37.

Kirby MA, Pelivanov I, Song S, et al. Optical coherence elastography in ophthalmology. J Biomed Opt. 2017;22(12):1–28.

Klein T, Wieser W, André R, Pfeiffer T, Eigenwillig C, Huber R. Multi-MHz FDML OCT: snapshot retinal imaging at 6.7 million axial-scans per second: SPIE; 2012.

Kumar A, Drexler W, Leitgeb RA. Subaperture correlation based digital adaptive optics for full field optical coherence tomography. Opt Express. 2013;21(9):10850–66.

Leitgeb R, Wojtkowski M, Kowalczyk A, Hitzenberger CK, Sticker M, Fercher AF. Spectral measurement of absorption by spectroscopic frequency-domain optical coherence tomography. Opt Lett. 2000;25(11):820–2.

Leitgeb R, Hitzenberger C, Fercher A. Performance of fourier domain vs. time domain optical coherence tomography. Opt Express. 2003;11(8):889–94.

Liu B, Brezinski ME. Theoretical and practical considerations on detection performance of time domain, Fourier domain, and swept source optical coherence tomography. J Biomed Opt. 2007;12(4):044007.

Liu YZ, South FA, Xu Y, Carney PS, Boppart SA. Computational optical coherence tomography [Invited]. Biomed Opt Express. 2017;8(3):1549–74.

Mrejen S, Spaide RF. Optical coherence tomography: imaging of the choroid and beyond. Surv Ophthalmol. 2013;58(5):387–429.

Nafar Z, Jiang M, Wen R, Jiao S. Visible-light optical coherence tomography-based multimodal retinal imaging for improvement of fluorescent intensity quantification. Biomed Opt Express. 2016;7(9):3220–9.

Nakamura Y, Makita S, Yamanari M, Itoh M, Yatagai T, Yasuno Y. High-speed three-dimensional human retinal imaging by line-field spectral domain optical coherence tomography. Opt Express. 2007;15(12):7103–16.

Popescu DP, Choo-Smith LP, Flueraru C, et al. Optical coherence tomography: fundamental principles, instrumental designs and biomedical applications. Biophys Rev. 2011;3(3):155.

Scarcelli G, Yun SH. In vivo Brillouin optical microscopy of the human eye. Opt Express. 2012;20(8):9197–202.

Spaide RF, Koizumi H, Pozzoni MC. Enhanced depth imaging spectral-domain optical coherence tomography. Am J Ophthalmol. 2008;146(4):496–500.

Yamanari M, Makita S, Yasuno Y. Polarization-sensitive swept-source optical coherence tomography with continuous source polarization modulation. Opt Express. 2008;16(8):5892–906.

Yi J, Liu W, Chen S, et al. Visible light optical coherence tomography measures retinal oxygen metabolic response to systemic oxygenation. Light Sci Appl. 2015;4(9):e334.

Peripapillary RNFL Imaging

Jin Wook Jeoung

Abstract

Glaucoma is an optic neuropathy characterized by progressive loss of retinal ganglion cells and their axons. Detection of glaucoma is based on the identification of abnormalities in the optic nerve head or the retinal nerve fiber layer (RNFL), either structural or functional. Several techniques including clinical examination, red-free fundus photography, and modern imaging devices are currently available for detecting and quantifying RNFL damage. Optical coherence tomography (OCT) is one of the most recent technologies allowing for quantitative assessment of the peripapillary RNFL. Several studies investigating the performance of OCT in glaucoma have shown promising results. However, as with other technologies, imaging may produce false identification of glaucoma; thus, clinicians should not depend solely on the results of one single imaging device. Recent studies also suggest that glaucoma imaging devices may serve as a useful adjunct in accurately and objectively assessing the degree of glaucomatous damage. Peripapillary RNFL imaging by OCT technology can provide useful measures that assist the clinician in the early detection of glaucoma. This chapter details OCT-based peripapillary RNFL imaging used for diagnosis of glaucoma and monitoring of disease progression.

Keywords

Glaucoma · Optical coherence tomography
Retinal nerve fiber layer

1 Introduction

Glaucoma is an optic neuropathy characterized by structural changes to the optic nerve head and retinal nerve fiber layer (RNFL), with corresponding visual field loss. RNFL loss is thought to precede measurable optic nerve head and visual field damage (Sommer et al. 1977, 1991). Thus, evaluation of peripapillary RNFL damage is an important method for detecting glaucomatous changes, particularly early in the glaucoma continuum.

Several techniques including clinical examination, red-free fundus photography, and modern imaging devices are available for detecting and quantifying RNFL damage. Optical coherence tomography (OCT) is one of the most recent technologies allowing for quantitative assessment of RNFL thickness. Moreover, OCT's diagnostic

J. W. Jeoung (✉)
Department of Ophthalmology, Seoul National University Hospital, Seoul National University College of Medicine, Jongno-gu, Seoul, Korea
e-mail: jwjung76@snu.ac.kr

K. H. Park, T.-W. Kim (eds.), *OCT Imaging in Glaucoma*,
https://doi.org/10.1007/978-981-16-1178-0_2

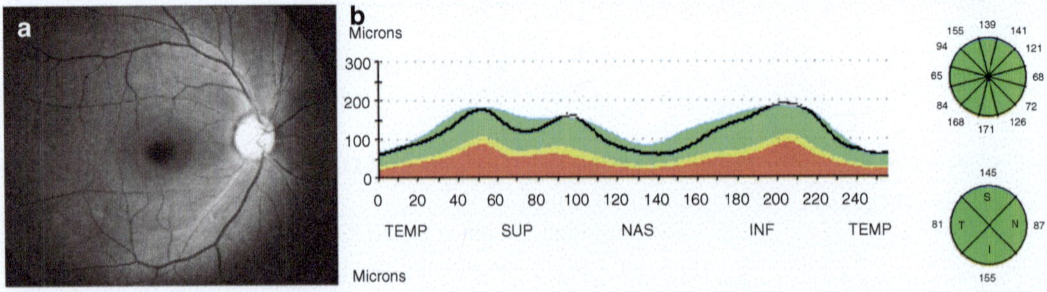

Fig. 1 RNFL images of a normal healthy eye. (**a**) Red-free RNFL photography. (**b**) OCT TSNIT (temporal–superior–nasal–inferior–temporal) RNFL thickness graph and OCT sector (clock-hour and quadrant) plots

classifications based on its internal normative database enables clinicians to assess structural glaucomatous damage more efficiently.

Recently, there has been considerable improvement in OCT technology. Spectral-domain OCT (SD-OCT), for example, offers several advantages over time-domain OCT (TD-OCT). With its faster scan speed, it allows for the acquisition of OCT data with fewer motion artifacts. Another advantage of SD-OCT over TD-OCT is the improved axial resolution (5–8 μm (SD-OCT) vs. 8–10 μm (TD-OCT) in tissue).

2 Histology and Anatomy of Retinal Nerve Fiber Layer (RNFL)

The RNFL contains the retinal ganglion cell axons covered by astrocytes and bundled by the Müller cell processes. The retinal nerve fibers are ophthalmoscopically detectable as bright and fine striations in the inner retinal layer (Hoyt et al. 1973; Airaksinen et al. 1984; Airaksinen and Nieminen 1985). According to an electron microscopic study, these fine striations appear to be bundles of axons compartmentalized within glial tunnels formed by the Müller cell processes (Radius and Anderson 1979).

The RNFL is distributed in a characteristic pattern. Axons arising from the temporal retina arc, above or below the macula, enter the superior temporal and inferior temporal areas, respectively, of the optic nerve head in an arcuate pattern. Those arising in the macular region pass directly to the temporal edge of the optic nerve, forming the papillomacular bundle.

Dividing the fundus into eight regions, the nerve fiber bundles are most visible in the temporal inferior region, followed by the temporal superior region, the nasal superior region, and finally the nasal inferior region (Jonas et al. 1989). It is least visible in the superior, inferior, temporal horizontal, and nasal horizontal regions. Figure 1 shows the RNFL images of a normal healthy eye.

3 Clinical Findings on Peripapillary RNFL in Glaucoma

Since Hoyt et al. (1973) initially described RNFL atrophy in glaucoma, evaluation of the RNFL has been essential to glaucomatous optic neuropathy diagnostics. For detection and quantification of RNFL damage, several techniques including red-free RNFL photography and modern imaging devices have been proposed. Clinically, RNFL atrophy can be divided into localized atrophy (wedge-shaped defect) and diffuse atrophy. The localized defects are not spindle-like defects but wedge-shaped ones that run toward or touch the optic disc border (Jonas and Dichtl 1996).

4 OCT Reproducibility for Peripapillary RNFL Measurements

OCT RNFL thickness measurements have been shown to be reproducible and reliable. Several studies evaluated the reproducibility of OCT RNFL thickness measurements from various SD-OCT devices. Leung et al. (2009) reported that the intravisit repeatability of Cirrus HD-OCT ranged between 5.12 and 15.02 μm, and the intervisit reproducibility ranged between 4.31 and 22.01 μm. Vizzeri et al. (2009) and González-García et al. (2009) showed excellent reproducibility levels that can be obtained by different SD devices (Cirrus and RTVue OCT). Vizzeri et al. (2009) showed that the coefficient of variation and intra-class correlation for average RNFL thickness were 1.5% and 0.96, respectively, in healthy eyes and 1.6% and 0.98, respectively, in glaucomatous eyes.

5 Glaucoma Diagnostic Performance of SD-OCT

Several studies investigating the performance of OCT in glaucoma have shown promising results. Earlier studies reported that RNFL thickness in the inferior region often had the best ability to discriminate normal eyes from eyes with early to moderate glaucoma, with sensitivities between 64% and 79% for specificities of 90% or higher (Bowd et al. 2001; Kanamori et al. 2003; Medeiros et al. 2004). Also, several studies have investigated the diagnostic capability of SD-OCT RNFL thickness measurements using an area-under-the-receiver-operating-characteristic curve (AUROC) for discrimination between healthy and glaucomatous eyes, which have shown that the AUROCs of the RNFL parameter ranged from 0.60 to 0.98, depending on the parameters and the characteristics of the population evaluated (Leite et al. 2010, 2011; Mwanza et al. 2012; Jeoung et al. 2013).

6 Diagnostic Accuracy in Preperimetric Glaucoma

In the study from Korea that enrolled 55 preperimetric glaucoma patients and 55 age- and sex-matched controls, the sensitivity of the Cirrus OCT parameters ranged from 21.0% to 87.1% with the criterion of abnormal at the 5% level (Jeoung and Park 2010). Based on the normative database, the highest Cirrus OCT sensitivity was obtained with the deviation-from-normal map (sensitivity 87.1% and specificity 61.8%). Another study by Jeoung et al. (2014) evaluated the diagnostic abilities of the speckle noise-reduced spectral-domain optical coherence tomography (SD-OCT; Spectralis OCT) and time-domain optical coherence tomography (TD-OCT; Stratus OCT) to detect localized retinal nerve fiber layer (RNFL) defects in patients with preperimetric open-angle glaucoma. They found that the AUROC for the best parameter from SD-OCT (inferotemporal sector, AUROC = 0.940) was significantly higher than that of TD-OCT (7 o'clock sector, AUROC = 0.881; $P = 0.009$), suggesting that speckle noise-reduced SD-OCT is better able to detect preperimetric localized RNFL defects than TD-OCT.

7 Instrument-Specific Maps and Interpretation

7.1 Cirrus HD-OCT

Cirrus OCT extracts from the data cube 256 A-scan samples along the path of the calculation circle. Based on the RNFL layer boundaries in the extracted circle scan image, the Cirrus OCT calculates the RNFL thickness at each point along the circle. Using these data, Cirrus OCT provides the 12-clock-hour thicknesses, 4-quadrant thicknesses, a global 360° average thickness, and TSNIT (temporal–superior–nasal–inferior–temporal) thickness profiles. For each parameter, the Cirrus OCT software provides a classification (within normal limits, borderline, or outside normal limits) based on comparison with an internal normative database.

The Cirrus OCT has a normative database generated from 284 healthy individuals with a mean age of 46.5 years. For the Cirrus normative database, 43% were Caucasians, 24% were Asians, 18% were African American, 12% were Hispanic, 1% were Indian, and 6% were of mixed ethnicity. The individuals were age-stratified into six groups: 18–29, 30–39, 40–49, 50–59, 60–69, and 70 and older (Chong and Lee 2012).

The Cirrus OCT printout also provides deviation-from-normal maps that are derived from superpixel average thickness measurements and report a statistical comparison against the normal thickness range for each superpixel, overlaid on the OCT fundus image. These maps apply the yellow and red colors of the age-matched normative data to superpixels whose average thickness falls in the yellow and red normal distribution percentiles (i.e., 1%–5% and <1% of normal distribution percentiles, respectively). Figures 2 and 3 demonstrate the Cirrus HD-OCT RNFL analysis printouts.

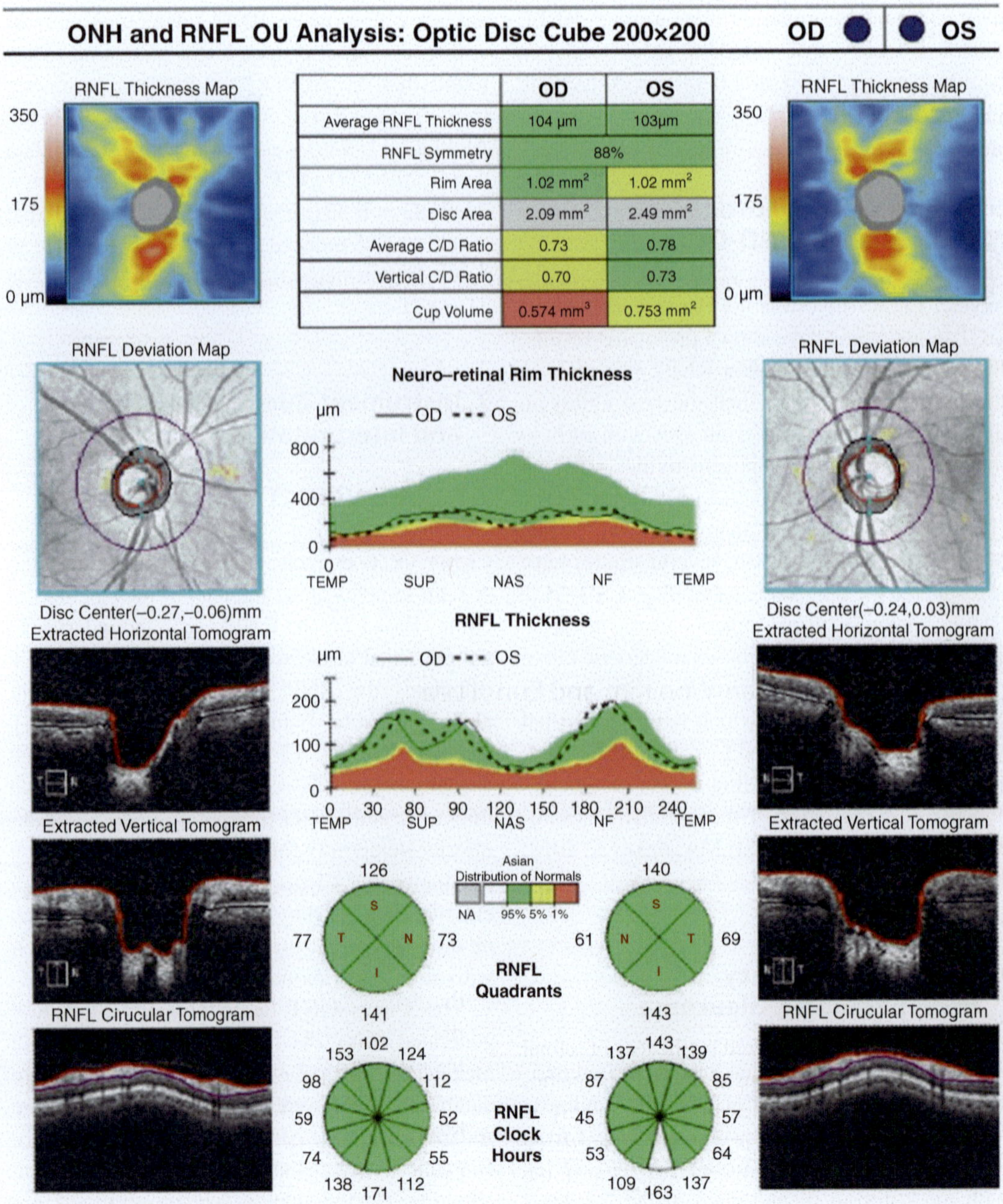

Fig. 2 Cirrus OCT retinal nerve fiber layer analysis. A case without glaucoma who has normal RNFL thickness on thickness maps, deviation maps, RNFL thickness plots, quadrant, and clock-hour plots

7.2 Spectralis OCT

The Spectralis OCT uses a superluminescent diode laser with a center wavelength of 840 nm. During OCT imaging, a scan circle with a diameter of approximately 3.46 mm was manually positioned at the center of the optic disc while the eye-tracking system was activated. This instrument combines confocal laser scanning ophthalmoscopy, which enables real-time three-dimensional tracking of eye movements, with real-time averaging of multiple B-scans acquired at an identical location of interest on the retina, to reduce speckle noise (Hangai et al. 2009). RNFL boundaries were automatically delineated according to software algorithms underneath the circumpapillary circle. The RNFL in each image was then automatically segmented. These values were averaged to yield a global average and sectoral (temporal, superotemporal, superonasal, nasal, inferonasal, and inferotemporal sectors) RNFL thickness measurement. Figure 4 shows a representative case of bilateral glaucoma with two different OCT printouts (Cirrus and Spectralis OCT).

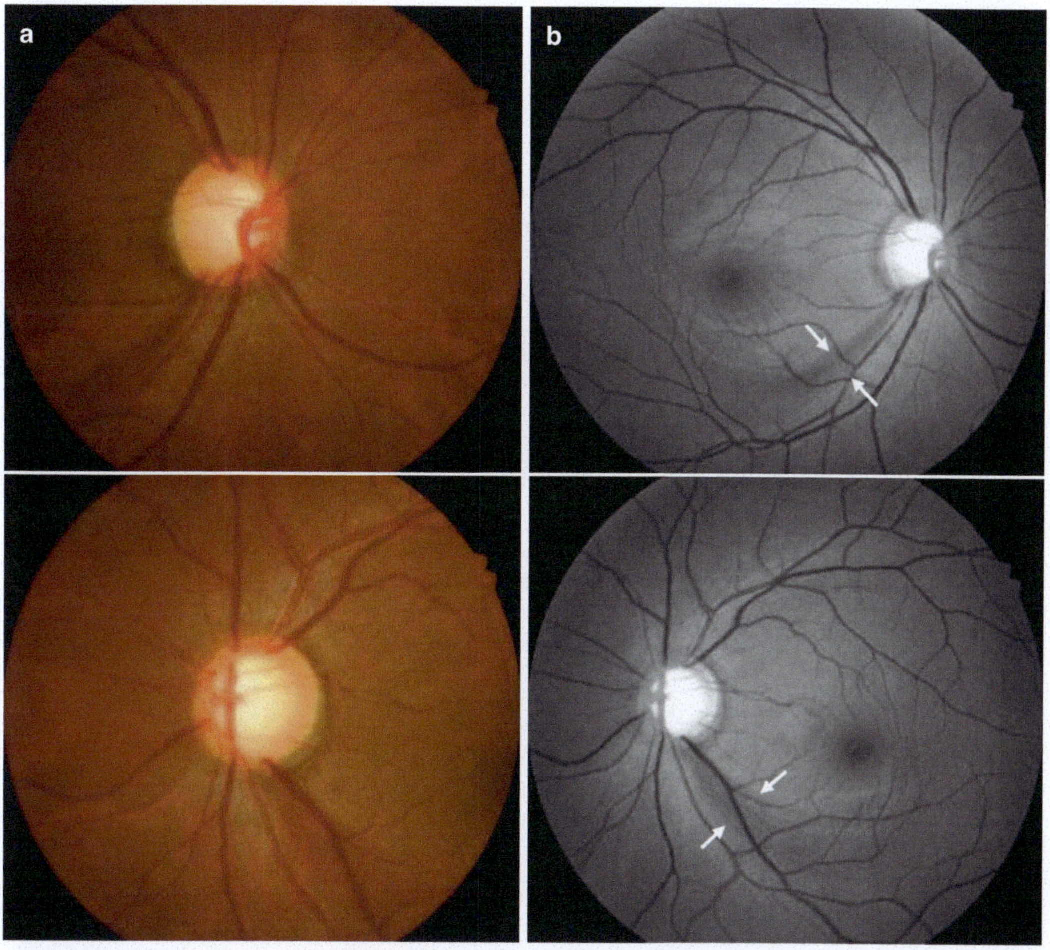

Fig. 3 Glaucoma Patient 1. (**a**, **b**) Optic disc photography and red-free RNFL photography show inferotemporal RNFL defects on both eyes. (**c**) The Cirrus OCT printout shows thinning of the RNFL in the inferotemporal region of both eyes

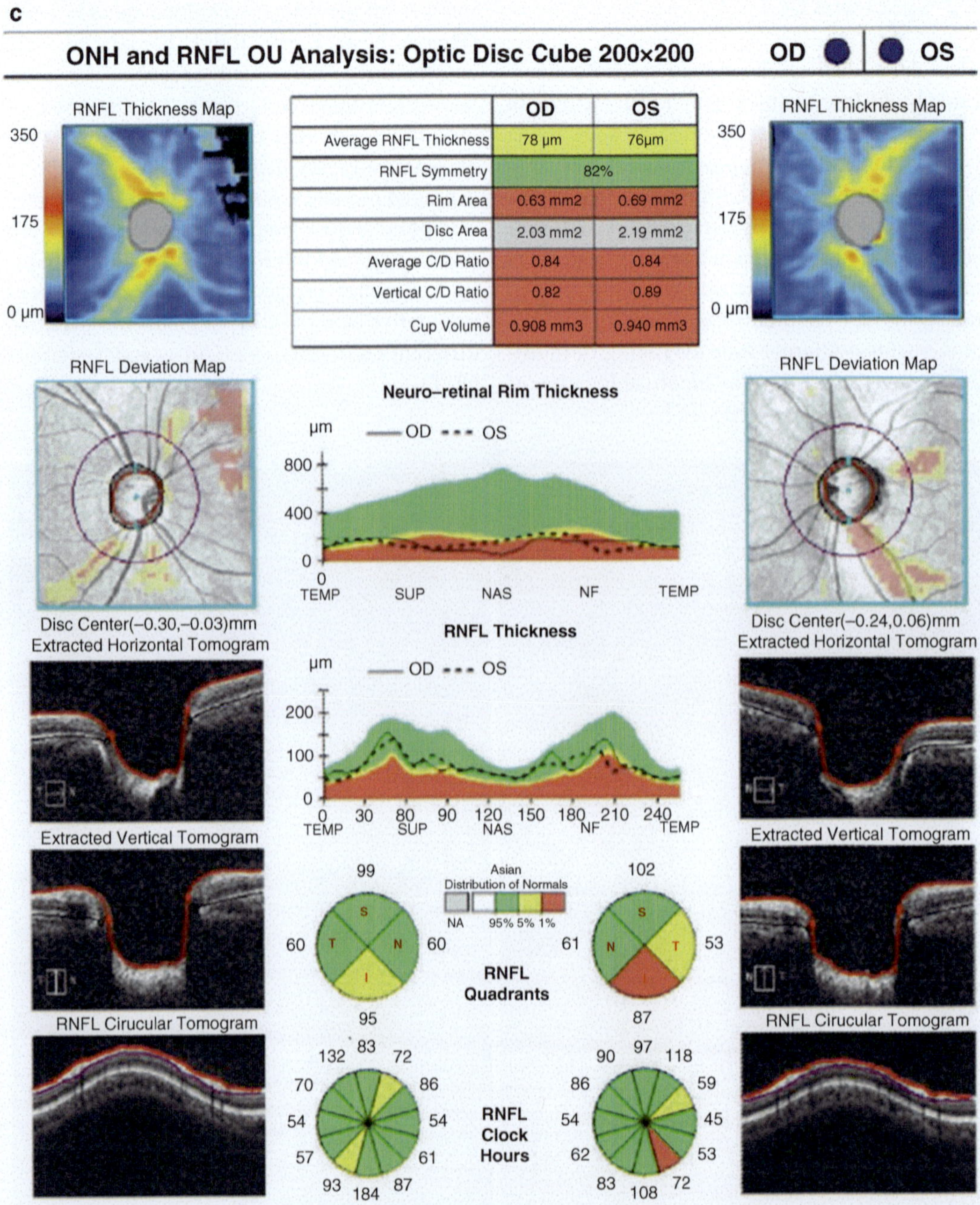

Fig. 3 (continued)

7.3 Topcon DRI-OCT

The DRI-OCT is an SS-OCT device that uses a wavelength-sweeping laser with a center wavelength of 1050 nm and a tuning range of 100 nm. In total, 100,000 A-scans with a 5 μm axial resolution in tissue are acquired per second. The DRI-OCT can provide a wide-field scan protocol (12 × 9 mm), which enables to obtain images of the macular and optic nerve head region in a single scan.

With the built-in analysis software, the RNFL boundary was automatically segmented and the RNFL thickness throughout the scan was calculated. The RNFL thickness map was generated within the 12 × 9 mm wide-field area with color scales that corresponded with numeric RNFL

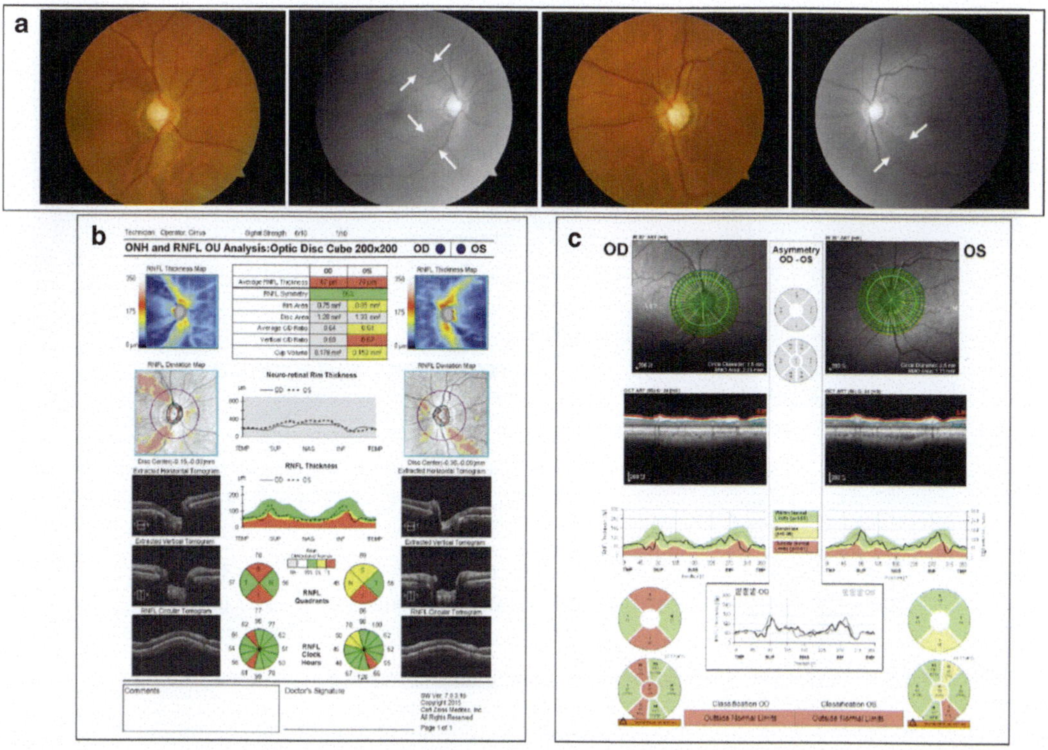

Fig. 4 Glaucoma Patient 2. (**a**) Optic disc photography and red-free RNFL photography show superotemporal and inferotemporal RNFL defects of the right eye and inferotemporal RNFL defect of the left eye. (**b**) Cirrus OCT RNFL analysis printout. (**c**) Spectralis OCT RNFL analysis printout

thickness measurements. Abnormal results based on a comparison of the RNFL and macular (GC-IPL + RNFL) thickness to the normative database are displayed on the SuperPixel deviation map. The uncolored pixels indicated the normal range, whereas the yellow- or red-colored pixels indicated abnormality at 1%–5% and <1% of the normal level, respectively. Figures 5 and 6 demonstrate the Topcon DRI-OCT maps.

8 Clinical Application of Peripapillary RNFL Imaging in Glaucoma

OCT RNFL thickness measurements are usually lower in glaucoma eyes than those in normal healthy eyes. It is well recognized that glaucomatous RNFL defects often occur at the superotemporal or inferotemporal parapapillary region, or both (Jonas and Dichtl 1996). OCT abnormal thinning of the RNFL in the superior or inferior regions can suggest the diagnosis of glaucoma.

OCT devices usually offer diagnostic classifications based on the internal normative databases. OCT color codes can provide important clues to differentiate glaucomatous eyes from healthy eyes. At the same time, careful interpretation of abnormal color codes is required because of false-positive possibilities. Kim et al. (2015) demonstrated the overall rate of false-positive diagnostic classification by SD-OCT RNFL maps as 30.8%. Longer axial length and smaller disc area were associated with abnormal RNFL diagnostic classification. Figure 7 shows the red-color regions of the RNFL (false-positive results) in a myopic healthy eye.

9 Wide-Field Map for Detection of Glaucoma

Recently, the swept-source OCT (SS-OCT) has been introduced, which has the advantages of higher speed and higher penetration with a longer wavelength than SD-OCT (Mansouri et al. 2014).

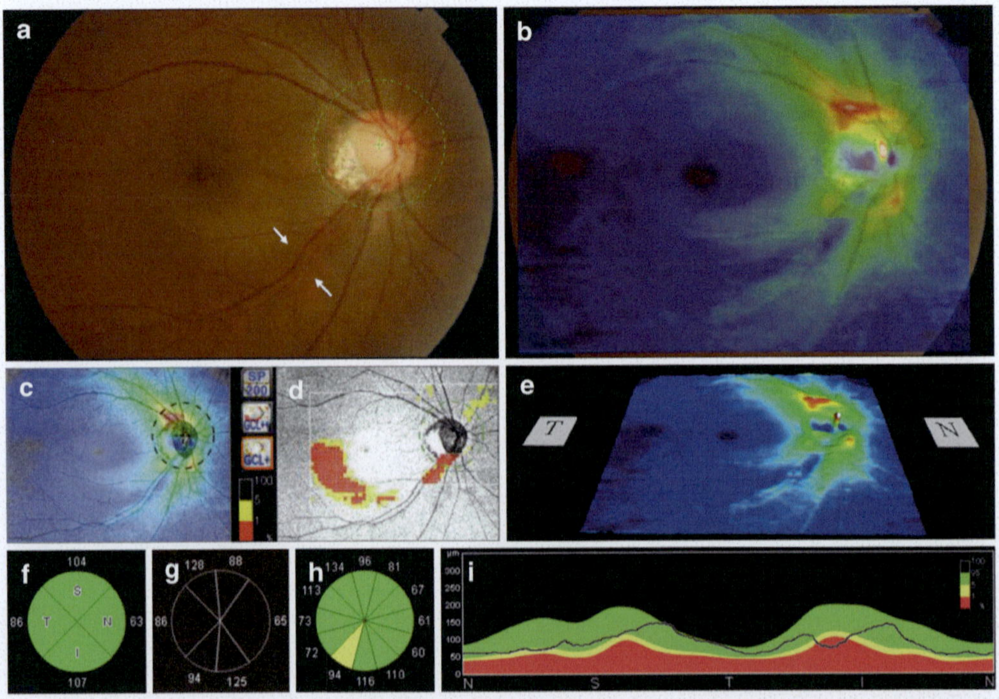

Fig. 5 Glaucoma Patient 3. Wide-field map of Topcon DRI OCT. (**a**) Fundus photography shows inferotemporal RNFL defect of the right eye. (**b**) OCT RNFL thickness map. (**c**, **d**, **e**) OCT thickness map, SuperPixel map (deviation from normal for GCIPL and RNFL thickness), and thickness surface map. (**f**, **g**, **h**, **i**) OCT Sector and RNFL thickness plots

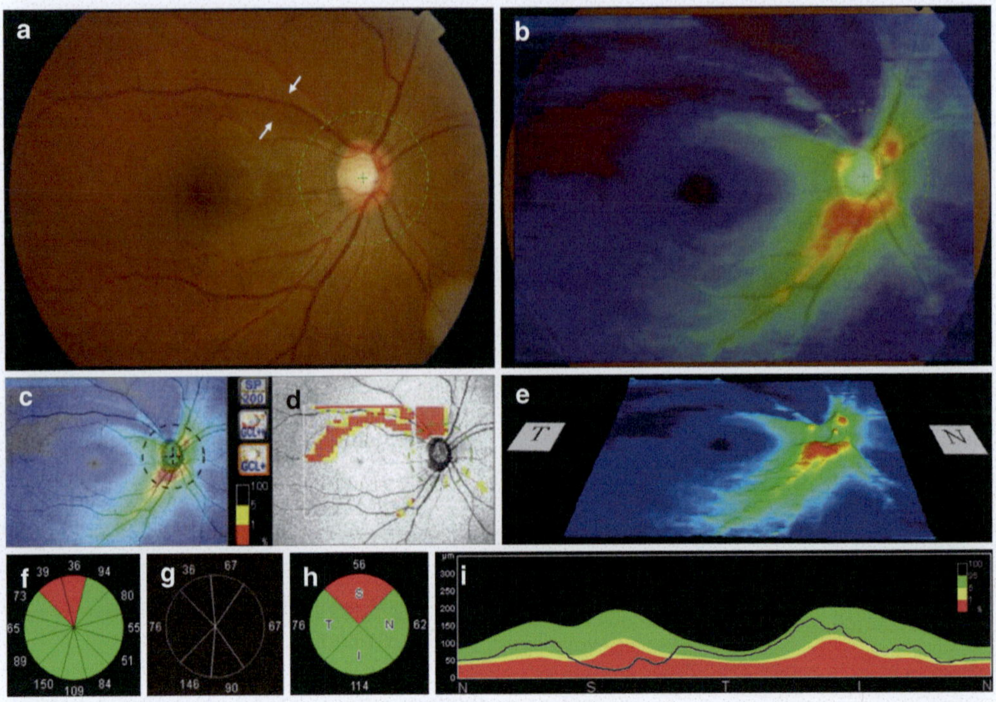

Fig. 6 Glaucoma Patient 4. Wide-field map of Topcon DRI OCT. (**a**) Fundus photography shows a superotemporal RNFL defect of the right eye. (**b**) OCT RNFL thickness map. (**c**, **d**, **e**) OCT thickness map, SuperPixel map (deviation from normal for GCIPL and RNFL thickness), and thickness surface map. (**f**, **g**, **h**, **i**) OCT Sector and RNFL thickness plots

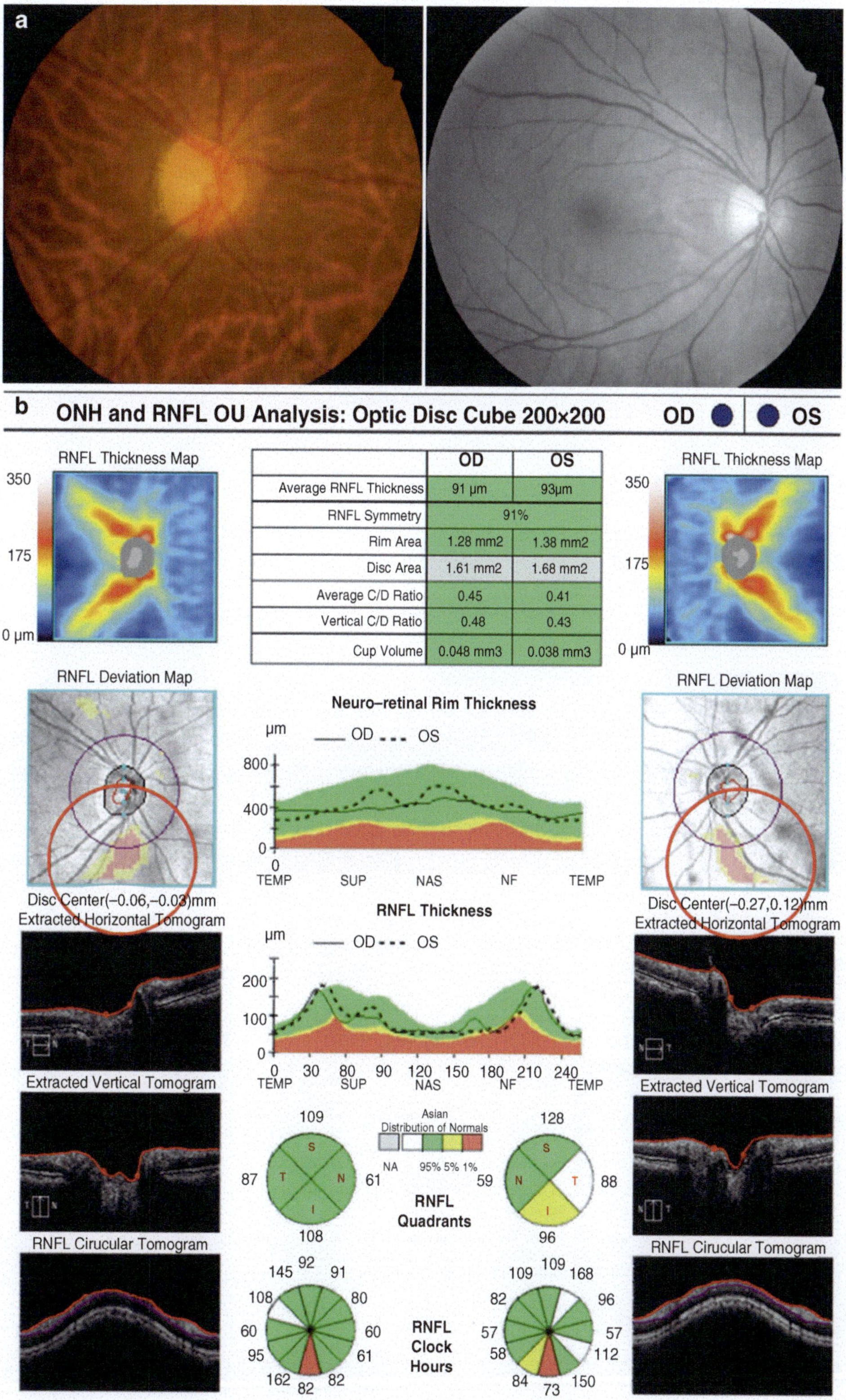

Fig. 7 A subject with the myopic healthy eye. (**a**) Optic disc photography and red-free RNFL photography. (**b**) The OCT printout shows red-color regions of the RNFL (false-positive results) in both eyes, based on the built-in normative database

Therefore, SS-OCT has been used in the glaucoma field to image deep ocular structures such as the choroid and lamina cribrosa, as well as RNFL thickness (Kim et al. 2016a, b). Also, SS-OCT can provide wide-field visualization for imaging of a larger, 12 × 9 mm area of the posterior pole including the optic nerve head and macula, with one single-scan protocol. A recent study reported that the wide-field RNFL thickness map using SS-OCT performed well in distinguishing eyes with preperimetric and early glaucoma from healthy eyes (Lee et al. 2017, 2018). The wide-field RNFL map of SS-OCT can be a useful tool for the early detection of glaucoma. Figure 8 demonstrates the clinical usefulness of wide-field maps for the detection of glaucoma.

10 Detecting Glaucoma Progression by Peripapillary RNFL Imaging

Evaluation of glaucoma progression is essential in the management of glaucoma. Recently, OCT has been widely used for detecting and monitoring structural progression in glaucoma. Assessment of progressive changes in the optic disc and RNFL is based on event analysis or trend analysis. Event-based analysis detects progression when a follow-up measurement exceeds a preestablished threshold for change from baseline. Trend-based analysis detects progression by evaluating the slope of the measured parameter over time (Bussel et al. 2014). Progression is commonly defined by trend-based analysis when a significant negative slope is detected using linear regression analysis.

Recently, commercially available software for change analysis has been introduced in OCT devices, which can provide a clinically important reference to evaluate glaucoma progression. The Guided Progression Analysis (GPA) of the Cirrus HD-OCT performs event analysis of the RNFL thickness maps and displays the area of change in the RNFL thickness change map (Fig. 9). In addition, this software reports trend and event analyses of the circumpapillary RNFL thickness profiles. Pixels exceeding the test-retest variability between a follow-up and the first and second baseline images are coded in yellow and in red if the same changes are evident on three consecutive images (Leung et al. 2012).

In Spectralis OCT, eye-tracking improves reproducibility (Langenegger et al. 2011), which in turn leads to more accurate detection of glaucoma progression. Spectralis also oversamples specific points and combines them to reduce speckle (or random noise), enhancing the visualization of structures of interest. This device provides an RNFL Change Report that includes individual baseline and follow-up scans for the overall and sectoral RNFL measurements and classifications (Abe et al. 2015). The OCT change report and trend report plot the serial exams over time to calculate the rate of change using linear regression analysis (Grewal and Tanna 2013) (Fig. 10).

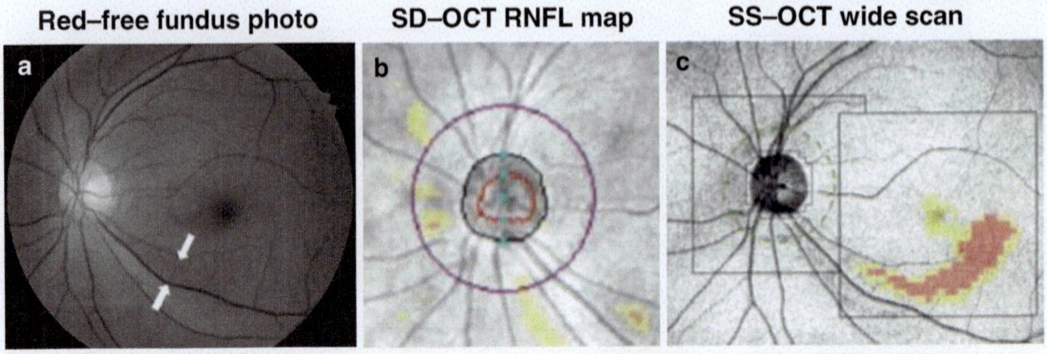

Fig. 8 A case with preperimetric glaucoma. (**a**) Conventional red-free photography revealed the inferotemporal retinal nerve fiber layer (RNFL) defect (white arrows). (**b**) SD-OCT RNFL map shows island-like isolated color patterns in the inferior and nasal areas. (**c**) The wide-field SuperPixel map (GCL+, equivalent with GCIPL in Cirrus OCT) of SS-OCT clearly showed an arcuate pattern of contiguous yellow/red abnormal pixels extending to the macular area

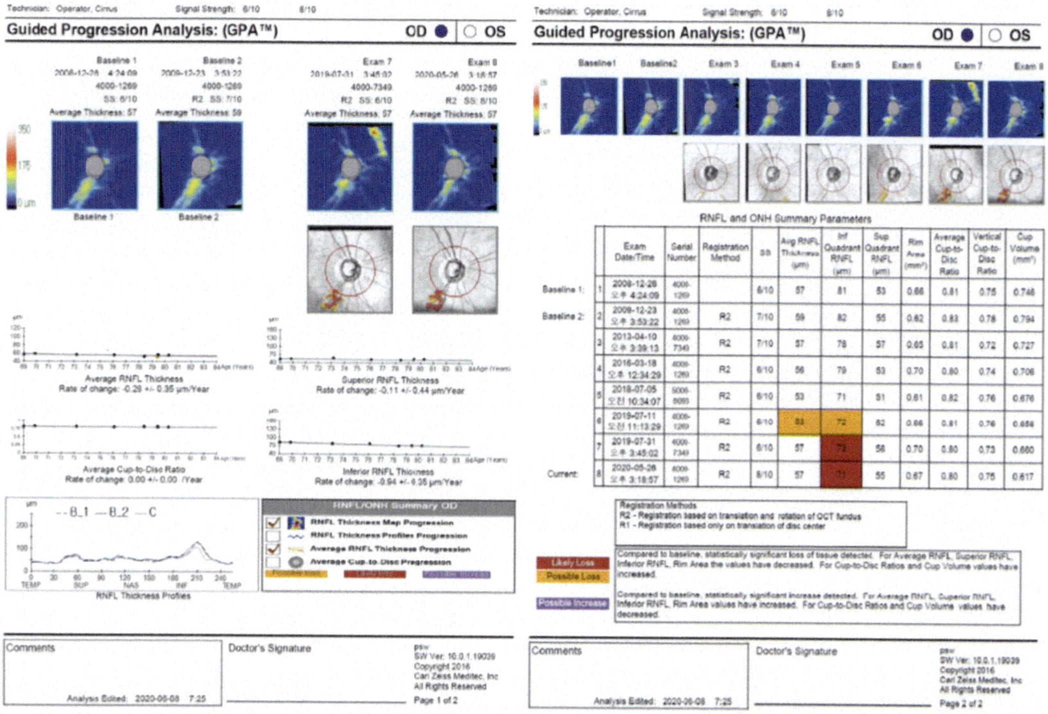

Fig. 9 Cirrus OCT guided progression analysis (GPA). Progression analysis report shows change plots over time and serial RNFL thickness maps. The OCT GPA report demonstrates the progressive RNFL thinning in the inferotemporal area

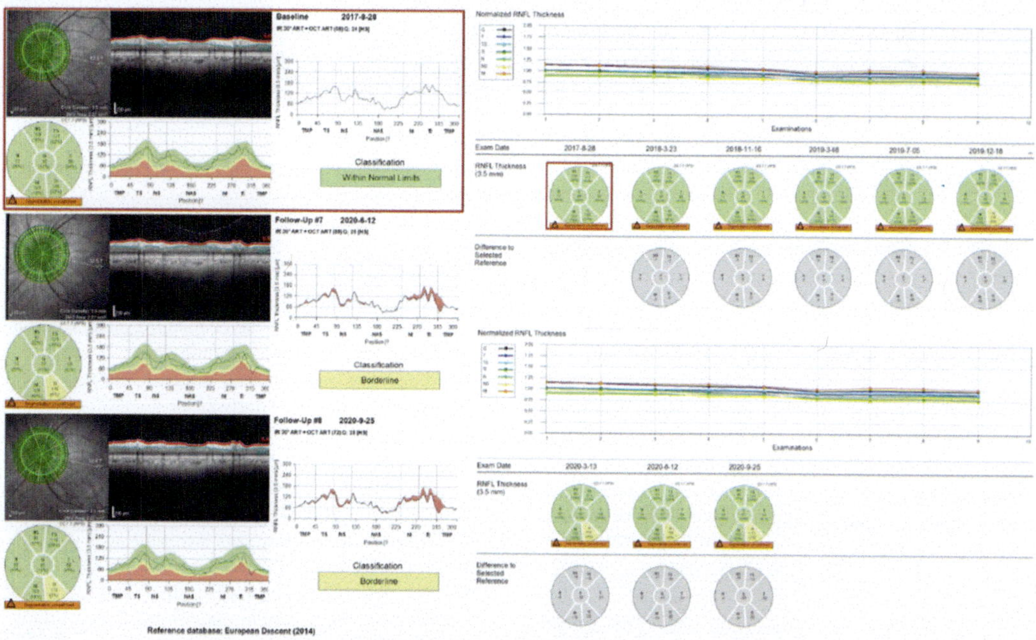

Fig. 10 Spectralis OCT scans of a glaucoma patient followed for 3 years. The RNFL change and trend reports show progressive loss of the retinal nerve fiber layer. (Courtesy of Kyeong Ik Na, M.D.)

References

Abe RY, Gracitelli CP, Medeiros FA. The use of spectral-domain optical coherence tomography to detect glaucoma progression. Open Ophthalmol J. 2015;9:78–88.

Airaksinen PJ, Nieminen H. Retinal nerve fiber layer photography in glaucoma. Ophthalmology. 1985;92(7):877–9.

Airaksinen PJ, Drance SM, Douglas GR, Mawson DK, Nieminen H. Diffuse and localized nerve fiber loss in glaucoma. Am J Ophthalmol. 1984;98(5):566–71.

Bowd C, Zangwill LM, Berry CC, Blumenthal EZ, Vasile C, Sanchez-Galeana C, et al. Detecting early glaucoma by assessment of retinal nerve fiber layer thickness and visual function. Invest Ophthalmol Vis Sci. 2001;42(9):1993–2003.

Bussel, II, Wollstein G, Schuman JS. OCT for glaucoma diagnosis, screening and detection of glaucoma progression. Br J Ophthalmol. 2014;98 Suppl 2(Suppl 2):ii15–9.

Chong GT, Lee RK. Glaucoma versus red disease: imaging and glaucoma diagnosis. Curr Opin Ophthalmol. 2012;23(2):79–88.

González-García AO, Vizzeri G, Bowd C, Medeiros FA, Zangwill LM, Weinreb RN. Reproducibility of RTVue retinal nerve fiber layer thickness and optic disc measurements and agreement with Stratus optical coherence tomography measurements. Am J Ophthalmol. 2009;147(6):1067–74, 74.e1.

Grewal DS, Tanna AP. Diagnosis of glaucoma and detection of glaucoma progression using spectral domain optical coherence tomography. Curr Opin Ophthalmol. 2013;24(2):150–61.

Hangai M, Yamamoto M, Sakamoto A, Yoshimura N. Ultrahigh-resolution versus speckle noise-reduction in spectral-domain optical coherence tomography. Opt Express. 2009;17(5):4221–35.

Hoyt WF, Frisén L, Newman NM. Fundoscopy of nerve fiber layer defects in glaucoma. Investig Ophthalmol. 1973;12(11):814–29.

Jeoung JW, Park KH. Comparison of Cirrus OCT and Stratus OCT on the ability to detect localized retinal nerve fiber layer defects in preperimetric glaucoma. Invest Ophthalmol Vis Sci. 2010;51(2):938–45.

Jeoung JW, Choi YJ, Park KH, Kim DM. Macular ganglion cell imaging study: glaucoma diagnostic accuracy of spectral-domain optical coherence tomography. Invest Ophthalmol Vis Sci. 2013;54(7):4422–9.

Jeoung JW, Kim TW, Weinreb RN, Kim SH, Park KH, Kim DM. Diagnostic ability of spectral-domain versus time-domain optical coherence tomography in preperimetric glaucoma. J Glaucoma. 2014;23(5):299–306.

Jonas JB, Dichtl A. Evaluation of the retinal nerve fiber layer. Surv Ophthalmol. 1996;40(5):369–78.

Jonas JB, Nguyen NX, Naumann GO. The retinal nerve fiber layer in normal eyes. Ophthalmology. 1989;96(5):627–32.

Kanamori A, Nakamura M, Escano MF, Seya R, Maeda H, Negi A. Evaluation of the glaucomatous damage on retinal nerve fiber layer thickness measured by optical coherence tomography. Am J Ophthalmol. 2003;135(4):513–20.

Kim DW, Jeoung JW, Kim YW, Girard MJ, Mari JM, Kim YK, et al. Prelamina and lamina cribrosa in glaucoma patients with unilateral visual field loss. Invest Ophthalmol Vis Sci. 2016a;57(4):1662–70.

Kim KE, Jeoung JW, Park KH, Kim DM, Kim SH. Diagnostic classification of macular ganglion cell and retinal nerve fiber layer analysis: differentiation of false-positives from glaucoma. Ophthalmology. 2015;122(3):502–10.

Kim YW, Jeoung JW, Kim DW, Girard MJ, Mari JM, Park KH, et al. Clinical assessment of lamina cribrosa curvature in eyes with primary open-angle glaucoma. PLoS One. 2016b;11(3):e0150260.

Langenegger SJ, Funk J, Töteberg-Harms M. Reproducibility of retinal nerve fiber layer thickness measurements using the eye tracker and the retest function of Spectralis SD-OCT in glaucomatous and healthy control eyes. Invest Ophthalmol Vis Sci. 2011;52(6):3338–44.

Lee WJ, Na KI, Kim YK, Jeoung JW, Park KH. Diagnostic ability of wide-field retinal nerve fiber layer maps using swept-source optical coherence tomography for detection of preperimetric and early perimetric glaucoma. J Glaucoma. 2017;26(6):577–85.

Lee WJ, Oh S, Kim YK, Jeoung JW, Park KH. Comparison of glaucoma-diagnostic ability between wide-field swept-source OCT retinal nerve fiber layer maps and spectral-domain OCT. Eye (Lond). 2018;32(9):1483–92.

Leite MT, Zangwill LM, Weinreb RN, Rao HL, Alencar LM, Sample PA, et al. Effect of disease severity on the performance of Cirrus spectral-domain OCT for glaucoma diagnosis. Invest Ophthalmol Vis Sci. 2010;51(8):4104–9.

Leite MT, Rao HL, Zangwill LM, Weinreb RN, Medeiros FA. Comparison of the diagnostic accuracies of the Spectralis, Cirrus, and RTVue optical coherence tomography devices in glaucoma. Ophthalmology. 2011;118(7):1334–9.

Leung CK, Cheung CY, Weinreb RN, Qiu Q, Liu S, Li H, et al. Retinal nerve fiber layer imaging with spectral-domain optical coherence tomography: a variability and diagnostic performance study. Ophthalmology. 2009;116(7):1257–63, 63.e1–2.

Leung CK, Yu M, Weinreb RN, Lai G, Xu G, Lam DS. Retinal nerve fiber layer imaging with spectral-domain optical coherence tomography: patterns of retinal nerve fiber layer progression. Ophthalmology. 2012;119(9):1858–66.

Mansouri K, Medeiros FA, Tatham AJ, Marchase N, Weinreb RN. Evaluation of retinal and choroidal thickness by swept-source optical coherence tomography: repeatability and assessment of artifacts. Am J Ophthalmol. 2014;157(5):1022–32.

Medeiros FA, Zangwill LM, Bowd C, Weinreb RN. Comparison of the GDx VCC scanning laser polarimeter, HRT II confocal scanning laser ophthalmoscope, and stratus OCT optical coherence tomograph for the detection of glaucoma. Arch Ophthalmol. 2004;122(6):827–37.

Mwanza JC, Durbin MK, Budenz DL, Sayyad FE, Chang RT, Neelakantan A, et al. Glaucoma diagnostic accuracy of ganglion cell-inner plexiform layer thickness: comparison with nerve fiber layer and optic nerve head. Ophthalmology. 2012;119(6):1151–8.

Radius RL, Anderson DR. The histology of retinal nerve fiber layer bundles and bundle defects. Arch Ophthalmol. 1979;97(5):948–50.

Sommer A, Miller NR, Pollack I, Maumenee AE, George T. The nerve fiber layer in the diagnosis of glaucoma. Arch Ophthalmol. 1977;95(12):2149–56.

Sommer A, Katz J, Quigley HA, Miller NR, Robin AL, Richter RC, et al. Clinically detectable nerve fiber atrophy precedes the onset of glaucomatous field loss. Arch Ophthalmol. 1991;109(1):77–83.

Vizzeri G, Weinreb RN, Gonzalez-Garcia AO, Bowd C, Medeiros FA, Sample PA, et al. Agreement between spectral-domain and time-domain OCT for measuring RNFL thickness. Br J Ophthalmol. 2009;93(6):775–81.

Macular Imaging

Ki Ho Park and Yong Woo Kim

Abstract

Innovative advances in optical coherence tomography (OCT) imaging facilitate precise exploration and monitoring of macular structures in glaucoma patients. Measurement of ganglion cell layer (GCL) and inner plexiform layer (IPL) thicknesses in the macula provides excellent diagnostic ability for glaucoma comparable to that of peripapillary retinal nerve fiber layer (RNFL) measurement. The thickness and deviation maps provided by OCT devices broadened our understanding of the patterns and temporal relationships of glaucomatous damage in the macular and peripapillary areas. This technology has enhanced the topographical analysis of structural damage to the macula and corresponding changes in the peripapillary region. The macular parameters can facilitate early detection of glaucomatous damage and discriminate meaningful progression in advanced as well as early stages of glaucoma. This chapter provides information from the basics to the latest updates on macular imaging in the field of glaucoma along with relevant clinical cases.

Keywords

Macular imaging · Ganglion cell layer · Inner plexiform layer · Temporal raphe sign · Macular vulnerability zone · Preperimetric glaucoma

1 Anatomy and Histology for Macular Imaging by OCT

The retina is a multi-layered structure made up of two synaptic (plexiform) layers sandwiched between three nuclear layers: the outer nuclear layer (ONL), inner nuclear layer (INL), and ganglion cell layer (GCL). The ONL contains the cell bodies of photoreceptors (rods and cones), and the INL contains the cell bodies of bipolar, horizontal, amacrine, and radial glial (Müller) cells. The GCL contains displaced amacrine and retinal ganglion cells (RGC). These three nuclear layers are separated by two synaptic (plexiform) layers. The outer plexiform layer (OPL) is located between the ONL and the INL, and is the place where the photoreceptors, horizontal and bipolar cell dendrites interact. The inner plexiform layer (IPL) lies between the INL and GCL and is where the bipolar cell axons, amacrine, and ganglion cells interact. The retinal nerve fiber layer (RNFL) consists primarily of RGC axons.

K. H. Park (✉) · Y. W. Kim
Department of Ophthalmology, Seoul National University Hospital, Seoul National University College of Medicine, Jongno-gu, Seoul, Korea
e-mail: kihopark@snu.ac.kr

K. H. Park, T.-W. Kim (eds.), *OCT Imaging in Glaucoma*,
https://doi.org/10.1007/978-981-16-1178-0_3

Optical coherence tomography (OCT) technology has attained improved axial resolution to 5–8 μm. This makes it possible to correlate OCT images in-vivo with histological features of the retina. Despite the fact that the OCT features of the outer retina are less well understood and remain controversial, the features of the inner retina appear to be well correlated with histology. Within the retina, the RNFL and the plexiform layers (both inner and outer) are seen as hyperreflective, while the GCL and the nuclear layers (both inner and outer) are hyporeflective. The retinal blood vessels can be seen in OCT images as circular hyperreflective structures in the inner retina, with a reduced reflectivity that extends into the deeper layers (vertical shadow). A representative OCT image of a human retina with annotated layers is provided in Fig. 1.

The macula is an oval-shaped pigmented area (*macula lutea*) in the center of the retina, about 5.5 mm in diameter in humans. It covers the region surrounding the fovea with the highest density of RGCs (over 30% of RGCs) despite occupying less than 2% of the retinal area. The macular structure is characterized by less variation among individuals, and therefore, is relatively less affected by ocular or demographic factors than is the peripapillary RNFL. Glaucoma is characterized by progressive loss of RGCs, with typical changes in the optic nerve head, resulting in progressive visual field defect in the corresponding area. It has long been well documented that early-glaucomatous damage can affect the macula (Anctil and Anderson 1984; Heijl and Lundqvist 1984). However, clinicians paid less attention to the macula until accurate measurements of each of the retinal layers of the macula became possible in-vivo. Lately, several commercially available OCT devices have made available various types of macular parameters. The two representative macular parameters are the combinations of measurements of the RNFL, GCL, and IPL: the ganglion cell-inner plexiform layer (GCIPL) thickness is the sum of the thicknesses of the GCL and IPL; the ganglion cell complex (GCC) thickness is the sum of the thicknesses of the RNFL, GCL, and IPL. These two parameters are the most commonly used and obviously essential for early detection and monitoring of glaucoma.

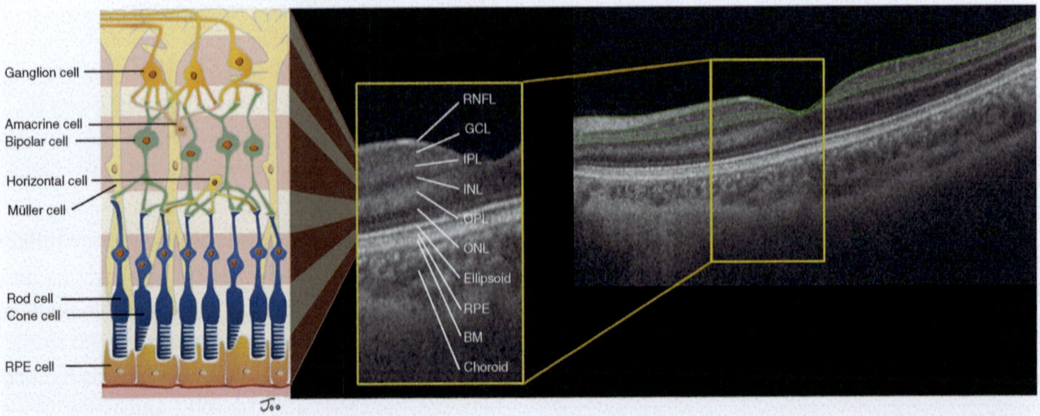

Fig. 1 Human macular structure. Retinal layers (Left) and representative human macular structure imaged by swept-source optical coherence tomography (SS-OCT) (Middle and Right). Retinal nerve fiber layer (RNFL), ganglion cell layer (GCL), and inner plexiform layer (IPL) are annotated in green solid lines. The foveal structure in the yellow inset is magnified and each retinal layer is annotated. RNFL, retinal nerve fiber layer; GCL, ganglion cell layer; IPL, inner plexiform layer; INL, inner nuclear layer; OPL, outer plexiform layer; ONL, outer nuclear layer; RPE, retinal pigment epithelium; BM, Bruch's membrane

2 Topographic Correlations among Optic Nerve Head, RNFL, and Macula

The axons of the RGC lie in the RNFL in bundles and enter the optic disc. The RNFL bundles each have their own course of travel to the optic disc. The RNFL at the temporal side of the fovea travels to the optic disc in an arcuate shape around the fovea. The axons of the RGC do not cross the horizontal meridian, so that a raphe with relatively few axons is formed in the temporal area (temporal raphe). According to this anatomy, most macular change in glaucomatous eyes appears in an arcuate-to-crescent shape, and is located mainly in the temporal macular regions along the horizontal raphe. The macular change also is usually located within the same hemifield on the continuum of the corresponding RNFL defect and optic disc damage (Fig. 2).

It is widely accepted that glaucomatous defect is most prevalent in the inferotemporal and superotemporal regions of the optic disc. The neural canal opening is connected to the superonasal region of the eyeball. This means that the center of the optic disc lies about 6° above the horizontal midline through the center of the fovea.

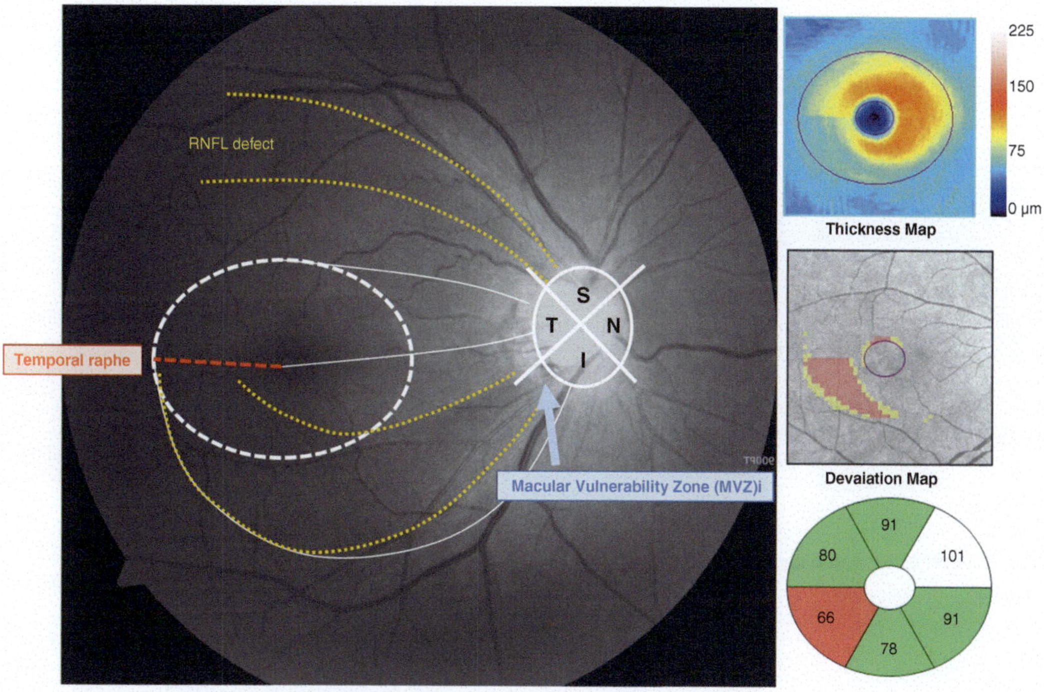

Fig. 2 Macular damage in glaucoma. The axons of the retinal ganglion cells (RGC) travel in the retinal nerve fiber layer (RNFL) in bundles and enter the optic disc. The RNFL at the temporal side of the fovea travels to the optic disc in an arcuate shape around the fovea. The RGC axons do not cross the horizontal meridian, so that a raphe with relatively few axons is formed in the temporal area (temporal raphe, red dotted line). RGC axons in the superior macula enter through the temporal border of the optic disc while RGC axons in the inferior macula enter through the inferotemporal border of the optic disc. This topographical relationship between the macula and the optic disc results in an overlap of the inferior macular region with the inferotemporal region of the optic disc, where glaucomatous defects dominate. Hood et al. designated this region the "macular vulnerability zone (MVZ)" of the optic disc (blue arrow). Case of 40-year-old male with primary open-angle glaucoma (POAG) in right eye. Note the inferotemporal and superotemporal RNFL defects in the red-free RNFL photography. Thickness and deviation maps for the ganglion cell-inner plexiform layer (GCIPL) from Cirrus HD-OCT (Carl Zeiss Meditec, Dublin, CA, USA) are provided. Macular damage is manifest in the inferotemporal macular region (inferotemporal GCIPL thickness = 66 μm), in an arcuate shape that does not cross the horizontal raphe. The superior RNFL defect does not invade the superior macular region, with the result that the superior macula is not damaged

Therefore, the RGC axons in the superior macula enter through the temporal border of the optic disc, while RGC axons in the inferior macula enter through the inferotemporal border of the optic disc. This topographical relationship between macula and optic disc results in an overlap of the inferior macular region with the inferotemporal region of the optic disc, where glaucomatous defects dominate. Hood et al. designated this region as the "macular vulnerability zone (MVZ)" of the optic disc (Fig. 2) (Hood et al. 2013; Hood 2017). Most of the RGCs in the inferior macular region project to the MVZ, which is the commonly affected region in glaucoma.

Kim et al. (2014a) further investigated the topographical relationship between localized peripapillary RNFL defect and macular GCIPL defect. They utilized the MATLAB program to construct a "GCIPL deviation frequency map" from 140 eyes of 140 open-angle glaucoma patients showing localized RNFL defect in one hemifield. According to the analysis from six different clock-hour locations of RNFL defect, the GCIPL defects had an arcuate shape that appeared as a continuation of the RNFL defect in the same hemisphere. The temporal macular region was the most frequently damaged site in either hemifield, and was larger in the inferior hemifield than in the superior (Fig. 3).

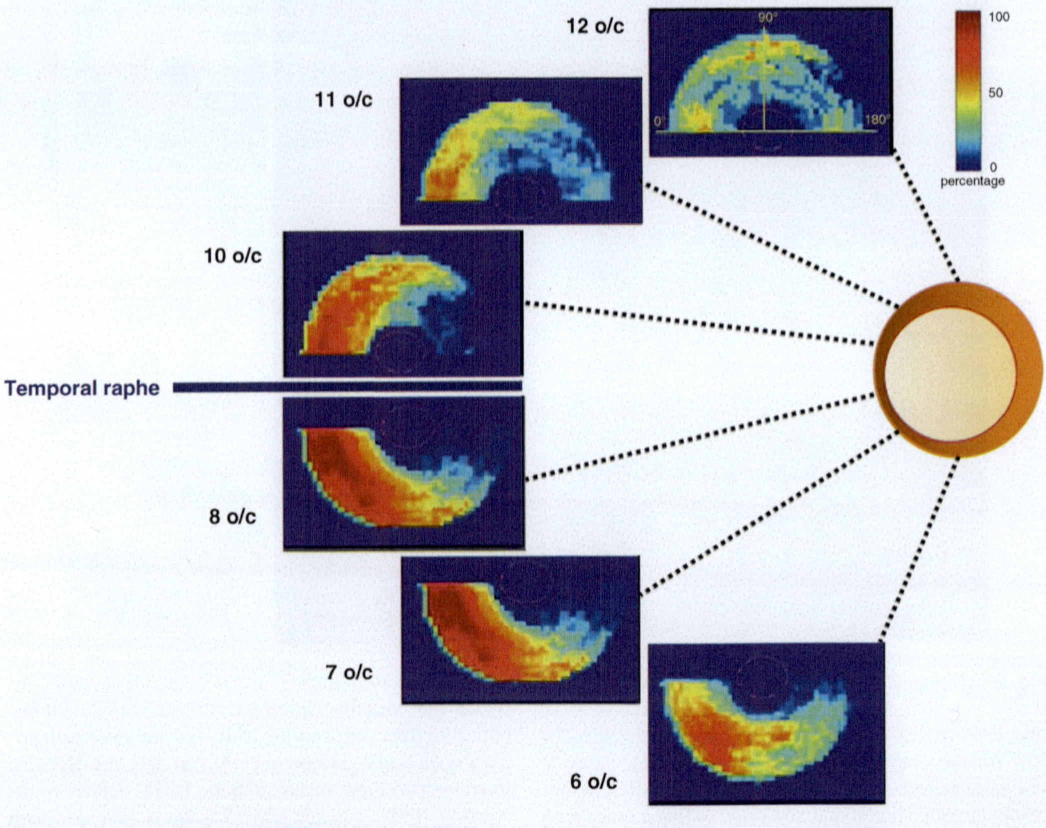

Fig. 3 Topographic relationship between localized peripapillary RNFL and macular GCIPL defects. A "GCIPL deviation frequency map" was constructed by superimposing the ganglion cell-inner plexiform layer (GCIPL) defects onto the deviation map corresponding to peripapillary retinal nerve fiber layer (RNFL) defects at different clock-hour locations (from 6 to 12 o'clock). The color-coded scale presents the frequency of GCIPL defects: the red-colored region indicates the highest GCIPL defect frequency, while the blue-colored region is close to zero. The GCIPL defects had an arcuate shape that appeared as a continuation of the RNFL defect in the same hemisphere. The temporal macular region was the most frequently damaged site in either hemifield, and was larger in the inferior hemifield than in the superior (adapted and modified from Kim et al. 2014a)

3 Diagnostic Accuracy of Macular Imaging

The macular parameters are known to have a high diagnostic utility for perimetric glaucoma comparable to those of peripapillary RNFL thickness or optic nerve head (ONH) parameters. In one study, the minimum (defined as the GCIPL thickness on the meridian showing the lowest average measurement) and inferotemporal GCIPL showed the highest sensitivity (94.8%) among GCIPL parameters, with comparable specificities (87.9 and 85.8%, respectively) (Mwanza et al. 2012). In another study, the GCC also showed good diagnostic utility for glaucoma comparable to that of peripapillary RNFL thickness, where global loss volume (percentage of global GCC loss over the entire GCC map) was found to be the best parameter (Tan et al. 2009).

3.1 Diagnostic Accuracy for Preperimetric and Early Glaucoma

Consistent with earlier studies investigating early-glaucomatous damage affecting the macula, the macular parameters have exhibited excellent RNFL-comparable diagnostic power for discriminating early-stage glaucoma (glaucoma suspect or preperimetric glaucoma). Mwanza et al. (2012) for the first time reported that minimum GCIPL thickness was found to be the best GCIPL parameter for discriminating early glaucoma (including both preperimetric and perimetric) from normal eyes. In a Korean study that had enrolled 92 preperimetric glaucoma patients and 92 age-matched controls, the inferotemporal GCIPL had comparable diagnostic power for glaucoma (area under receiver operating characteristic curves [AUROC] = 0.823), which results were not significantly different from those of the best parameter for peripapillary RNFL (7 o'clock sector, AUROC = 0.764) and ONH (rim area, 0.767) (Kim et al. 2014b). As the angular distance between the fovea and an RNFL defect increases, the sensitivity of macular GCIPL parameters for detection of RNFL defects deteriorates (Kim et al. 2014b; Hwang et al. 2014).

3.2 Diagnostic Accuracy in Myopic Eyes

Myopic eyes have divergent optic disc shapes such as are manifested in tilted disc, peripapillary atrophy, or posterior staphyloma. These structural variations make diagnosis and monitoring of glaucoma challenging in myopic eyes (Tan et al. 2019). Macular inner retinal thickness is known to be less affected by the degree of myopia and myopia-related ONH structural change relative to peripapillary RNFL thickness (Kim et al. 2015a; Jeong et al. 2016). In this context, macular GCIPL thickness can be an effective alternative method to evaluate glaucomatous damage in myopic eyes. A Korean study that included open-angle glaucoma patients with either highly myopic or non-highly myopic eyes reported that the best parameters for discriminating normal eyes from glaucomatous ones were inferior RNFL (0.906) and inferotemporal GCIPL (0.852) thickness in the highly myopic group, and average RNFL (0.920) and minimum GCIPL (0.908) thickness in the non-highly myopic group (Choi et al. 2013). Another Korean study further investigated inferotemporal GCIPL thickness's diagnostic utility in a myopic preperimetric glaucoma population, and found it to be the best parameter, having a significantly greater diagnostic power than the other parameters including average RNFL or GCIPL thickness, rim area, inferior RNFL thickness, and minimum GCIPL thickness (Seol et al. 2015). A recent study using swept-source OCT (SS-OCT, deep range imaging [DRI] OCT, Topcon, Tokyo, Japan) demonstrated that inferotemporal GCL+ (identical with GCIPL thickness) and GCL++ (identical with GCC thickness) had the greatest AUROC for myopic glaucoma (Kim et al. 2020). In this study, macular GCL++ thickness (87.6%) and GCL+ thickness (87.5%) showed greater AUROC than did macular GCIPL thickness based on spectral-domain OCT (Cirrus HD-OCT, Carl Zeiss Meditec, Dublin, CA, USA).

However, it should be noted that the macular parameters are not always dispositive in myopic eyes. The current normative database in most commercially available OCT devices does not fully represent the myopic population, with the result that the prevalence of false-positive red signs can reach 40.4% (Kim et al. 2015b). Myopic macular degeneration can cause abnormal thinning (due to patch atrophy) or thickening (due to retinoschisis) of the retinal layers, and these structural abnormalities may deteriorate the accuracy of OCT devices' automated segmentation (Tan et al. 2019; Ruiz-Medrano et al. 2019). Therefore, before interpreting macular parameters in glaucoma diagnostics, it would be prudent to carefully examine the entire macular structure and OCT scan quality rather than rely solely on the color-coded map and thickness profile.

4 Instrument-Specific Maps and Interpretation

4.1 Cirrus HD-OCT

Cirrus HD-OCT is an SD-OCT with a speed of 68,000 scans/s (latest model: Cirrus HD 6000) (Cirrus HD-OCT User Manual). It provides GCIPL thickness in a Ganglion Cell Analysis (GCA) printout. The GCIPL thickness is measured within a horizontally oval 4.8 × 4.0 mm area excluding a central perifoveal ellipse of 1.2 × 1.0 mm area: global average, minimum, and 6 wedge-shaped sectoral GCIPL thicknesses are provided in the GCA printout (Fig. 4). The normative database for macular measurements consists of 282 normal subjects aged between 19 and 84 years (mean: 46.5 years). Only 28 subjects aged 70–79 years and 3 subjects above age 80 are included therein, so caution is needed when interpreting patient data in these age ranges (Cirrus HD-OCT User Manual). There is no normative database for subjects younger than 19 years. Cirrus HD-OCT additionally provides an "Asian normative database" consisting of 315 individuals from Japan, China, and India (aged 19–79). All of these normative databases are adjusted only by age, and the color-coded maps in the GCA printouts do not take into account differences that may be present due to ethnicity, axial length, refraction, optic disc area, or signal strength (Cirrus HD-OCT User Manual).

Besides thickness measurements, the GCA printout provides additional GCIPL thickness and deviation maps. The thickness map provides the raw measurement thickness profiles on a color-scaled map. The deviation map shows regions wherein GCIPL thickness has fallen below the 5% limit based on the normative database with the yellow- (percentile values <5%) and red-color superpixels (percentile values <1%).

4.1.1 Temporal Raphe Sign

Temporal raphe sign (or GCIPL hemifield test) is determined to be positive in subjects who have a straight line on the horizontal raphe longer than one-half of the length between the inner and outer annulus in the temporal elliptical area of the GCIPL color thickness map (Fig. 5). This sign is known to be more effective than other macular parameters in discriminating early-glaucomatous changes (AUROC 0.967 in preperimetric glaucoma and 0.962 in perimetric glaucoma) (Kim et al. 2015c). This method is easy to apply in clinical practice and is advantageous for discrimination of glaucomatous change in highly myopic eyes that have a depigmented fundus and where RNFL defects are difficult to find (Kim et al. 2016). Temporal raphe sign positivity at the baseline has been associated with faster conversion to glaucoma in elderly subjects with a large cup-to-disc ratio (Ha et al. 2020).

4.1.2 PanoMap

Cirrus HD-OCT integrates the optic disc cube and macular cube scans into a single image and provides a combined wide-field OCT map, the so-called PanoMap (Fig. 6). The integration of the RNFL and GCIPL maps is useful for understanding the topographic patterns of glaucomatous structural damage in the early stages of glaucoma. By this method, Kim et al. (2017a) demonstrated that no single case of peripapillary RNFL defect in the MVZ was found without inferior macular GCIPL loss. However, there

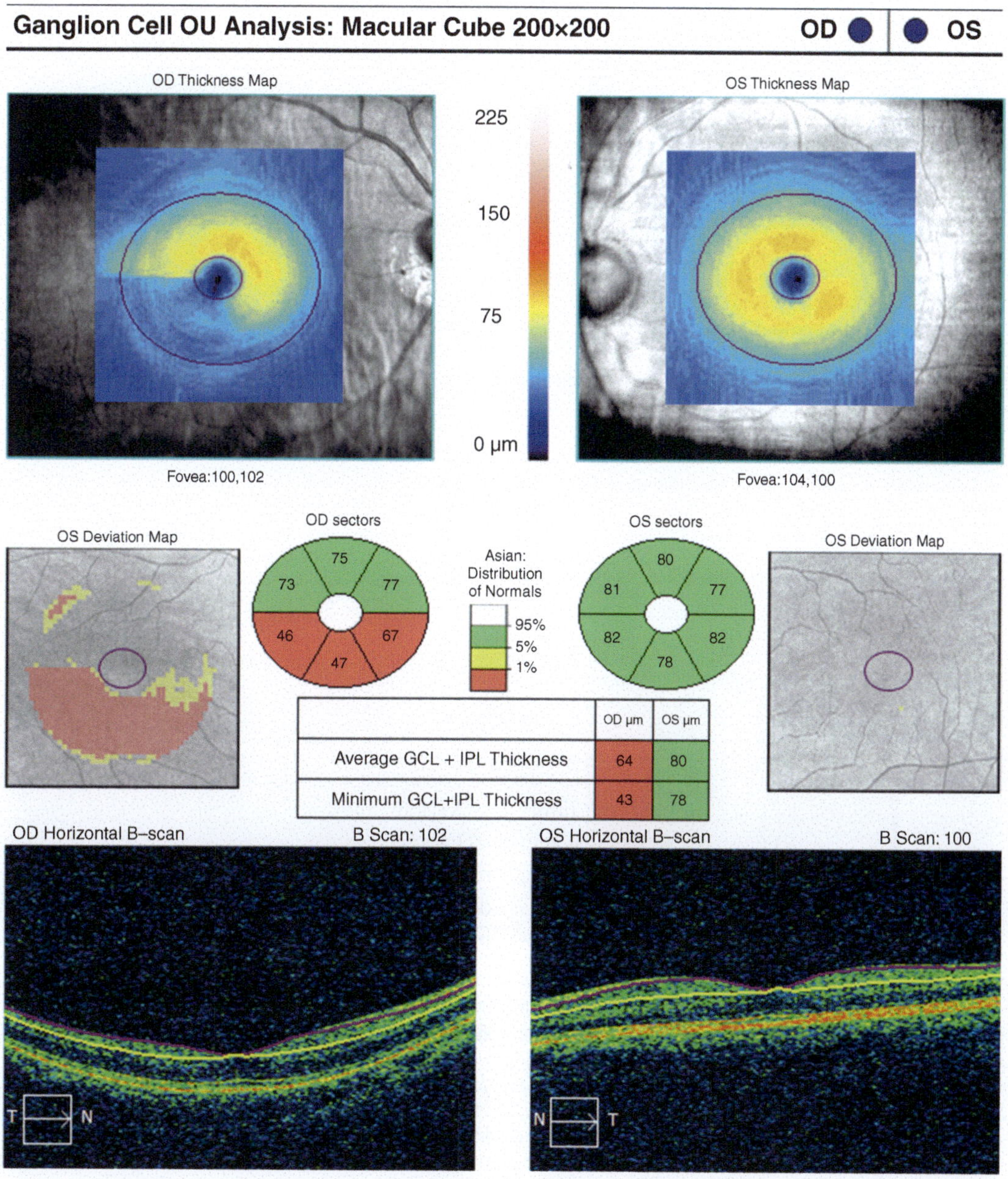

Fig. 4 Cirrus HD-OCT: Ganglion Cell Analysis. Typical printout of Ganglion Cell Analysis (GCA) from Cirrus HD-OCT. The thickness map (horizontally oval 4.8 × 4.0 mm area excluding central perifoveal ellipse 1.2 × 1.0 mm sized area) is provided in the first row. In the second row are the deviation maps showing regions where GCIPL thickness fell below the 5% limit based on the normative database with the yellow- (percentile values <5%) and red-color superpixels (percentile values <1%). Thickness measurements (average, minimum, and six sectoral measurements) with color-coded maps based on the internal normative database are provided in the center

were a few cases of inferior macular GCIPL loss without peripapillary RNFL defect in the MVZ. This finding suggests that inferior macular GCIPL loss may precede peripapillary RNFL defect in the MVZ. In Kim et al.'s (2017b) subsequent longitudinal observation of deviation maps of macular GCIPL and peripapillary RNFL from 151 eyes with early-stage glaucoma, macular

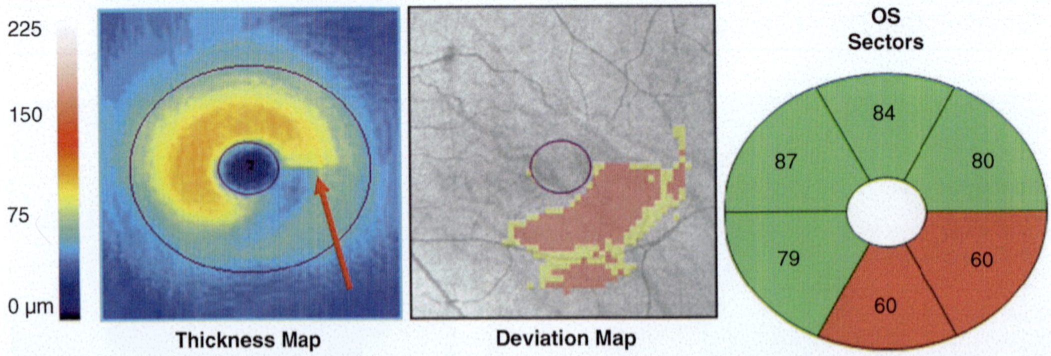

Fig. 5 Temporal Raphe sign. Temporal raphe sign (or GCIPL hemifield test) is determined to be positive in subjects who have a straight line longer than one-half of the length between the inner and outer annulus in the temporal elliptical area of the GCIPL color thickness map (red arrow). In this case, the patient has an inferotemporal retinal nerve fiber layer (RNFL) defect and a corresponding inferotemporal ganglion-cell inner plexiform layer (GCIPL) defect

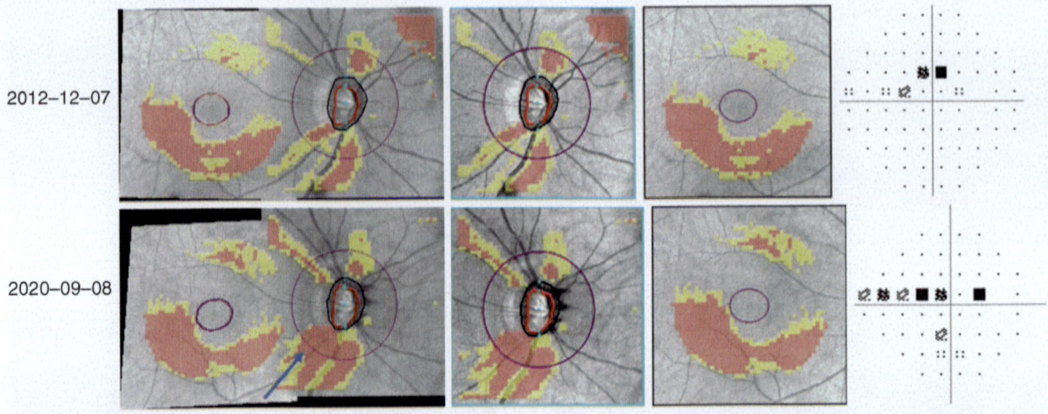

Fig. 6 PanoMap: combined GCA and RNFL deviation map. Cirrus HD-OCT PanoMap Analysis integrates data from optic disc cube and macular cube scans into a single image and provides a wide-field perspective for comprehensive posterior segment analysis. A case of 27-year-old male with myopia (spherical equivalence –5 diopters, axial length = 25.65 mm) and open-angle glaucoma in his right eye. At baseline (2012-12-07), the patient had inferoinferior retinal nerve fiber layer (RNFL) and inferotemporal ganglion-cell inner plexiform layer (GCIPL) defects. The automated perimetry showed a few superior paracentral scotomas (mean deviation, –2.14 dB). Eight years later (2020-09-08), the patient showed progressive thinning of the RNFL in the macular vulnerability zone (MVZ) (blue arrow) with increased nasal and paracentral scotomas

GCIPL change was frequently detected before corresponding peripapillary RNFL change (Fig. 6). Another study, this one from Australia, further demonstrated an association between lower intraocular pressure and glaucomatous structural change manifesting at the macular GCIPL before manifesting at the peripapillary RNFL (Marshall et al. 2019). These findings highlight the importance of macular imaging in glaucoma patients, as peripapillary RNFL analysis alone can overlook macular damage. The PanoMap is also known to be helpful in the detection of early-stage structural progression by inspecting various progression patterns of RNFL and GCIPL from a single combined image (Lee et al. 2018a, b).

4.2 Spectralis OCT

Spectralis OCT (Heidelberg Engineering GmbH, Heidelberg, Germany) has Glaucoma Module Premium Edition (GMPE) software that provides a Posterior Pole Asymmetry Analysis consisting of 61 horizontal B-scans, each comprised of 768 A-scans that are acquired along the Bruch's membrane opening (BMO)-fovea axis (Heidelberg Engineering). It provides a thickness map, a thickness deviation map, and a color-coded classification chart for the total retina, RNFL, GCL, and IPL (Fig. 7). On the thickness deviation map, the red and yellow areas represent percentile values <1% and <5%, respectively, while the blue and purple areas represent percentile values >95% and >99%, respectively. The green areas represent a percentile value of 5–95%. There is no RNFL color-coded classification chart, because the macular RNFL is anatomically thin, which limits the reliability of measurements in this location, and also because RNFL defects are typically most prominent beyond the confines of the GCL-optimized grid (Heidelberg Engineering).

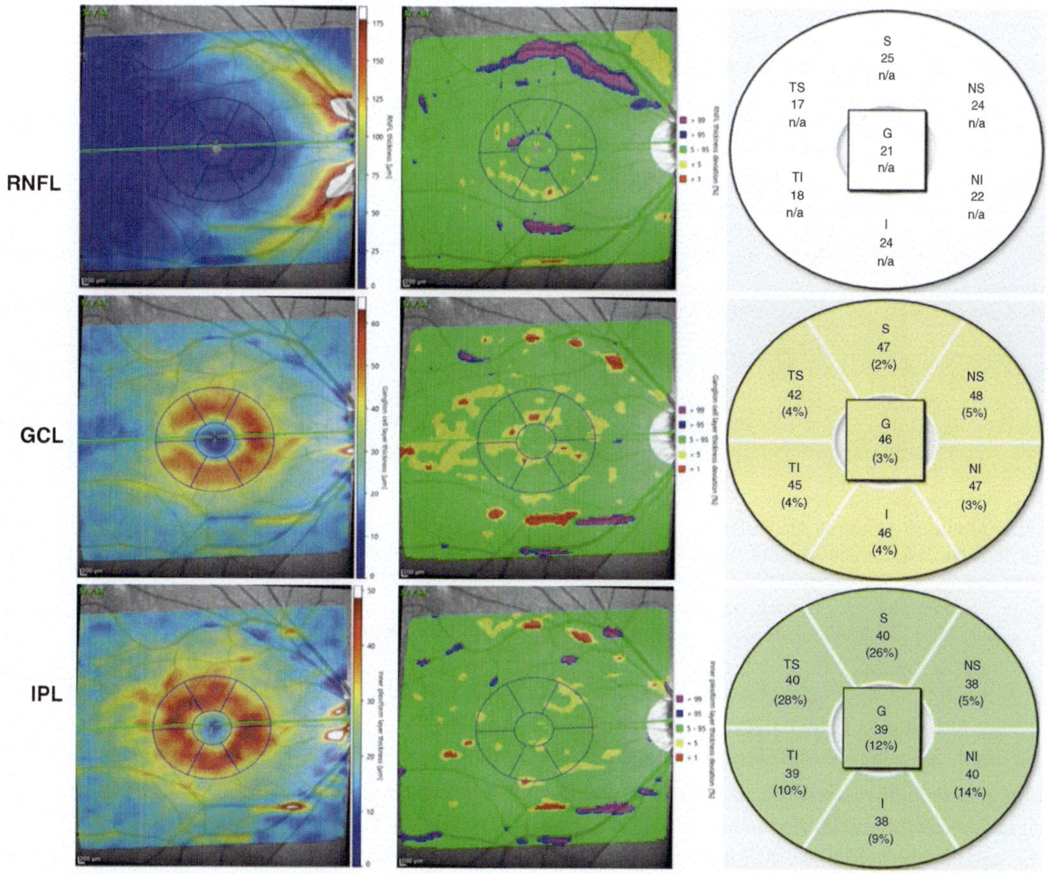

Fig. 7 Spectralis OCT: thickness and deviation maps. Spectralis OCT provides a thickness map, thickness deviation map, and color-coded classification chart for the total retina, retinal nerve fiber layer (RNFL), ganglion cell layer (GCL), and inner plexiform layer (IPL). In the thickness deviation map, the red and yellow areas represent percentile values <1% and <5%, respectively, while the blue and purple areas represent percentile values >95% and >99%, respectively. The green areas represent a percentile value of 5–95%. There is no RNFL color-coded classification chart, because the macular RNFL is anatomically thin, which limits the reliability of measurements in this location, and also because RNFL defects are typically most prominent beyond the confines of the GCL-optimized grid

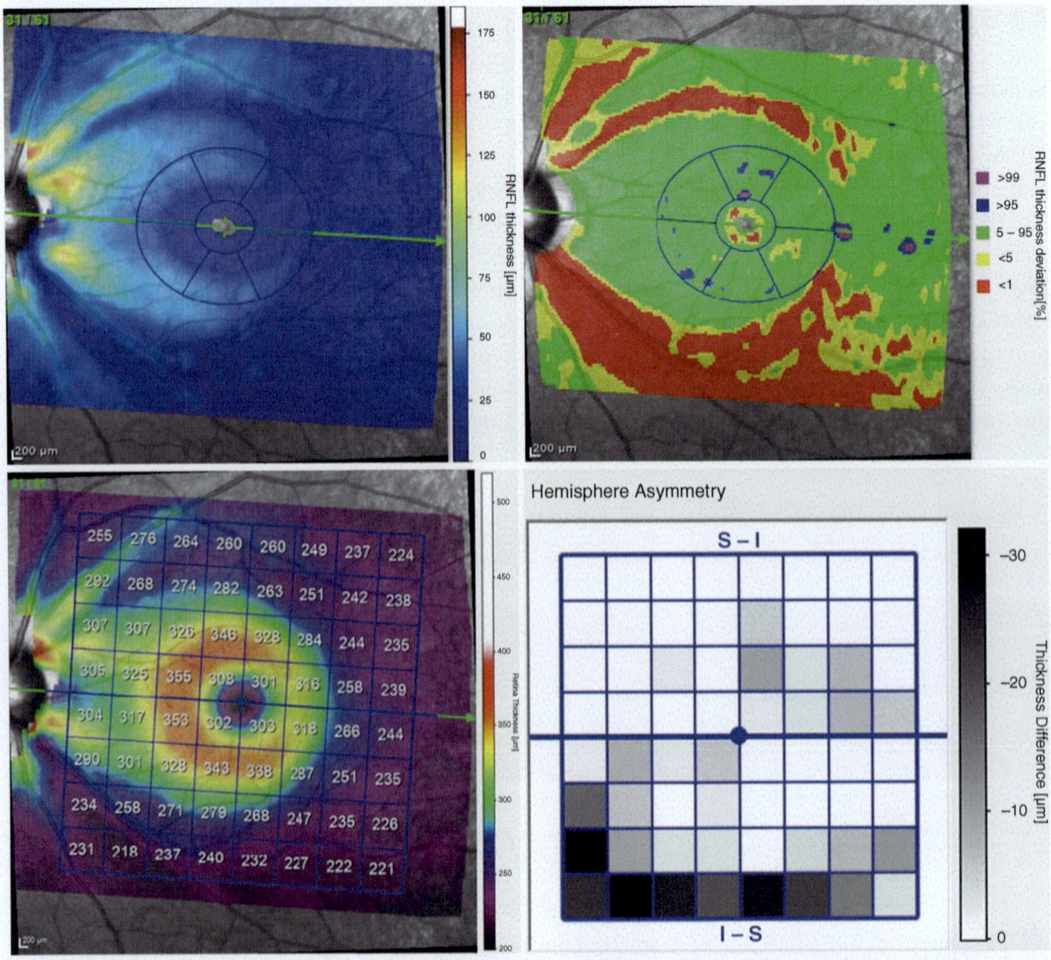

Fig. 8 Posterior pole asymmetry analysis. Spectralis OCT provides a retinal thickness asymmetry graph between the inferior and superior macula hemisphere of each eye. A case of 28-year-old male with open-angle glaucoma on his left eye. The patient had mild superotemporal and more severe inferotemporal retinal nerve fiber layer (RNFL) defects. The thickness asymmetry graph (bottom right) revealed asymmetrical retinal thinning in the inferior region

Total retinal thickness is further displayed on a color-coded map (Fig. 8). A thickness asymmetry graph between the inferior and superior macular hemispheres of each eye, and between the right and left eyes, is also available. The darker the square, the larger the difference in thickness between that square and the corresponding square in the opposite hemisphere or eye, with jet-black squares indicating a difference >30 μm.

4.3 DRI OCT Triton

DRI OCT Triton (Topcon, Tokyo, Japan) is a swept-source OCT using a longer, 1,050 nm wavelength light-source that enables a deeper imaging range and better tissue penetration. It provides a faster scanning speed of 100,000 A-scans/s, which significantly reduces motion artifacts with short capture times and collects

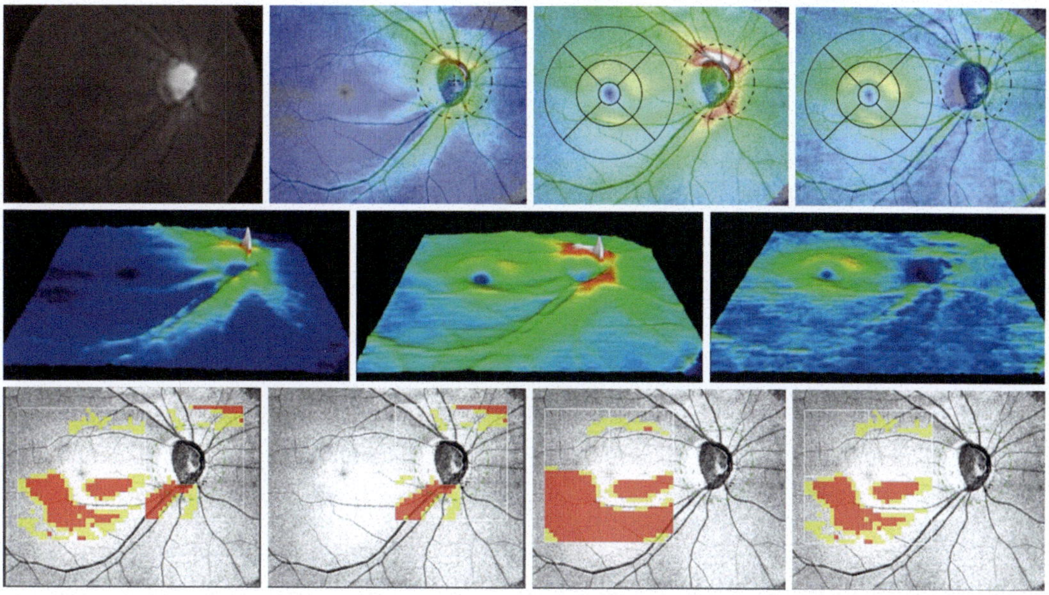

Fig. 9 DRI OCT Triton: wide-field map. The 3D Wide scan in DRI OCT Triton provides a 12 × 9 mm wide-field thickness map (first row), a thickness surface map (second row), and SuperPixel maps (third row) for the retinal nerve fiber layer (RNFL) (second column), GCL++ (third column), and GCL+ layers (fourth column). SuperPixel maps can be displayed as a combination of RNFL with either GCL++ or GCL+ (first column). The thickness surface map (second row) is displayed in 3D for selected layers (RNFL, GCL++, or GCL+, respectively), and can be rotated or zoomed-in and -out by mouse operation. The SuperPixel-200 map consists of 26 × 26 grids within a 5.2 × 5.2 mm^2 peripapillary area and 30 × 30 grids within a 6.0 × 6.0 mm^2 macular area, thereby providing a significance map based on the built-in normative database. The side length of each grid is 200 μm. The uncolored pixels indicate the normal range, whereas the yellow- and red-colored pixels indicate abnormality at P = 1–5% and P < 1% of the normal level, respectively

more OCT data in a single scan. The 3D Wide scan in DRI OCT Triton provides a 12 × 9 mm wide-field thickness map, a thickness surface map, and SuperPixel maps for the RNFL, GCL++, and GCL+ layers. The thickness surface map (second row) is displayed in 3D for selected layers (RNFL, GCL++, or GCL+) and can be rotated or zoomed-in and -out by mouse operation (Fig. 9). The SuperPixel-200 map consists of 26 × 26 grids within a 5.2 × 5.2 mm^2 peripapillary area and 30 × 30 grids within a 6.0 × 6.0 mm^2 macular area, thereby providing a significance map (identical with the deviation map in Cirrus OCT) based on the built-in normative database. The side length of each grid is 200 μm. Uncolored pixels indicate the normal range, whereas yellow- and red-colored pixels indicate abnormality at P = 1–5% and P < 1% of the normal level, respectively.

The inferior GCL++ (AUROC = 0.809) and inferotemporal GCL+ thickness (AUROC = 0.809) showed the greatest diagnostic ability for detection of preperimetric glaucoma from healthy eyes (Lee et al. 2017a). In addition, inferotemporal GCL++ (AUROC = 0.865) and GCL+ thicknesses (AUROC = 0.865) showed the best diagnostic power for early-perimetric glaucoma (Lee et al. 2017a). The wide-field thickness map showed comparable diagnostic power for preperimetric and early-perimetric glaucoma with Cirrus HD-OCT (Lee et al. 2018c). A recent study that enrolled 150 myopic primary open-angle glaucoma (POAG) eyes and 100 healthy myopic eyes reported that the RNFL/GCL++/GCL+ wide-field thickness (thickness surface) map showed better accuracy for glaucomatous defects in both the superotemporal and inferotemporal regions than did the Cirrus HD-OCT thickness map (Kim et al. 2020). This possibly was due to the difference in the measurement regions between the two devices. The measurement area of the macular parameter is within a 6 mm diameter circle for DRI OCT Triton and within a 4.8 × 4.0 mm elliptical annulus for Cirrus HD-OCT. A wider scan range in SS-OCT may be more advantageous for diagnosis of POAG in myopic eyes. Furthermore, the difference in the segmentation algorithms between the two OCT devices may influence the diagnostic power for myopic POAG (Kim et al. 2020; Pierro et al. 2012).

5 Detecting Glaucoma Progression

Monitoring of macular parameters facilitates detection of structural progression in glaucomatous eyes and prediction of subsequent visual field defect. The rate of GCIPL thinning reportedly is significantly faster in glaucomatous eyes with progression (Lee et al. 2017b, c). The mean rate of GCIPL thinning has been found to be significantly faster, even, in pseudoexfoliative glaucoma (–1.46 μm/year) than in open-angle glaucoma (–0.49 μm/year) or normal eyes (–0.31 μm/year) (Lee et al. 2019). A trend-based analysis (>5 years) of macular GCIPL and peripapillary RNFL from 163 POAG patients revealed that progressive macular GCIPL and peripapillary RNFL thinning were mutually predictive, and that both were indicative of visual field progression (Hou et al. 2018). Another retrospective cohort study, this one from Korea, also demonstrated that eyes with progressive GCIPL and RNFL thinning showed a significant higher risk of developing visual field defects (Shin et al. 2020).

Trend-based analysis of GCIPL is also known to be useful in detecting progression even in advanced-glaucoma eyes. Peripapillary RNFL is likely to reach the measurement floor in advanced-glaucoma eyes, which makes it less valuable for detection of progression in these eyes. However, recent studies reported significant rates of change for macular GCIPL but no significant changes for peripapillary RNFL or rim area in advanced-glaucoma eyes (Shin et al. 2017; Lavinsky et al. 2018). This suggests that damage impacting the macular GCIPL occurs at a different rate than in the case of the peripapillary RNFL.

References

Anctil JL, Anderson DR. Early foveal involvement and generalized depression of the visual field in glaucoma. Arch Ophthalmol. 1984;102(3):363–70.

Choi YJ, Jeoung JW, Park KH, Kim DM. Glaucoma detection ability of ganglion cell-inner plexiform layer thickness by spectral-domain optical coherence tomography in high myopia. Invest Ophthalmol Vis Sci. 2013;54(3):2296–304.

Cirrus HD-OCT User Manual 2660021159751 Rev. A 2015-08. Appendix A. https://www.zeiss.co.uk/content/dam/Meditec/gb/Chris/Refractive-Business-Builder/2018Updates/UserGuides/oct_usermanual.pdf. Accessed 25 Oct 2020.

Ha A, Kim YK, Kim JS, Jeoung JW, Park KH. Temporal raphe sign in elderly patients with large optic disc cupping: its evaluation as a predictive factor for glaucoma conversion. Am J Ophthalmol. 2020;219:205–14.

Heidelberg Engineering. Spectralis Glaucoma Toolkit. 10-4. https://business-lounge.heidelbergengineering.com/us/en/products/spectralis/glaucoma-module/downloads/#downloads. Accessed 25 Oct 2020.

Heijl A, Lundqvist L. The frequency distribution of earliest glaucomatous visual field defects documented by automatic perimetry. Acta Ophthalmol. 1984;62(4):658–64.

Hood DC. Improving our understanding, and detection, of glaucomatous damage: An approach based upon optical coherence tomography (OCT). Prog Retin Eye Res. 2017;57:46–75.

Hood DC, Raza AS, de Moraes CG, Liebmann JM, Ritch R. Glaucomatous damage of the macula. Prog Retin Eye Res. 2013;32:1–21.

Hou HW, Lin C, Leung CK. Integrating macular ganglion cell inner plexiform layer and parapapillary retinal nerve fiber layer measurements to detect glaucoma progression. Ophthalmology. 2018;125(6):822–31.

Hwang YH, Jeong YC, Kim HK, Sohn YH. Macular ganglion cell analysis for early detection of glaucoma. Ophthalmology. 2014;121(8):1508–15.

Jeong JH, Choi YJ, Park KH, Kim DM, Jeoung JW. Macular ganglion cell imaging study: covariate effects on the spectral domain optical coherence tomography for glaucoma diagnosis. PLoS One. 2016;11(8):e0160448.

Kim KE, Park KH, Yoo BW, Jeoung JW, Kim DM, Kim HC. Topographic localization of macular retinal ganglion cell loss associated with localized peripapillary retinal nerve fiber layer defect. Invest Ophthalmol Vis Sci. 2014a;55(6):3501–8.

Kim MJ, Jeoung JW, Park KH, Choi YJ, Kim DM. Topographic profiles of retinal nerve fiber layer defects affect the diagnostic performance of macular scans in preperimetric glaucoma. Invest Ophthalmol Vis Sci. 2014b;55(4):2079–87.

Kim MJ, Park KH, Yoo BW, Jeoung JW, Kim HC, Kim DM. Comparison of macular GCIPL and peripapillary RNFL deviation maps for detection of glaucomatous eye with localized RNFL defect. Acta Ophthalmol. 2015a;93(1):e22–8.

Kim KE, Jeoung JW, Park KH, Kim DM, Kim SH. Diagnostic classification of macular ganglion cell and retinal nerve fiber layer analysis: differentiation of false-positives from glaucoma. Ophthalmology. 2015b;122(3):502–10.

Kim YK, Yoo BW, Kim HC, Park KH. Automated detection of hemifield difference across horizontal raphe on ganglion cell—inner plexiform layer thickness map. Ophthalmology. 2015c;122(11):2252–60.

Kim YK, Yoo BW, Jeoung JW, Kim HC, Kim HJ, Park KH. Glaucoma-diagnostic ability of ganglion cell-inner plexiform layer thickness difference across temporal raphe in highly myopic eyes. Invest Ophthalmol Vis Sci. 2016;57(14):5856–63.

Kim YK, Jeoung JW, Park KH. Inferior macular damage in glaucoma: its relationship to retinal nerve fiber layer defect in macular vulnerability zone. J Glaucoma. 2017a;26(2):126–32.

Kim YK, Ha A, Na KI, Kim HJ, Jeoung JW, Park KH. Temporal relation between macular ganglion cell-inner plexiform layer loss and peripapillary retinal nerve fiber layer loss in glaucoma. Ophthalmology. 2017b;124(7):1056–64.

Kim YW, Lee J, Kim JS, Park KH. Diagnostic accuracy of wide-field map from swept-source optical coherence tomography for primary open-angle glaucoma in myopic eyes. Am J Ophthalmol. 2020;218:182–91.

Lavinsky F, Wu M, Schuman JS, Lucy KA, Liu M, Song Y, et al. Can macula and optic nerve head parameters detect glaucoma progression in eyes with advanced circumpapillary retinal nerve fiber layer damage? Ophthalmology. 2018;125(12):1907–12.

Lee WJ, Na KI, Kim YK, Jeoung JW, Park KH. Diagnostic ability of wide-field retinal nerve fiber layer maps using swept-source optical coherence tomography for detection of preperimetric and early perimetric glaucoma. J Glaucoma. 2017a;26(6):577–85.

Lee WJ, Kim YK, Park KH, Jeoung JW. Evaluation of ganglion cell-inner plexiform layer thinning in eyes with optic disc hemorrhage: a trend-based progression analysis. Invest Ophthalmol Vis Sci. 2017b;58(14):6449–56.

Lee WJ, Kim YK, Park KH, Jeoung JW. Trend-based analysis of ganglion cell-inner plexiform layer thickness changes on optical coherence tomography in glaucoma progression. Ophthalmology. 2017c;124(9):1383–91.

Lee WJ, Kim TJ, Kim YK, Jeoung JW, Park KH. Serial combined wide-field optical coherence tomography maps for detection of early glaucomatous structural progression. JAMA Ophthalmol. 2018a;136(10):1121–7.

Lee WJ, Na KI, Ha A, Kim YK, Jeoung JW, Park KH. Combined use of retinal nerve fiber layer and ganglion cell-inner plexiform layer event-based progression analysis. Am J Ophthalmol. 2018b;196:65–71.

Lee WJ, Oh S, Kim YK, Jeoung JW, Park KH. Comparison of glaucoma-diagnostic ability between wide-field swept-source OCT retinal nerve fiber layer maps and spectral-domain OCT. Eye. 2018c;32(9):1483–92.

Lee WJ, Baek SU, Kim YK, Park KH, Jeoung JW. Rates of ganglion cell-inner plexiform layer thinning in normal, open-angle glaucoma and pseudoexfoliation glaucoma eyes: a trend-based analysis. Invest Ophthalmol Vis Sci. 2019;60(2):599–604.

Marshall HN, Andrew NH, Hassall M, Qassim A, Souzeau E, Ridge B, et al. Macular ganglion cell-inner plexiform layer loss precedes peripapillary retinal nerve fiber layer loss in glaucoma with lower intraocular pressure. Ophthalmology. 2019;126(8):1119–30.

Mwanza JC, Durbin MK, Budenz DL, Sayyad FE, Chang RT, Neelakantan A, et al. Glaucoma diagnostic accuracy of ganglion cell-inner plexiform layer thickness: comparison with nerve fiber layer and optic nerve head. Ophthalmology. 2012;119(6):1151–8.

Pierro L, Gagliardi M, Iuliano L, Ambrosi A, Bandello F. Retinal nerve fiber layer thickness reproducibility using seven different OCT instruments. Invest Ophthalmol Vis Sci. 2012;53(9):5912–1920.

Ruiz-Medrano J, Montero JA, Flores-Moreno I, Arias L, García-Layana A, Ruiz-Moreno JM. Myopic maculopathy: Current status and proposal for a new classification and grading system (ATN). Prog Retin Eye Res. 2019;69:80–115.

Seol BR, Jeoung JW, Park KH. Glaucoma detection ability of macular ganglion cell-inner plexiform layer thickness in myopic preperimetric glaucoma. Invest Ophthalmol Vis Sci. 2015;56(13):8306–13.

Shin JW, Sung KR, Lee GC, Durbin MK, Cheng D. Ganglion cell-inner plexiform layer change detected by optical coherence tomography indicates progression in advanced glaucoma. Ophthalmology. 2017;124(10):1466–74.

Shin JW, Sung KR, Song MK. Ganglion cell-inner plexiform layer and retinal nerve fiber layer changes in glaucoma suspects enable prediction of glaucoma development. Am J Ophthalmol. 2020;210:26–34.

Tan O, Chopra V, Lu AT, Schuman JS, Ishikawa H, Wollstein G, et al. Detection of macular ganglion cell loss in glaucoma by Fourier-domain optical coherence tomography. Ophthalmology. 2009;116(12):2305–14. e1–2.

Tan NYQ, Sng CCA, Jonas JB, Wong TY, Jansonius NM, Ang M. Glaucoma in myopia: diagnostic dilemmas. Br J Ophthalmol. 2019;103(10):1347–55.

Early Diagnosis and Detection of Progression

Yong Woo Kim

Abstract

Glaucoma is one of the leading causes of blindness. It is a progressive disease with differing rates of progression among individuals. Since the severity of the disease at presentation is a major risk factor for glaucoma blindness, early diagnosis and detection of progression is critical to prevention of blindness due to glaucoma. This chapter provides an overview on the utility of optical coherence tomography (OCT) imaging for early detection of glaucomatous structural damage and progression, with relevant clinical cases. The OCT devices enable not only thickness measurement of each retinal layer but also topographical analysis of glaucomatous damage based on deviation and/or thickness maps. Clinicians can use built-in Guided Progression Analysis (GPA) software to detect structural change and estimate the rate of progression. This chapter offers the latest knowledge along with practical tips for interpreting OCT printouts for early diagnosis and monitoring of glaucomatous damage.

Y. W. Kim (✉)
Department of Ophthalmology, Seoul National University Hospital, Jongno-gu, Seoul, Korea
e-mail: yongwookim@snu.ac.kr

Keywords

Optical coherence tomography · Early diagnosis · Progression analysis · RNFL thickness · Neuroretinal rim thickness
Macular GCIPL thickness

1 Early Diagnosis of Glaucoma

1.1 OCT Thickness Analysis

Optical coherence tomography (OCT) devices can provide objective and reproducible thicknesses of each retinal layer including the retinal nerve fiber layer (RNFL), ganglion cell layer (GCL), and inner plexiform layer (IPL). The measurement data are compared with the internally built-in normative database and color coded accordingly as green (normal range), yellow (< 5 percentile), red (< 1 percentile), or white (thicker than normal range). These thickness profiles can be utilized to detect early-glaucomatous structural damage.

1.1.1 RNFL Thickness

OCT-measured peripapillary RNFL thickness has been shown to be effective in discriminating preperimetric glaucoma from glaucoma-suspect eyes (Lisboa et al. 2012). Figure 1 provides a representative case of early diagnosis of glaucoma from peripapillary RNFL thickness. The infero-

K. H. Park, T.-W. Kim (eds.), *OCT Imaging in Glaucoma*,
https://doi.org/10.1007/978-981-16-1178-0_4

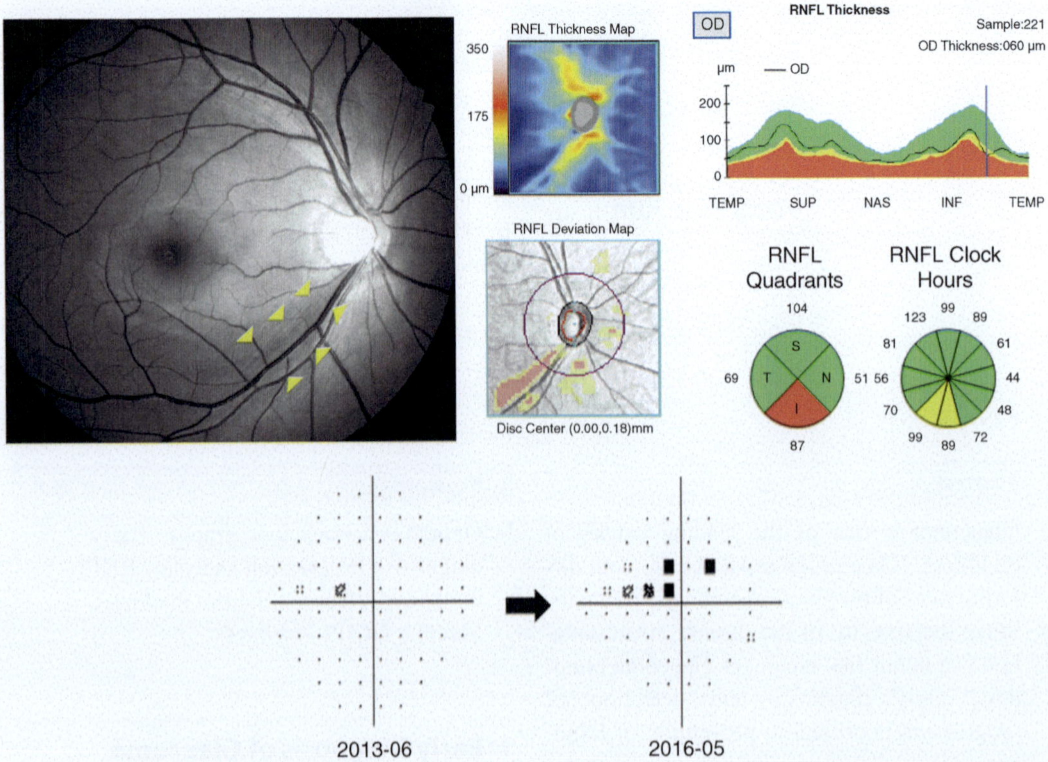

Fig. 1 Peripapillary RNFL thinning in preperimetric glaucoma. Optic disc cube scan of 40-year-old male with preperimetric glaucoma. The inferotemporal retinal nerve fiber layer (RNFL) defect in the red-free RNFL photography is well reflected in the optical coherence tomography (OCT) thickness profiles. The sectoral analysis of RNFL thickness revealed the red-color code (less than 1 percentile relative to normative database) in the inferior quadrant. The 12-hour sectoral analysis revealed the yellow-color code (less than 5 percentile of normative database) in the 6 and 7 o'clock sectors. Subsequent visual field loss appeared after 3 years, showing a superior arcuate defect

temporal RNFL defect in the red-free RNFL photography is well reflected in the OCT thickness profiles. The sectoral analysis of RNFL thickness returned the red-color code for the inferior quadrant. The 12 clock-hour sectoral analysis returned the yellow-color code for the 6 and 7 o'clock sectors. The patient, who had a within normal range visual field, showed progressive visual field defect in the corresponding superior hemifield. As shown in Fig. 1, peripapillary RNFL thickness effectively detects early structural glaucomatous damage prior to the presence of visual field defect. However, several studies have reported unsatisfactory sensitivity of peripapillary RNFL thickness, when averaged in quadrants or clock-hour sectors, for detection of localized RNFL defects in preperimetric glaucoma (Jeoung and Park 2010; Rao et al. 2013; Jeoung et al. 2014). One reported sensitivity for localized RNFL defect was 59.5% (Jeoung et al. 2014). Earlier studies reported that RNFL defects with narrow angular width are less likely to be detected on sector maps (Jeoung and Park 2010; Nukada et al. 2011). This phenomenon often occurs when clinicians solely look at the color coded sector map but not the TSNIT thickness profile graph from the OCT printout. Jeoung et al. (2014) demonstrated substantial improvement of sensitivity (up to 83.8%) for localized RNFL defect when using the TSNIT thickness graph. Figure 2 provides a representative case of preperimetric glaucoma with inferotemporal RNFL defect. In this case, the quadrant map showed "within normal range" and the 12 clock-

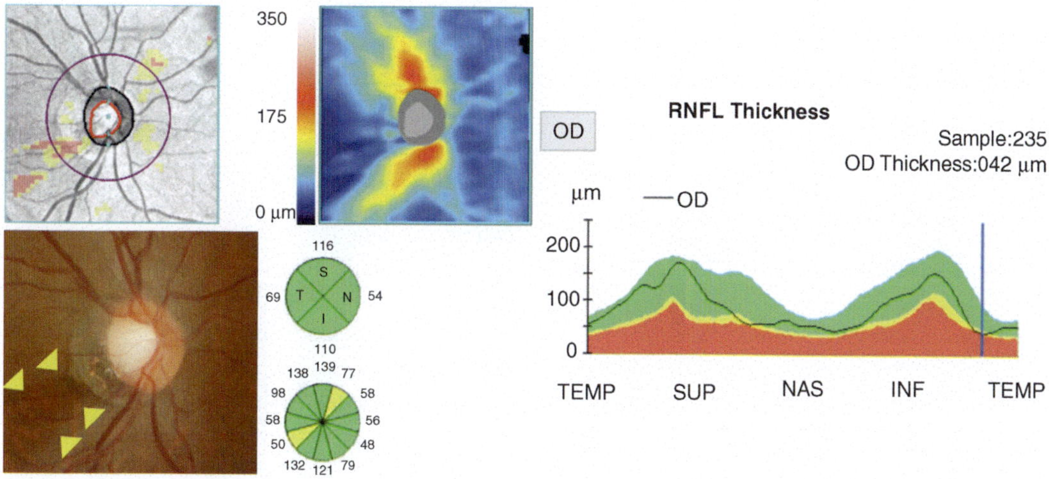

Fig. 2 TSNIT graph for early detection of glaucoma. Optic disc cube scan of 45-year-old female with preperimetric glaucoma on right eye. Note the optic disc rim narrowing and retinal nerve fiber layer (RNFL) defect (yellow triangle) in the inferotemporal region. The quadrant map showed within the normal range, and the 12-hour sector map showed only yellow color in the 8 o'clock sector. However, the TSNIT thickness graph clearly demonstrated a focal defect (thickness 42 µm) in the inferotemporal region (light blue solid line)

hour sector map showed "only yellow color" at the 8 o'clock sector. However, the TSNIT thickness graph clearly demonstrated the focal defect in the inferotemporal region.

1.1.2 Macular Parameters

The latest OCT devices provide measurement of macular ganglion cell complex (GCC, sum of macular RNFL, GCL, and IPL thickness) or ganglion cell-inner plexiform layer (GCIPL) thickness (sum of macular GCL and IPL). The macular parameters are also known to be effective in discriminating early-glaucomatous structural damage from healthy eyes. Several studies have reported that macular GCIPL or GCC showed comparable diagnostic ability for early glaucoma (Mwanza et al. 2012; Akashi et al. 2013; Jeoung et al. 2013). Mwanza et al. (2012) reported that minimum GCIPL thickness was the best parameter for discriminating early-glaucomatous change from normal eyes. Inferotemporal macular GCIPL thickness is known to be the best parameter for discriminating myopic preperimetric glaucoma from healthy myopic eyes (Seol et al. 2015). A representative case of preperimetric glaucoma with macular damage in the inferotemporal region is provided in Fig. 3. This case featured the inaugural use of the 12 × 9 mm^2-sized wide-field map from swept-source OCT (SS-OCT), which enables combined macular parameter/peripapillary RNFL thickness analysis.

However, some researchers have reported that macular GCIPL thickness showed only moderate diagnostic ability for discriminating preperimetric glaucoma from healthy eyes, and in fact, that it had even less diagnostic power than that of peripapillary RNFL or optic nerve head (ONH) parameters (Rao et al. 2013; Lisboa et al. 2013; Begum et al. 2014). This phenomenon possibly arose from the fact that macular scanning is limited to a 6 × 6 mm^2 area centered around the fovea, and as such, cannot detect any localized RNFL defect beyond this scanning area. It has been demonstrated that the diagnostic utility of GCIPL improves significantly if the RNFL defect is closer to the fovea (Kim et al. 2014; Hwang et al. 2014). A recent study compared the diagnostic ability of macular parameters between spectral-domain OCT (Cirrus HD-OCT, Carl Zeiss Meditec, Inc., Dublin, CA, USA) and swept-source OCT (SS-OCT, Triton DRI OCT, Topcon, Tokyo, Japan) for glaucomatous structural damage in myopic eyes. It confirmed that

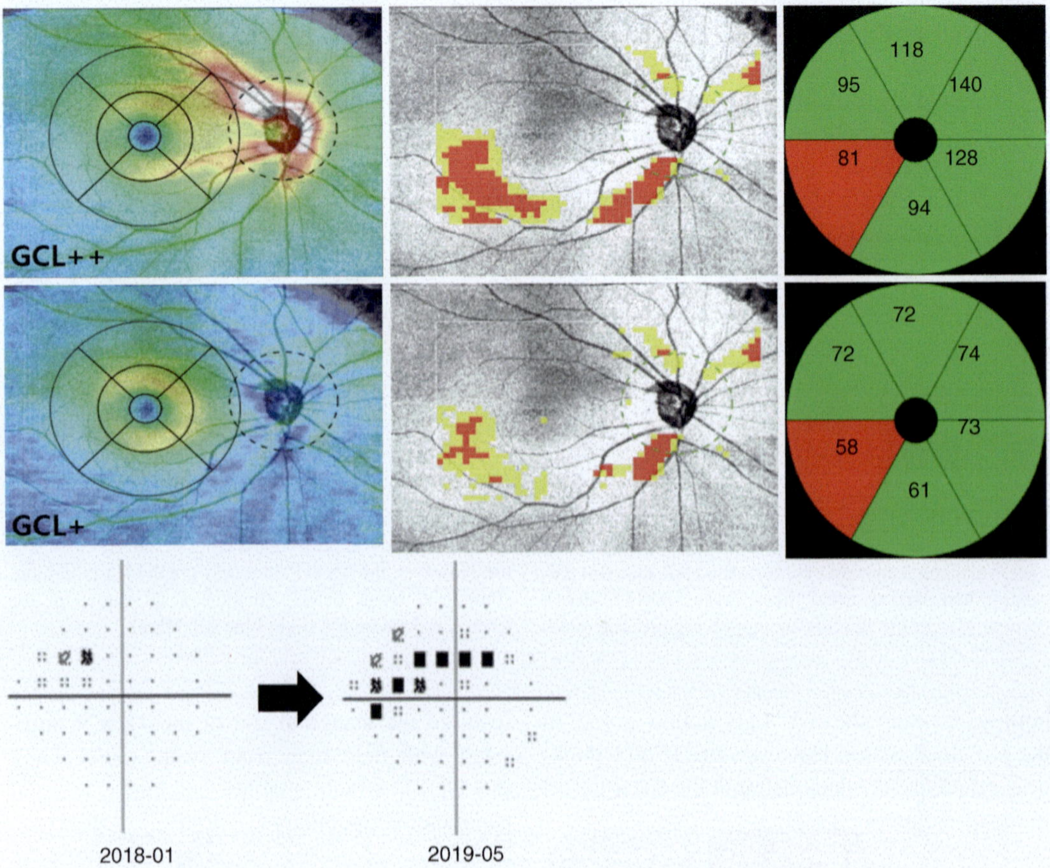

Fig. 3 Macular damage in preperimetric glaucoma. Wide-field analysis for macular and peripapillary region of 54-year-old female with preperimetric glaucoma. The 12×9 mm^2-sized wide-field maps for GCL++ (upper row) and GCL+ (bottom row) from swept-source optical coherence tomography (SS-OCT) are provided. The wide-field map can also provide a combined SuperPixel map of peripapillary retinal nerve fiber layer (RNFL) and macular GCL++/GCL+ map (second column). Note the significant thinning in the inferotemporal sectors of both GCL++ and GCL+ at the baseline, and the progressive superior visual field defect 1 year later. GCL++: sum of macular retinal nerve fiber layer (RNFL), ganglion cell layer (GCL), and inner plexiform layer (IPL); GCL+: sum of macular GCL and IPL

SS-OCT, with a larger macular scan area than that of SD-OCT, had better glaucoma-diagnostic performance (Kim et al. 2020a).

1.1.3 Neuroretinal Rim Parameters

The neuroretinal rim parameters such as Bruch's membrane opening minimum rim width (BMO-MRW) in Spectralis OCT (Heidelberg Engineering, Heidelberg, Germany) or three-dimensional neuroretinal rim thickness (3D-NRT) in Cirrus HD-OCT (Carl Zeiss Meditec, Dublin, CA, USA) are other essential OCT parameters for glaucoma diagnosis. The BMO-MRW is defined as the minimum distance between the Bruch's membrane opening (BMO) and the internal limiting membrane. Cirrus HD-OCT detects the minimum area of a surface from the optic disc margin (defined as the BMO) to the vitreoretinal interface (VRI) based on 3D volume scan data. The 3D-NRT is defined as the distance between the BMO and VRI, which is associated with the minimum cross-sectional rim area in the given direction. These parameters are known to have comparable diagnostic ability for glaucoma (Chauhan et al. 2013; Kim and Park 2018). Figure 4 shows a representative case of early glaucoma with BMO-MRW thinning.

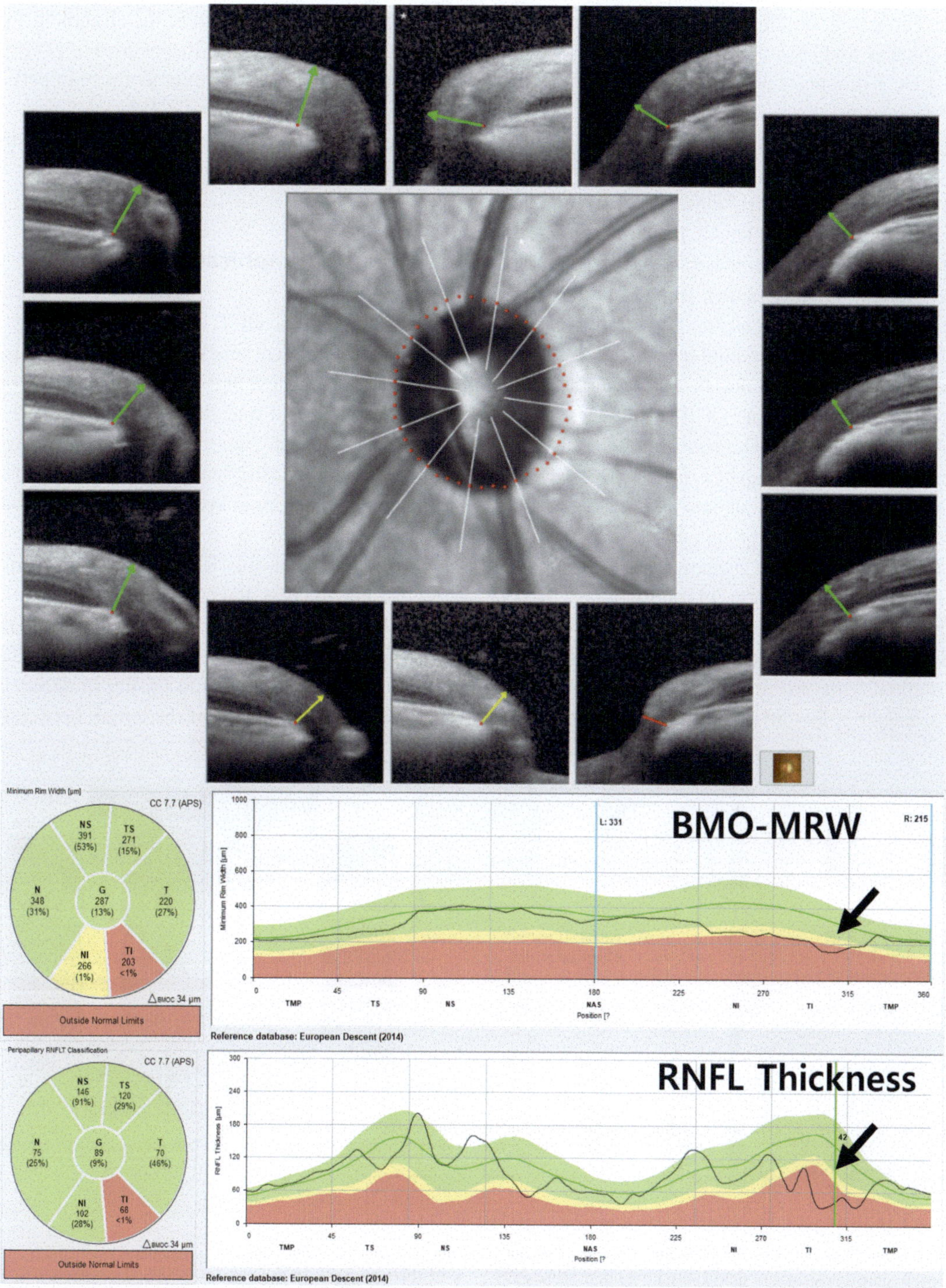

Fig. 4 BMO-MRW thinning in early glaucoma. Left eye of 43-year-old female with early open-angle glaucoma (mean deviation of visual field, –0.41 dB). Note the Bruch's membrane opening minimum rim width (BMO-MRW) as well as the decreased retinal nerve fiber layer (RNFL) thickness in the inferotemporal region

There is no doubt that the peripapillary RNFL thickness and macular parameters are essential for OCT diagnosis and monitoring of glaucoma. However, false-positive signs for these parameters are encountered in real clinical practice. False-positive rates have been reported to be as high as 30.8% for peripapillary RNFL thickness and 40.4% for macular GCIPL thickness (Kim et al. 2011, 2015a). In these studies, greater axial length and small disc area were associated with false-positive red signs for peripapillary RNFL thickness, and greater axial length and fovea-disc angle were determined to be risk factors for false positivity in macular GCIPL thickness (Kim et al. 2011, 2015a). The neuroretinal rim parameters, alternatively, can be referenced as to reduce false positives in glaucoma diagnosis, particularly in myopic eyes (Kim and Park 2018; Malik et al. 2016). Figure 5 shows the examples of false-positive red signs of peripapillary RNFL thickness in a myopic eye. The BMO-MRW from Spectralis OCT, however, revealed an intact neuroretinal rim within the normal range. This parameter is less affected by temporal migration of major vessels or scan-circle misalignment in myopic eyes. In this light, the neuroretinal rim parameters can be used complementarily to peripapillary RNFL or macular GCIPL thicknesses in detecting early-glaucomatous damage with improved specificity.

1.2 OCT Topographical Analysis

Recent advances in OCT scanning speed have enabled topographical analysis of glaucomatous damage from thickness or deviation maps of peripapillary RNFL and macular GCIPL. The peripapillary RNFL deviation map significantly improved the diagnostic sensitivity for glaucoma and provided additional spatial information for RNFL damage (Leung et al. 2010). Another study reported that the RNFL thickness map demonstrated the best diagnostic ability in detecting localized RNFL defects (Hwang et al. 2013). The temporal raphe sign from the macular GCIPL thickness map, a straight line on the horizontal raphe longer than one-half of the length between

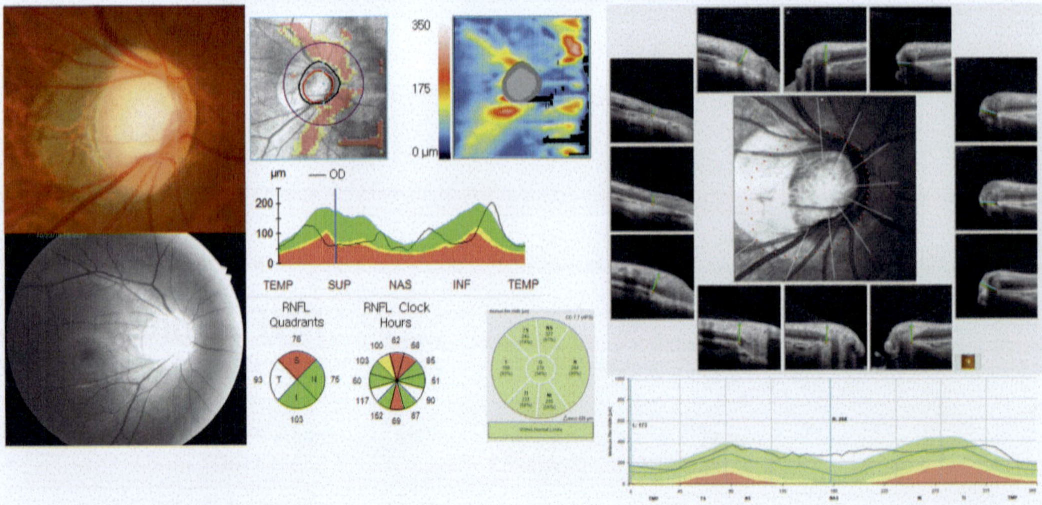

Fig. 5 False positives of RNFL thickness in myopic eyes. Cirrus HD-OCT (Carl Zeiss Meditec, Inc., Dublin, CA, USA) and Spectralis OCT (Heidelberg Engineering, Heidelberg, Germany) scan of 27-year-old healthy male with high myopia in right eye. His refraction was −11 diopters and the axial length was 30.47 mm. Optic disc and red-free retinal nerve fiber layer (RNFL) photography showed no abnormalities (left column). The RNFL deviation map as well as the quadrant and clock-hour maps showed red signs (central column). However, the Bruch's membrane opening minimum rim width (BMO-MRW) from Spectralis OCT was revealed to be within the normal range. The red-sign indications of RNFL thickness may have originated from migration of RNFL peaks and major vessels in the temporal direction

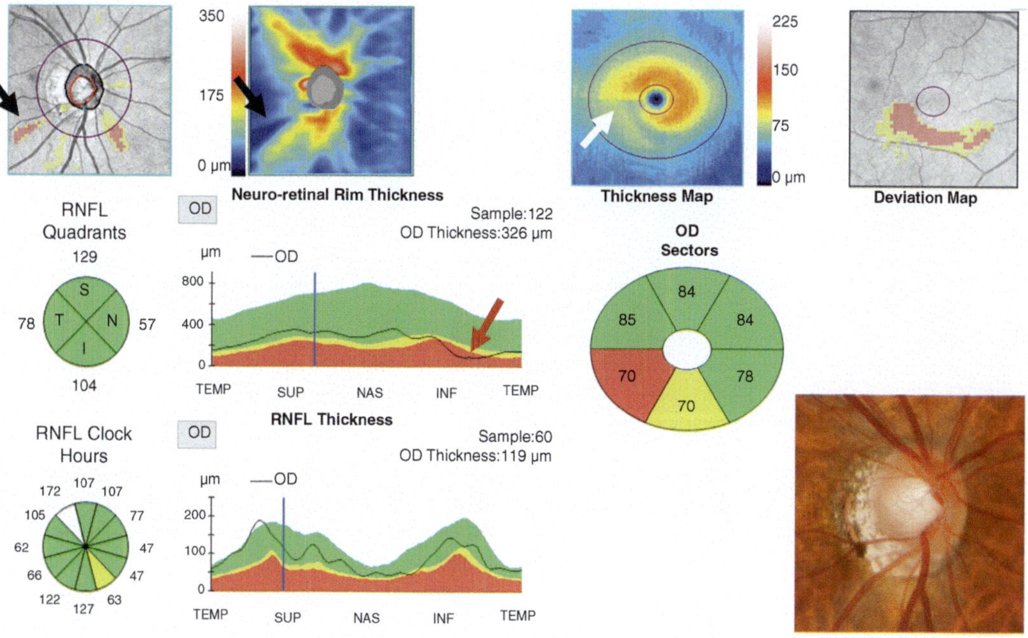

Fig. 6 Utility of OCT thickness map in detecting early-glaucomatous damage. Optic disc and macular cube scans of 40-year-old male with preperimetric glaucoma in right eye. The retinal nerve fiber layer (RNFL) quadrant and clock-hour thickness maps showed no red signs. However, the RNFL thickness and deviation maps showed RNFL defect in the inferotemporal region (black arrows). This finding is further confirmed by the three-dimensional neuroretinal rim thickness (3D-NRT, dark red arrow) and the macular ganglion cell-inner plexiform layer (GCIPL) thinning in the inferotemporal region. Note the straight line on the horizontal raphe longer than one-half of the length between the inner and outer annulus in the temporal elliptical area on the GCIPL thickness map (temporal raphe sign, white arrow)

the inner and outer annulus in the temporal elliptical area, can discriminate glaucomatous damage even in challenging cases such as highly myopic eyes (Kim et al. 2015b, 2016). Figure 6 shows a representative case that highlights the usefulness of the peripapillary RNFL thickness map in detecting early-glaucomatous change. In this case, the quadrant and clock-hour RNFL maps as well as the TSNIT thickness graph showed normal ranges of measurements, but the RNFL thickness map exhibited the localized defect in the inferotemporal region. The 3D-NRT and GCIPL thickness maps further confirmed the structural damage in this case.

The latest commercially available SS-OCT (DRI OCT Triton, Topcon, Tokyo, Japan) can capture a wider area of the retina (12×9 mm^2) in a single scan, thus providing a "wide-field map." The wide-field thickness and SuperPixel map has been shown to be effective in discriminating preperimetric and early-perimetric glaucoma from healthy eyes (Lee et al. 2017a). The wide-field Superpixel map was superior even to that of the RNFL deviation map from Cirrus HD-OCT (Lee et al. 2018a). The wide-field thickness surface map is displayed in 3D for selected layers (RNFL, GCL++, or GCL+) and can be rotated or zoomed in and out by mouse operation. This map enables detection of localized RNFL defects intuitively easy. Figure 7 shows the benefits of the wide-field map when detecting a localized superior-hemifield RNFL defect that most conventional SD-OCT macular scans would not find.

2 Detection of Progression

Glaucoma progression varies greatly from person to person, ranging from rapid to slow (Heijl et al. 2009, 2013). It can continue to show progression

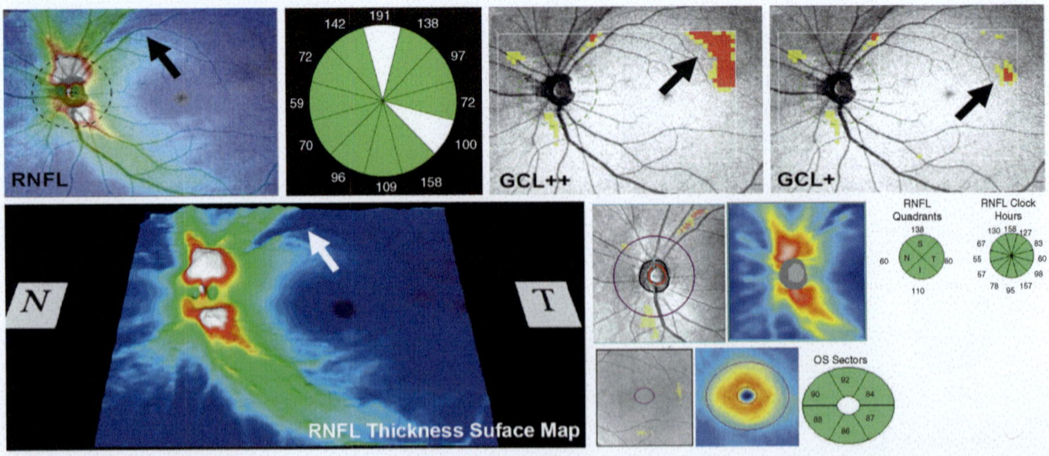

Fig. 7 Utility of wide-field map in detecting early-glaucomatous damage. Wide-field map scanned from 49-year-old male with early glaucoma in left eye (mean deviation of visual field, –3.11 dB). The wide-field map detected the localized retinal nerve fiber layer (RNFL) defect in the superotemporal region (black and white arrows). However, scans from the same eye by spectral-domain OCT (Cirrus HD-OCT, Carl Zeiss Meditec, Inc., Dublin, CA, USA) did not detect any structural damage, due possibly to the limited scan area (green box)

despite treatment, even within the normal range of intraocular pressure (Collaborative Normal-Tension Glaucoma Study Group 1998). Therefore, tonometry alone cannot be sufficient in monitoring glaucoma. OCT is a reliable tool for detection of structural progression and monitoring of the rate of change. Although glaucoma progression analysis is focused mainly on the peripapillary RNFL, recent OCT devices, such as BMO-MRW and 3D-NRT, also provide tools for monitoring of macular GCIPL or neuroretinal rim thickness.

2.1 RNFL Progression Analysis

Progressive RNFL thinning in glaucoma can be assessed on OCT scans either by comparing RNFL thickness between the baseline and selected follow-up images (event-based analysis) or by estimating the rate of RNFL thinning in a linear regression model from a series of OCT scans (trend-based analysis). While these kinds of analysis can be done manually by individual clinicians, they can be prohibitively time-consuming in a busy clinical setting. The latest OCT devices provide automated proprietary software tools for progression analysis, but different OCT brands have slightly different features. Guided Progression Analysis (GPA™) from Cirrus HD-OCT is unique in that it provides topographical event-based RNFL thickness change over the 6 × 6 mm^2 peripapillary region (Fig. 8). It allows the user to analyze between 3 and 8 exams and determines if statistically significant change has occurred. The earliest two exams are set as the baselines, and later exams are compared with them for determination of any significant change. Follow-up scans are aligned to the baselines based on the blood vessels or center of optic disc identified in the *en face* images (Cirrus HD-OCT User Manual). In event-based analysis, "Possible Loss" is declared and encoded in yellow when the individual plot has changed, relative to the two baseline exams, by a greater extent than the test-retest variability for a single visit. "Likely Loss" is declared and encoded in red when significant change has been detected on two visits in a row. "Possible Increase" is declared and encoded in lavender when the rate of gain is significant. In trend-based analysis, the slope is estimated by linear regression and is displayed in "μm/year" with the 95% confidence interval. This will be provided whenever at least 4 exams spanning at least 2 years are loaded. The linear regression line is plotted on each graph whenever

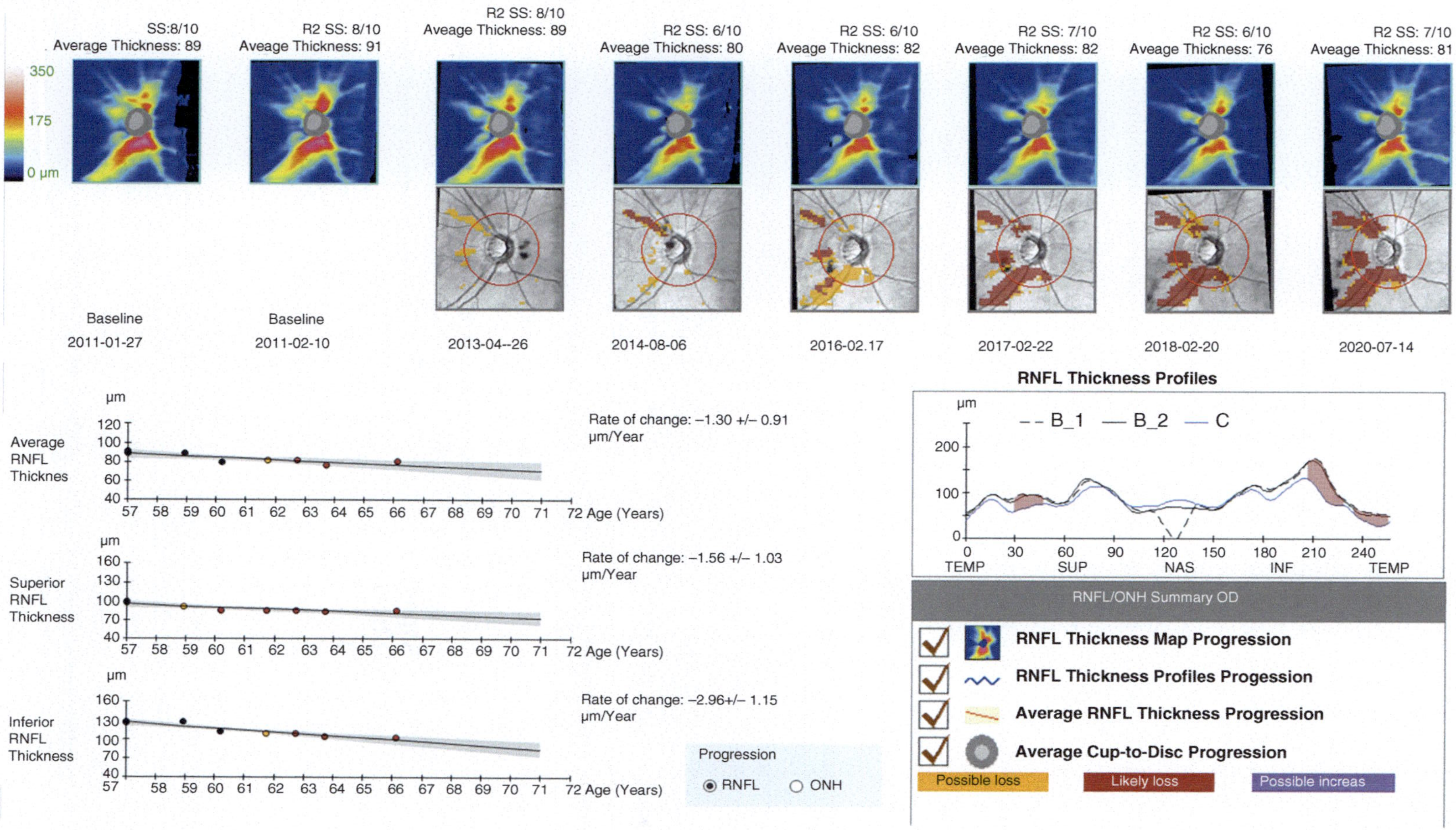

Fig. 8 RNFL progression analysis. Guided Progression Analysis (GPA™) from Cirrus HD-OCT detects event-based RNFL thickness change over the 6 × 6 mm^2 peripapillary region and estimates trend-based rates of change for average, superior, and inferior peripapillary RNFL thicknesses. The serial optic disc scans from a 57-year-old female with open-angle glaucoma and a history of recurrent disc hemorrhage showed significant progression ("Likely Loss") at the superotemporal, inferotemporal, and temporal regions. The rate of average retinal nerve fiber layer (RNFL) thinning was –1.30 ± 0.91 μm/year

there is both "Likely Loss" and a significant linear trend ($P < 5\%$). Other OCT brands can also automatically estimate and report the slope of RNFL thinning with statistical significance. Statistically significant *P*-values do not always mean that there is clinically significant "progression." Even small, clinically insignificant changes can be statistically significant in a series of large-scale OCT scans; and, vice versa, if the number of OCT images is small and of poor quality, a clinically significant change can be determined as insignificant ($P > 0.05$).

Monitoring of peripapillary RNFL thickness with OCT has been shown to be effective in detecting glaucomatous damage prior to the appearance of visual field defect (Kuang et al. 2015). Furthermore, OCT has been reported to be more sensitive than standard automated perimetry in detecting progression in the early stages of glaucoma (Wollstein et al. 2005; Zhang et al. 2017). It is therefore imperative to monitor progressive RNFL thinning by OCT, the findings of which are informative for prediction of future visual field loss in glaucoma (Yu et al. 2016; Lin et al. 2017).

2.2 GCIPL Progression Analysis

Progression analysis for macular GCIPL is also available in both event- and trend-based modes. Glaucoma patients who had shown progression on serial red-free RNFL photographs or automated perimetry had a significantly faster thinning rate of macular GCIPL than that of non-progressors (Lee et al. 2017b, c). In a dynamic range-normalized analysis, the rate of peripapillary RNFL thinning was faster than that of macular GCIPL (Hammel et al. 2017). Nevertheless, progressive macular GCIPL thinning and progressive peripapillary RNFL thinning were found to be mutually predictive, and were both indicative of visual field progression (Hou et al. 2018; Shin et al. 2020). In this sense, integrating progressive peripapillary RNFL and macular GCIPL thinning may be advantageous to progression analysis in glaucoma (Lee et al. 2018b, c; Wu et al. 2020).

Monitoring the macular GCIPL thickness in a topographical manner has improved our understanding of macular damage patterns in glaucoma. Macular GCIPL defect in one study was most commonly found in the inferotemporal region relative to the fovea (Shin et al. 2018). In that investigation, GPA™ analysis showed that the region toward the fovea and optic disc from the initial inferotemporal GCIPL defect was the most frequent site for progression. The most common pattern of progressive thinning, meanwhile, was widening of GCIPL defect, followed by deepening and newly developed GCIPL (Shin et al. 2018).

Monitoring macular GCIPL is advantageous to detection of progression in advanced glaucoma eyes when peripapillary RNFL thickness reaches the measurement floor (Hammel et al. 2017; Shin et al. 2017; Lavinsky et al. 2018). Figure 9 demonstrates the utility of monitoring progressive macular GCIPL thinning in advanced glaucoma eyes. The macular damage that causes GCIPL thinning might occur in the later stages of disease and at a different rate relative to peripapillary RNFL thinning. But given that a floor effect on macular GCIPL may also exist, the utility of macular GCIPL monitoring in advanced glaucoma may be limited for some patients.

2.3 BMO-MRW Progression Analysis

Spectralis OCT provides progression analysis reporting for BMO-MRW. Figure 10 shows a representative case with progressive BMO-MRW thinning in an open-angle glaucoma eye with recurrent disc hemorrhage. In a longitudinal analysis of glaucoma eyes with disc hemorrhage, the BMO-MRW showed progressive thinning, and the inferotemporal sector showed the highest rate of change (Cho and Kee 2020). Cirrus HD-OCT's 3D-NRT also showed a faster rate of thinning at the site of hemorrhage than in the other sectors (Kim et al. 2020b). The clinical utility of analyzing progressive change of neuroretinal rim parameters requires further elucidation in terms of glaucoma monitoring.

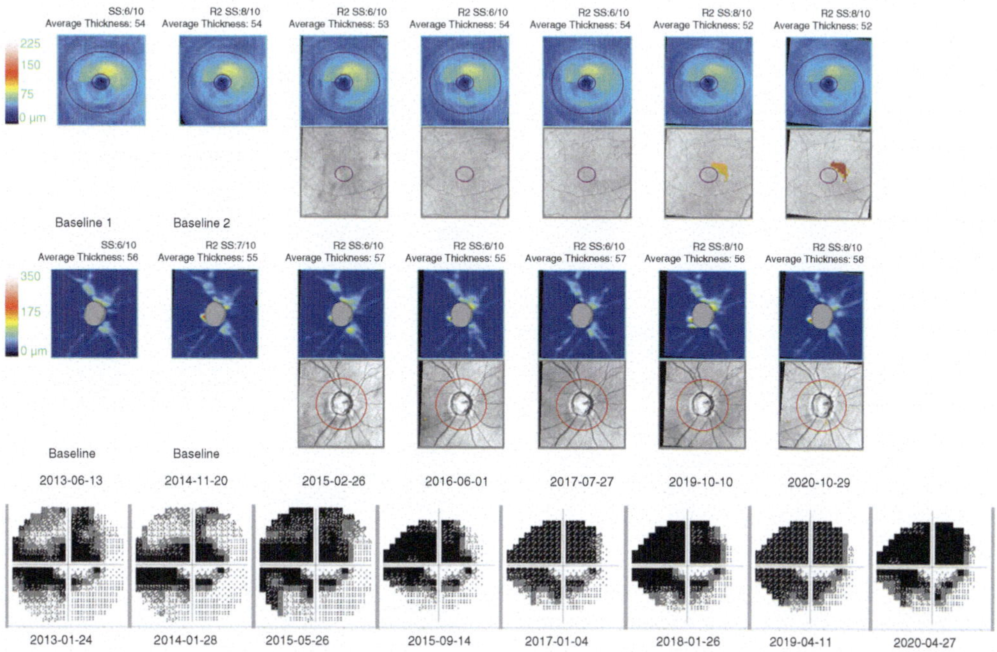

Fig. 9 GCIPL progression analysis. Guided Progression Analysis (GPA™) of macular ganglion cell-inner plexiform layer (GCIPL) and peripapillary retinal nerve fiber layer (RNFL) thicknesses from 53-year-old male with advanced glaucoma (baseline mean deviation of visual field [VF], –18.79 dB). Note the progressive thinning of the macular GCIPL ("Likely Loss" at superior parafovea) and note also the fact that the diffuse atrophied RNFL reached to the measurement floor and did not show any significant change ("floor effect"). The VF progressed significantly from –18.79 to –23.17 dB during the observation period

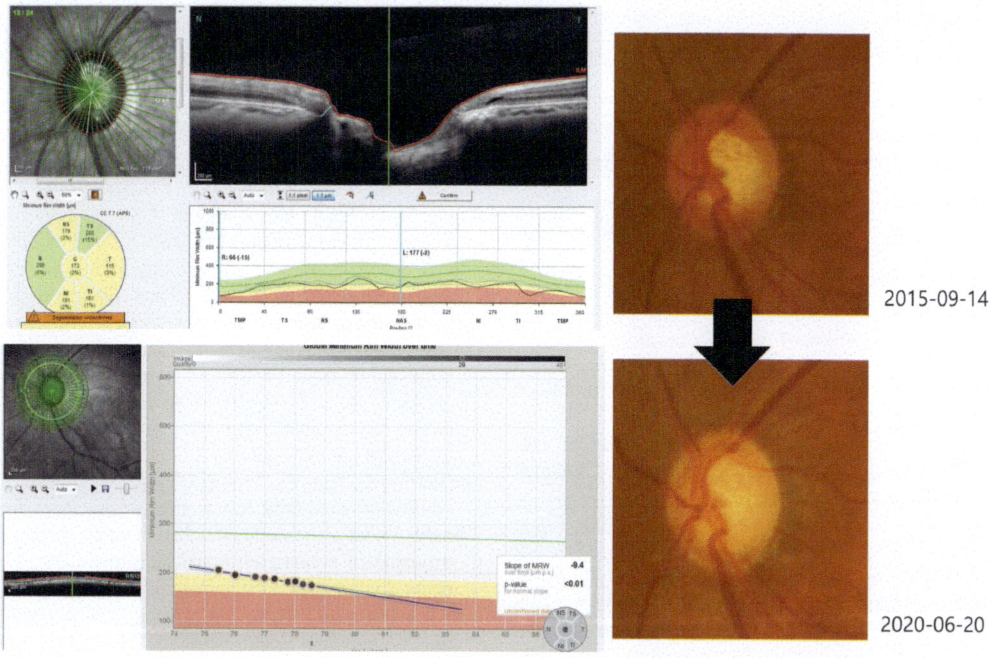

Fig. 10 BMO-MRW progression analysis. Spectralis OCT scan from 57-year-old female with open-angle glaucoma and history of recurrent disc hemorrhage in inferotemporal region of left eye. The progression analysis demonstrated significant thinning of the BMO-MRW (rate of change, –9.4 µm/year, $P < 0.01$)

References

Akashi A, Kanamori A, Nakamura M, Fujihara M, Yamada Y, Negi A. Comparative assessment for the ability of Cirrus, RTVue, and 3D-OCT to diagnose glaucoma. Invest Ophthalmol Vis Sci. 2013;54(7):4478–84.

Begum VU, Addepalli UK, Yadav RK, et al. Ganglion cell-inner plexiform layer thickness of high definition optical coherence tomography in perimetric and preperimetric glaucoma. Invest Ophthalmol Vis Sci. 2014;55(8):4768–75.

Chauhan BC, O'Leary N, AlMobarak FA, et al. Enhanced detection of open-angle glaucoma with an anatomically accurate optical coherence tomography-derived neuroretinal rim parameter. Ophthalmology. 2013;120(3):535–43.

Cho HK, Kee C. Comparison of rate of change between bruch's membrane opening minimum rim width and retinal nerve fiber layer in eyes showing optic disc hemorrhage. Am J Ophthalmol. 2020;217:27–37.

Cirrus HD-OCT User Manual 2660021159751 Rev. A 2015-08. Appendix A.

Collaborative Normal-Tension Glaucoma Study Group. Comparison of glaucomatous progression between untreated patients with normal-tension glaucoma and patients with therapeutically reduced intraocular pressures. Am J Ophthalmol. 1998;126(4):487–97.

Hammel N, Belghith A, Weinreb RN, Medeiros FA, Mendoza N, Zangwill LM. Comparing the rates of retinal nerve fiber layer and ganglion cell-inner plexiform layer loss in healthy eyes and in glaucoma eyes. Am J Ophthalmol. 2017;178:38–50.

Heijl A, Bengtsson B, Hyman L, Leske MC. Natural history of open-angle glaucoma. Ophthalmology. 2009;116(12):2271–6.

Heijl A, Buchholz P, Norrgren G, Bengtsson B. Rates of visual field progression in clinical glaucoma care. Acta Ophthalmol. 2013;91(5):406–12.

Hou HW, Lin C, Leung CK. Integrating macular ganglion cell inner plexiform layer and parapapillary retinal nerve fiber layer measurements to detect glaucoma progression. Ophthalmology. 2018;125(6):822–31.

Hwang YH, Kim YY, Kim HK, Sohn YH. Ability of cirrus high-definition spectral-domain optical coherence tomography clock-hour, deviation, and thickness maps in detecting photographic retinal nerve fiber layer abnormalities. Ophthalmology. 2013;120(7):1380–7.

Hwang YH, Jeong YC, Kim HK, Sohn YH. Macular ganglion cell analysis for early detection of glaucoma. Ophthalmology. 2014;121(8):1508–15.

Jeoung JW, Park KH. Comparison of Cirrus OCT and Stratus OCT on the ability to detect localized retinal nerve fiber layer defects in preperimetric glaucoma. Invest Ophthalmol Vis Sci. 2010;51(2):938–45.

Jeoung JW, Choi YJ, Park KH, Kim DM. Macular ganglion cell imaging study: glaucoma diagnostic accuracy of spectral-domain optical coherence tomography. Invest Ophthalmol Vis Sci. 2013;54(7):4422–9.

Jeoung JW, Kim TW, Weinreb RN, Kim SH, Park KH, Kim DM. Diagnostic ability of spectral-domain versus time-domain optical coherence tomography in preperimetric glaucoma. J Glaucoma. 2014;23(5):299–306.

Kim YW, Park KH. Diagnostic accuracy of three-dimensional neuroretinal rim thickness for differentiation of myopic glaucoma from myopia. Invest Ophthalmol Vis Sci. 2018;59(8):3655–66.

Kim NR, Lim H, Kim JH, Rho SS, Seong GJ, Kim CY. Factors associated with false positives in retinal nerve fiber layer color codes from spectral-domain optical coherence tomography. Ophthalmology. 2011;118(9):1774–81.

Kim MJ, Jeoung JW, Park KH, Choi YJ, Kim DM. Topographic profiles of retinal nerve fiber layer defects affect the diagnostic performance of macular scans in preperimetric glaucoma. Invest Ophthalmol Vis Sci. 2014;55(4):2079–87.

Kim KE, Jeoung JW, Park KH, Kim DM, Kim SH. Diagnostic classification of macular ganglion cell and retinal nerve fiber layer analysis: differentiation of false-positives from glaucoma. Ophthalmology. 2015a;122(3):502–10.

Kim YK, Yoo BW, Kim HC, Park KH. Automated detection of hemifield difference across horizontal raphe on ganglion cell-inner plexiform layer thickness map. Ophthalmology. 2015b;122(11):2252–60.

Kim YK, Yoo BW, Jeoung JW, Kim HC, Kim HJ, Park KH. Glaucoma-diagnostic ability of ganglion cell-inner plexiform layer thickness difference across temporal raphe in highly myopic eyes. Invest Ophthalmol Vis Sci. 2016;57(14):5856–63.

Kim YW, Lee J, Kim JS, Park KH. Diagnostic accuracy of wide-field map from swept-source optical coherence tomography for primary open-angle glaucoma in myopic eyes. Am J Ophthalmol. 2020a;218:182–91.

Kim YW, Lee WJ, Seol BR, Kim YK, Jeoung JW, Park KH. Rate of three-dimensional neuroretinal rim thinning in glaucomatous eyes with optic disc haemorrhage. Br J Ophthalmol. 2020b;104(5):648–54.

Kuang TM, Zhang C, Zangwill LM, Weinreb RN, Medeiros FA. Estimating lead time gained by optical coherence tomography in detecting glaucoma before development of visual field defects. Ophthalmology. 2015;122(10):2002–9.

Lavinsky F, Wu M, Schuman JS, et al. Can macula and optic nerve head parameters detect glaucoma progression in eyes with advanced circumpapillary retinal nerve fiber layer damage? Ophthalmology. 2018;125(12):1907–12.

Lee WJ, Na KI, Kim YK, Jeoung JW, Park KH. Diagnostic Ability of wide-field retinal nerve fiber layer maps using swept-source optical coherence tomography for detection of preperimetric and early perimetric glaucoma. J Glaucoma. 2017a;26(6):577–85.

Lee WJ, Kim YK, Park KH, Jeoung JW. Evaluation of ganglion cell-inner plexiform layer thinning in eyes with optic disc hemorrhage: a trend-based progression analysis. Invest Ophthalmol Vis Sci. 2017b;58(14):6449–56.

Lee WJ, Kim YK, Park KH, Jeoung JW. Trend-based analysis of ganglion cell-inner plexiform layer thickness changes on optical coherence tomography in glaucoma progression. Ophthalmology. 2017c;124(9):1383–91.

Lee WJ, Oh S, Kim YK, Jeoung JW, Park KH. Comparison of glaucoma-diagnostic ability between wide-field swept-source OCT retinal nerve fiber layer maps and spectral-domain OCT. Eye (Lond). 2018a;32(9):1483–92.

Lee WJ, Kim TJ, Kim YK, Jeoung JW, Park KH. Serial combined wide-field optical coherence tomography maps for detection of early glaucomatous structural progression. JAMA Ophthalmol. 2018b;136(10):1121–7.

Lee WJ, Na KI, Ha A, Kim YK, Jeoung JW, Park KH. Combined use of retinal nerve fiber layer and ganglion cell-inner plexiform layer event-based progression analysis. Am J Ophthalmol. 2018c;196:65–71.

Leung CK, Lam S, Weinreb RN, et al. Retinal nerve fiber layer imaging with spectral-domain optical coherence tomography: analysis of the retinal nerve fiber layer map for glaucoma detection. Ophthalmology. 2010;117(9):1684–91.

Lin C, Mak H, Yu M, Leung CK. Trend-based progression analysis for examination of the topography of rates of retinal nerve fiber layer thinning in glaucoma. JAMA Ophthalmol. 2017;135(3):189–95.

Lisboa R, Leite MT, Zangwill LM, Tafreshi A, Weinreb RN, Medeiros FA. Diagnosing preperimetric glaucoma with spectral domain optical coherence tomography. Ophthalmology. 2012;119(11):2261–9.

Lisboa R, Paranhos A Jr, Weinreb RN, Zangwill LM, Leite MT, Medeiros FA. Comparison of different spectral domain OCT scanning protocols for diagnosing preperimetric glaucoma. Invest Ophthalmol Vis Sci. 2013;54(5):3417–25.

Malik R, Belliveau AC, Sharpe GP, Shuba LM, Chauhan BC, Nicolela MT. Diagnostic accuracy of optical coherence tomography and scanning laser tomography for identifying glaucoma in myopic eyes. Ophthalmology. 2016;123(6):1181–9.

Mwanza JC, Durbin MK, Budenz DL, et al. Glaucoma diagnostic accuracy of ganglion cell-inner plexiform layer thickness: comparison with nerve fiber layer and optic nerve head. Ophthalmology. 2012;119(6):1151–8.

Nukada M, Hangai M, Mori S, et al. Detection of localized retinal nerve fiber layer defects in glaucoma using enhanced spectral-domain optical coherence tomography. Ophthalmology. 2011;118(6):1038–48.

Rao HL, Addepalli UK, Chaudhary S, et al. Ability of different scanning protocols of spectral domain optical coherence tomography to diagnose preperimetric glaucoma. Invest Ophthalmol Vis Sci. 2013;54(12):7252–7.

Seol BR, Jeoung JW, Park KH. Glaucoma detection ability of macular ganglion cell-inner plexiform layer thickness in myopic preperimetric glaucoma. Invest Ophthalmol Vis Sci. 2015;56(13):8306–13.

Shin JW, Sung KR, Lee GC, Durbin MK, Cheng D. Ganglion cell-inner plexiform layer change detected by optical coherence tomography indicates progression in advanced glaucoma. Ophthalmology. 2017;124(10):1466–74.

Shin JW, Sung KR, Park SW. Patterns of progressive ganglion cell-inner plexiform layer thinning in glaucoma detected by OCT. Ophthalmology. 2018;125(10):1515–25.

Shin JW, Sung KR, Song MK. Ganglion cell-inner plexiform layer and retinal nerve fiber layer changes in glaucoma suspects enable prediction of glaucoma development. Am J Ophthalmol. 2020;210:26–34.

Wollstein G, Schuman JS, Price LL, et al. Optical coherence tomography longitudinal evaluation of retinal nerve fiber layer thickness in glaucoma. Arch Ophthalmol. 2005;123(4):464–70.

Wu K, Lin C, Lam AK, Chan L, Leung CK. Wide-field trend-based progression analysis of combined retinal nerve fiber layer and ganglion cell inner plexiform layer thickness: a new paradigm to improve glaucoma progression detection. Ophthalmology. 2020;127(10):1322–30.

Yu M, Lin C, Weinreb RN, Lai G, Chiu V, Leung CK. Risk of visual field progression in glaucoma patients with progressive retinal nerve fiber layer thinning: a 5-year prospective study. Ophthalmology. 2016;123(6):1201–10.

Zhang X, Dastiridou A, Francis BA, et al. Comparison of glaucoma progression detection by optical coherence tomography and visual field. Am J Ophthalmol. 2017;184:63–74.

Lamina Cribrosa Imaging

Tae-Woo Kim and Eun Ji Lee

Abstract

Glaucoma is characterized by the loss of retinal ganglion cells and axons. Although the pathogenesis of glaucomatous optic neuropathy is not fully elucidated, it is generally considered that axonal damage is the earliest event in the process of cell death. Since lamina cribrosa (LC) is the putative site of axonal injury, understanding the changes in the LC and its effect on the axons are essential to understand the pathophysiology of glaucomatous optic neuropathy.

With the emergence of spectral domain optical coherence tomography (SD-OCT), it became feasible to image the LC in patients. Using this noninvasive technique, various observations have been reported including dynamic features along the course of disease and according to the variation of intraocular pressure. These data help understand the optic nerve head biomechanics in the development and progression of glaucoma. Although the image quality of LC obtained by OCT is not fully satisfactory, postprocessing technique is available to better visualize the LC. Yet, LC imaging is not widely used in the clinical practice. As research continues, it is expected that LC imaging will soon be implemented in the glaucoma diagnosis and patient management.

Keywords

Lamina cribrosa · Glaucoma · Lamina cribrosa curvature index · Focal lamina cribrosa defect

1 Histology of Lamina Cribrosa

Lamina cribrosa (LC) is the sieve-like connective tissue sheets which contains about 500–600 perforations (Ogden et al. 1988). The optic nerve axon bundles pass through the pores within the LC. The LC pores in the superior and inferior part are larger than those in the nasal and temporal quadrants (Morrison et al. 1989; Quigley and Addicks 1981; Radius and Gonzales 1981).

The lamina beams are composed of elastin, collagen (types I, III, IV, V and VI), laminin, and fibronectin (Goldbaum et al. 1989; Hernandez et al. 1986). The elastin is responsible for elastic property of elastic tissue (Mecham 1991). In young adults, elastin fibers are thin, long, and run longitudinally in the lamina beams (Hernandez et al. 1986). With aging, the density of elastin in the lamina increases and the elastin fibers thicken markedly to form long, tubular structures

T.-W. Kim (✉) · E. J. Lee
Seoul National University College of Medicine, Seoul National University Bundang Hospital, Seongnam, Korea
e-mail: twkim7@snu.ac.kr

K. H. Park, T.-W. Kim (eds.), *OCT Imaging in Glaucoma*,
https://doi.org/10.1007/978-981-16-1178-0_5

(Hernandez et al. 1989). The change in the elastin with aging probably changes the degree of elastic property of the lamina.

The beams are dense in the mid horizontal area of the optic nerve head and elevated compared to superior and inferior region, forming a bowtie-shaped ridge (Park et al. 2012a). In glaucomatous eyes, the laminar sheets are compressed and gross configuration shows backward bowing at late stage (Quigley et al. 1983).

2 LC Imaging Using OCT

LC can be visualized using spectral domain (SD)-OCT or swept source (SS)-OCT. The LC appears as a highly reflective plate in OCT images (Fig. 1). On enface OCT images, lamina pores are visible. Since the LC is located in the deep optic nerve head, LC imaging has lower signal-to-noise ratio than surface structure imaging such as retinal nerve fiber layer. To alleviate this prob-

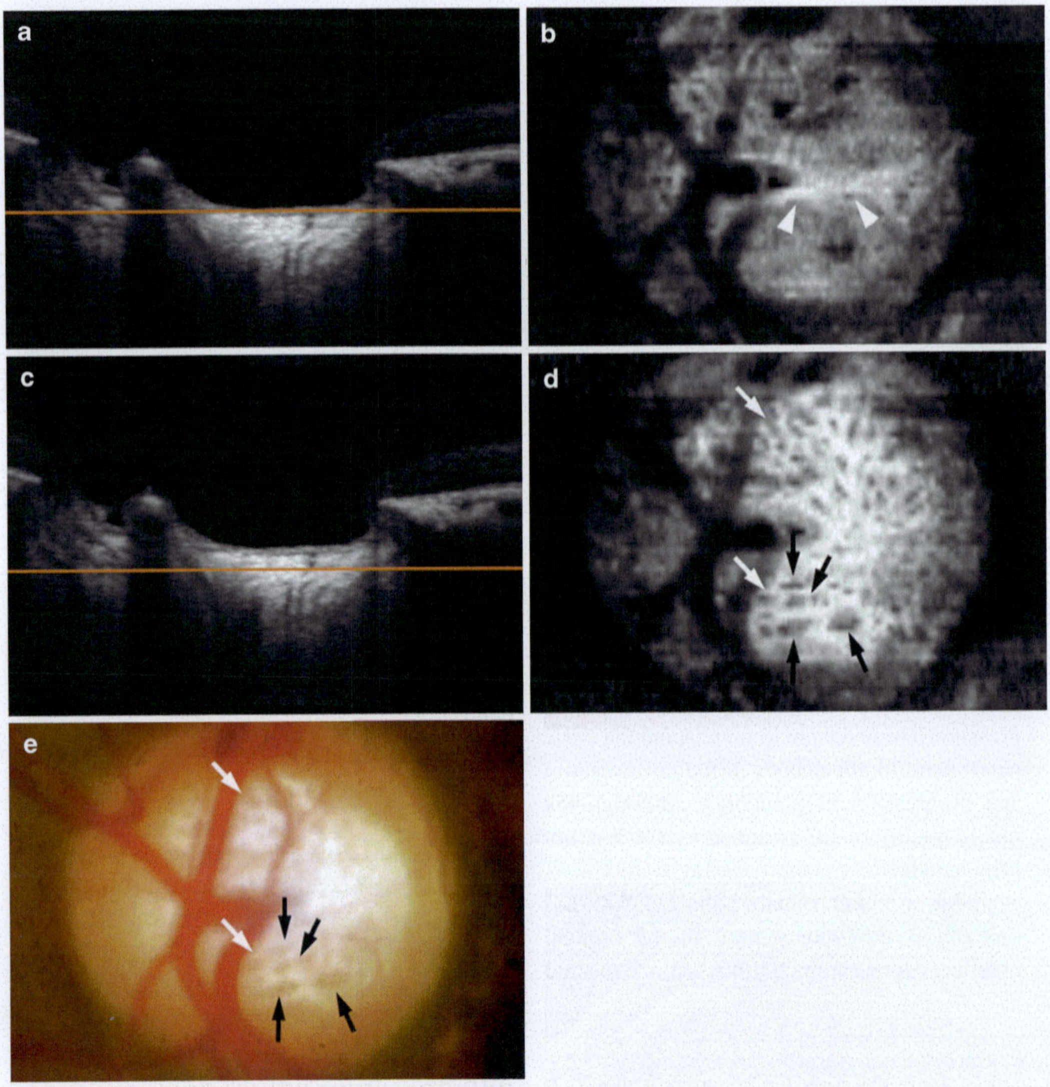

Fig. 1 Lamina cribrosa (LC) image obtained by spectral domain OCT (Spectralis, Heidelberg). B-scan (**a**, **c**) and enface (**b**, **d**) images at prelaminar (**a**, **b**) and LC (**c**, **d**) in a glaucomatous eye. The low reflective dots in the enface image through the LC consist of multiple pores that correspond to the laminar pores in the fundus photography (**e**, black arrows). Owing to the curved nature of the lamina, the enface image through the prelaminar tissue contains some lamina tissue in the central area (arrowheads). Adopted and modified from Lee et al. (2011)

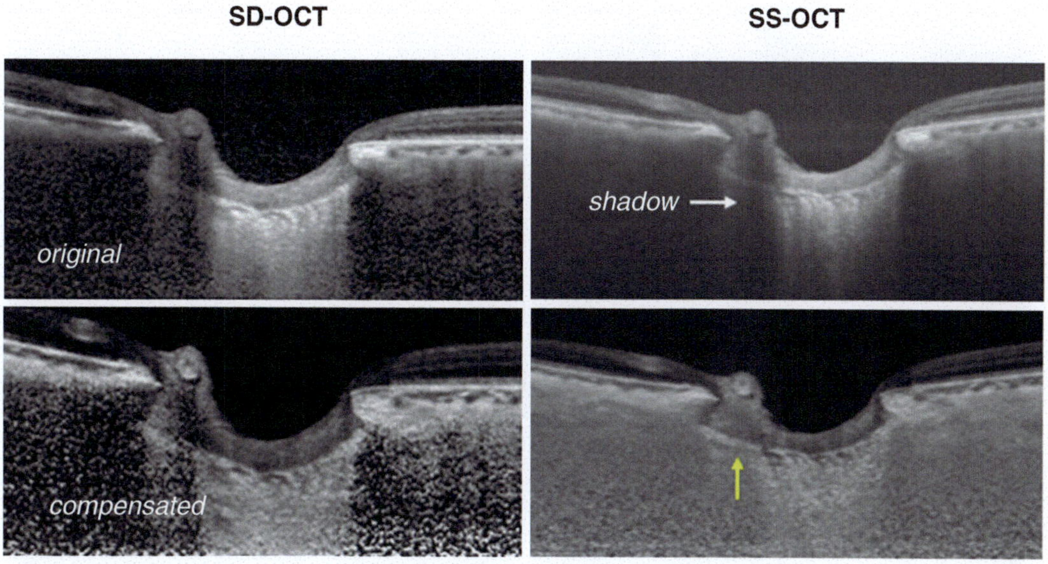

Fig. 2 Lamina cribrosa (LC) images obtained from SD-OCT (Spectralis, Heidelberg) and SS-OCT (Triton, Topcon). Images postprocessed by adaptive compensation are shown in the bottom. The LC surface is more clearly visible after adaptive compensation especially in the region of vascular shadow (yellow arrow)

lem, multiple separate scans are obtained at each scan position with the aid of eye tracking system and the result is averaged. The larger the image frames averaged, the higher the image quality. However, it requires longer time to obtain greater number of frames, which often lead to patient's poor cooperation. About 20–42 frames are generally used for SD-OCT in LC imaging (Lee et al. 2011, 2013a).

Swept Source (SS)-OCT is a newer generation of OCT that uses a short cavity swept laser with a tunable wavelength of operation. It has a longer central wavelength (1050 nm) compared to conventional SD-OCT (840 nm), providing deeper penetration. Due to this capability, high quality images can be obtained by averaging small number of image frames than SD-OCT. This enables the LC imaging to be completed within shorter period of time using SS-OCT compared to SD-OCT.

To further improve the visualization of LC, the OCT images can be postprocessed using an adaptive compensation technique which was developed by Girard and Mari et al. In this algorithm, standard compensation operations are performed until an energy threshold is reached, at which stage the compensation process is stopped to limit noise over-amplification in the deeper portion of the OCT image. This method is robust in that it can remove the shadows of blood vessels. Using this technique, the anterior surface of the LC can be more readily delineated (Fig. 2) (Girard et al. 2015).

3 Protocols to Image the LC

LC image can be evaluated using raster scans or radial scans. Each method has advantages over the other methods. Radial scan has advantage to see the LC insertion along the meridians. However, because of the bowtie-shaped central ridge of the LC (Park et al. 2012a), LC shape typically appears as a W-shape in vertical scans, and varies largely along the meridians (Fig. 3A). This large variability along the meridian makes it difficult to assess the LC shape using a simple parameter on images obtained by radial scans. Raster scans obtain multiple horizontal scans parallel to each other. The LC has a relatively regular configuration in the horizontal plane, with a flat or U-shaped appearance with different regional

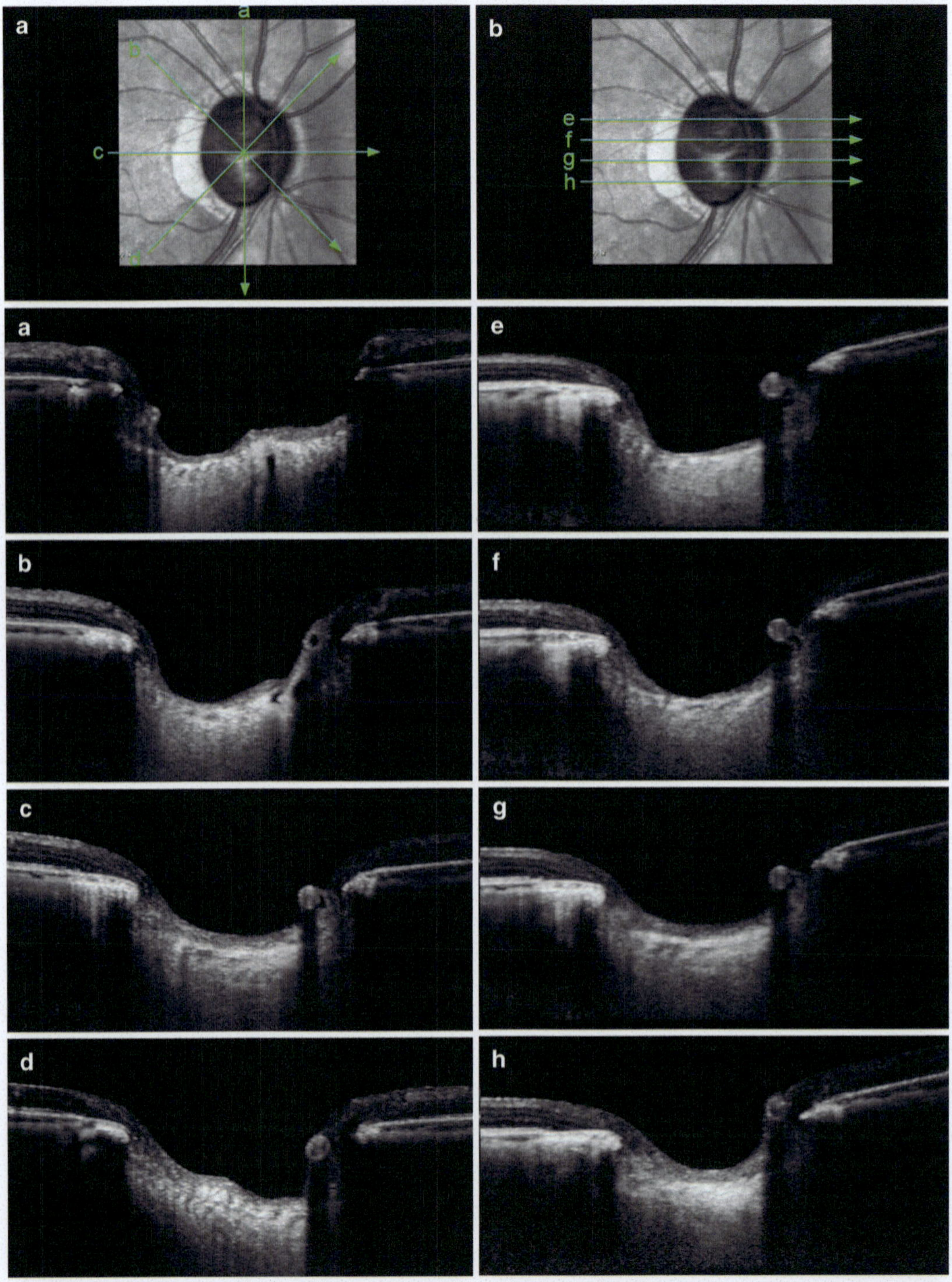

Fig. 3 Comparison of the patterns of the lamina cribrosa (LC) shape in radial (**A**), and raster (**B**) B-scans. Note that the largely different patterns of LC shape in radial scans (**A**). In contrast, the LC has a relatively regular configuration in the horizontal scans, with a flat or U-shaped appearance with different regional steepness (**B**). Note the central ridge (yellow arrow) in the vertical B-scan from 12 to 6 o/c. Adopted and modified from Lee et al. (2019)

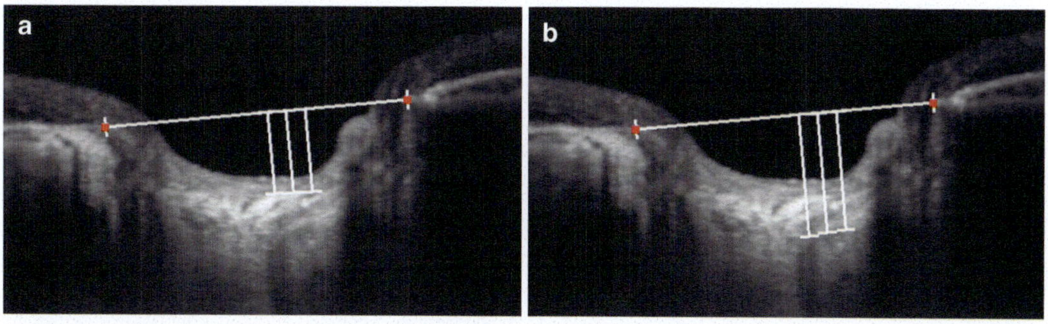

Fig. 4 Measuring the LC depth (**a**) and LC thickness. Distance to the posterior border of the LC is measured (**b**). From both measurements, the LC thickness can be calculated

steepness (Fig. 3B). Therefore, the LC shape can be readily evaluated on horizontal scans using LC curvature index (LCCI). Moreover, measuring LCCI on horizontal scans allows separate assessment of the LC morphologies in the superior and inferior region, which are often different in an individual eye (Kim et al. 2019a).

4 Indices to Evaluate LC Morphology

4.1 LC Thickness

LC thickness can be measured as the distance between the anterior and posterior LC surface (Fig. 4). Although it is measurable in many eyes, the posterior LC border is often difficult to delineate hampering the measurement of LC thickness. The LC thickness is relevant with glaucoma pathophysiology because it is associated with translaminar pressure gradient.

The LC forms the border between the intraocular space and the retrobulbar space. In general, the intraocular pressure is higher than CSF pressure. Therefore, a pressure gradient exists across the LC. At a given pressure difference between both sides of lamina, the pressure gradient is greater when the lamina is thinner (Jonas et al. 2004). An abnormal pressure gradient influences the physiology of the optic nerve fibers, with their orthograde and retrograde axoplasmic flow (Anderson and Hendrickson 1974; Quigley and Anderson 1976). Therefore, it is possible that eyes with thinner LC are more susceptible to glaucoma.

4.2 LC Depth

LC depth from Bruch's membrane opening (BMO) has been suggested as a parameter to evaluate LC morphology. Since Bruch's membrane opening is clearly visualized in most OCT images, BMO can be used as a reliable reference (Fig. 4). However, LC depth from BMO has a limitation. LC is sustained by load-bearing connective tissues of the peripapillary sclera. Thus, it would be more reasonable to assess LC morphology (and changes with IOP) from the scleral plane or directly within the LC. When the LC depth is measured from the BMO level would inappropriately include the choroidal thickness. Since the choroidal thickness varies among individuals and with aging within an individual patient (Rhodes et al. 2015), LC depth measurement form BMO may provide a biased assessment. To overcome this limitation, Vianna et al. (2017) suggested anterior scleral opening as a more reliable reference structure to measure the LC position. The measured depth is not influenced by the choroidal thickness. However, the anterior scleral opening is often difficult to reliable detect in OCT images.

4.3 LC Curvature Index (LCCI)

Since LC deformation occurs as a posterior bowing pattern, measuring the LC curve can be used to evaluate the LC strain. Differing methods have been suggested to evaluate the LC curve. Lee et al. suggested a simple parameter which was

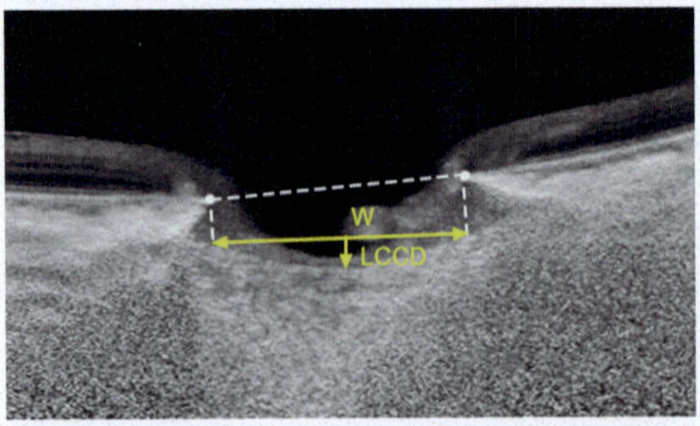

Fig. 5 Measurement of the lamina cribrosa curvature index (LCCI using a horizontal raster scan). The LC curvature depth (LCCD) was measured at the maximally depressed point as the distance from the reference line which connects two points at the anterior LC surface below the Bruch's membrane opening. The LCCI was measured by dividing the LC curve depth (LCCD) by the width of the reference line (W) and multiplying by 100. Adopted and modified from Lee et al. (2017)

named as LC curvature index (LCCI) (Lee et al. 2017). The LCCI was measured by measuring the LC depth from a reference line which was made by connecting two peripheral points on the anterior LC surface. The measured LC curve depth was divided by the width of the reference line and multiply by 100 (Fig. 5).

Another method that can be used in assessing the LC curve has been suggested by Kim et al. 2016a. They calculated the difference of mean mean depth from a reference line set in the LC surface and the LC insertion depth. To do this, they first measured the area demarcated by the reference line, two vertical lines from the LC insertion to the reference line, and the anterior LC surface. Then, the area was divided by the distance between the two LC insertions for the measurement of mean depth.

4.4 LC Insertion Depth

Posterior migration of the LC insertion has been recognized in histologic studies. Using a high quality LC images particularly with postprocessing by adaptive compensation, the LC insertion can be identified. The LC insertion depth can be measured from the anterior scleral opening level. Lee et al. (2014a) demonstrated that LC insertion depth was greater in eyes with POAG compared to healthy eyes, which accords to the histologic findings (Fig. 6). The utility of LC insertion depth in the clinical practice remains to be explored.

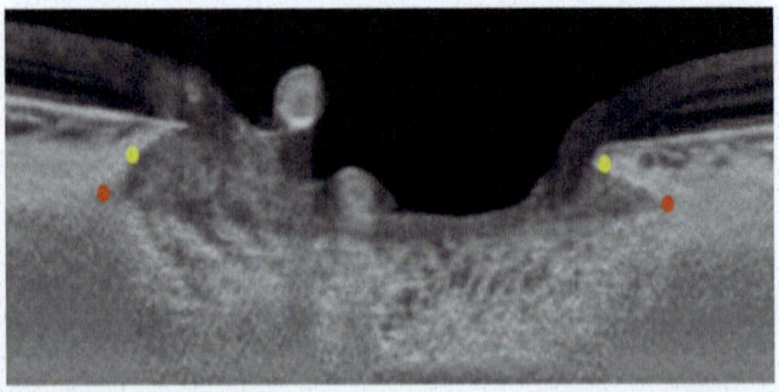

Fig. 6 LC insertion depth can be measured as the distance from the anterior scleral opening (yellow circles) to the LC insertion point (red circles)

5 Findings in Glaucoma

5.1 Thinner LC

LC thickness correlated significantly with visual field mean deviation (Inoue et al. 2009). Lee et al. (2011) demonstrated that LC thickness is smaller in eyes with glaucoma compared to healthy eyes.

Park et al. demonstrated that LC was thinner in the POAG and NTG groups than in the normal control group. Interestingly, they found that the lamina was also significantly thinner in patients with NTG and disc hemorrhage than in those with NTG but no disc hemorrhage (Park et al. 2012b).

A thinner LC would be associated with steeper translaminar pressure gradients when other conditions are equal (Jonas et al. 2004; Burgoyne et al. 2005). Therefore, it is not surprising that LC is thinner in eyes with glaucoma.

5.2 Dynamic Behavior According to IOP Change

Experimental glaucoma model studies demonstrated that LC morphology changes according to the variation of intraocular pressure. As it became possible to image the LC in patients, reduction of anterior LC depth and flattening of

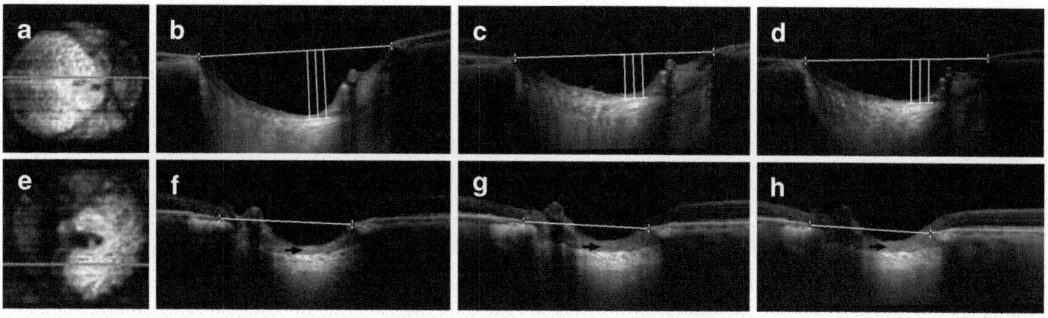

Fig. 7 Enface (**a**, **e**) and B-scan images obtained preoperatively (**b**, **f**) and at 1 (**c**, **g**) and 6 months (**d**, **h**) postoperatively in 15- (top) and 80-year-old (bottom) patients. Note the reduction of LC depth and LC curvature. The changes are seen more clearly in young patient. Adopted and modified from Lee et al. (2012)

the LC curve after IOP lowering treatment has been demonstrated (Fig. 7) (Lee et al. 2012, 2013b, 2016a, 2020; Barrancos et al. 2014; Krzyzanowska-Berkowska et al. 2018). Further, redisplacement of the anterior LC surface to the posterior direction has been demonstrated when the IOP re-elevated after bleb failure in patients who underwent trabeculectomy (Lee et al. 2013a). The anterior displacement of the anterior LC surface or flattening of the LC curve after IOP lowering is more prominent in young patients (Lee et al. 2012; Esfandiari et al. 2018), but also seen in elderly patients. The difference according to age suggests that the LC is more compliant and resilient according to IOP change in younger ages.

Theoretically, LC depth change can occur in opposite direction (i.e., posterior displacement upon IOP lowering). Finite element analysis has shown that anteroposterior displacement of the LC varied greatly depending on the properties of the lamina and sclera (Sigal et al. 2011). When the peripapillary sclera is more compliant than LC, IOP elevation can expand the canal, which in turn pulls the lamina taut from the sides. In this case, the LC depth may decrease when the IOP is increased. However, there has been little report which demonstrated this phenomenon in patients.

5.3 Greater LCCI

They demonstrated that LC curvature as assessed by LCCI also changes depending on the IOP change (Lee et al. 2016a). In addition, the LCCI performed better than LC depth measured from Bruch's membrane opening in discriminating between healthy and glaucomatous eyes (Lee et al. 2017). This finding suggests that the LC curvature may better characterize the glaucomatous LC deformation. This is probably because the LCCI is not affected by choroidal thickness. Kim et al. demonstrated that the LC curvature assessed by mean LC depth was greater in POAG eyes with high IOP than those with low IOP (Kim et al. 2016a).

The greater LCCI is associated with location of damage in individual patients. In unilateral glaucoma patients, glaucomatous eyes have greater LCCI than fellow healthy eyes (Kim et al. 2019b). Moreover, LCCI was greater in the hemifield corresponding with the location of RNFL defects compared to the opposite hemifield in glaucomatous eyes with hemifield optic nerve damage (Kim et al. 2019a).

5.4 Focal Lamina Defects

Several studies have demonstrated localized structural alteration of the peripheral LC, including focal LC defect and pit (Fig. 8). The focal LC defects were topographically correlated with localized neuroretinal rim loss, retinal nerve fiber layer defects, visual field defects, and parapaillary choroidal dropout (Park et al. 2013; You et al. 2013; Park et al. 2017a).

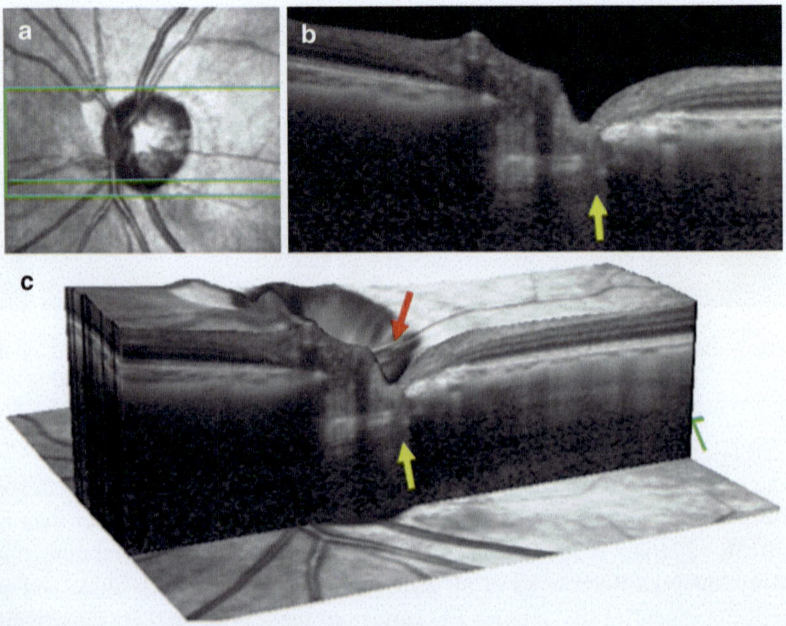

Fig. 8 Focal lamina cribrosa (LC) defect is seen in the B-scan (**b**) and reconstructed 3D images (**c**) at the location indicated in infrared photograph (green horizontal line in the inferior periphery, **a**) (yellow arrows). Focal neuroretinal rim is seen over the focal LC defect (red arrow)

5.5 Findings in Eyes with Disc Hemorrhage

Disc hemorrhage is often found in glaucoma patients and associated with glaucoma progression. The pathophysiology of disc hemorrhage is largely unveiled. Several LC imaging studies have suggested that LC deformation is associated with disc hemorrhage. Lee et al. demonstrated the structural alteration in the LC images obtained before and after DH, which were separated about 1 or 2 years (Fig. 9) (Lee et al. 2014b). This finding suggests that the DH may result from the disruption of capillaries in the laminar beams during the development of focal LC defect. In line with this finding, cross sectional studies demonstrated the association of DH and focal LC defects (Park et al. 2013; Kim and Park 2016; Kim et al. 2016b). Kim et al. have shown that the size of DH which corresponds to focal LC defect location tends to be larger than DH without correspondence (Kim et al. 2016b).

5.6 Association with Rate of Glaucoma Progression

Several characteristics of LC identified by OCT imaging have been found to be associated with rate of glaucoma progression. First, focal defects of the LC have been shown to be associated with the rate of glaucoma progression. Faridi et al. have shown that eyes with focal LC defects tend to progress faster than those without (Faridi et al. 2014). Park et al. demonstrated that glaucoma eyes with DH at the site of focal LC defects showed frequent and faster visual field progression compared with DH not accompanied by LC alterations or LC alterations not accompanied by DH (Park et al. 2017b). They reported in a separate article that the presence of focal LC defects was related to the rate of inferior RNFL thinning while a deeper and thinner LC was related to the rate of superior RNFL thinning (Park et al. 2017c).

Lee et al. investigated the relationship between LC change behavior and rate of glaucoma progression after trabeculectomy. They found that eyes with sustained LCD reduction over a long period had a slow rate of progressive RNFL thinning after trabeculectomy. A large LCD reduction in the early postoperative period was not associated with the long-term rate of progression if it was not maintained during subsequent follow-up (Lee and Kim 2015).

The LCCI has also been shown to be associated with the rate of visual field deterioration in POAG eyes (Ha et al. 2018). In addition, the

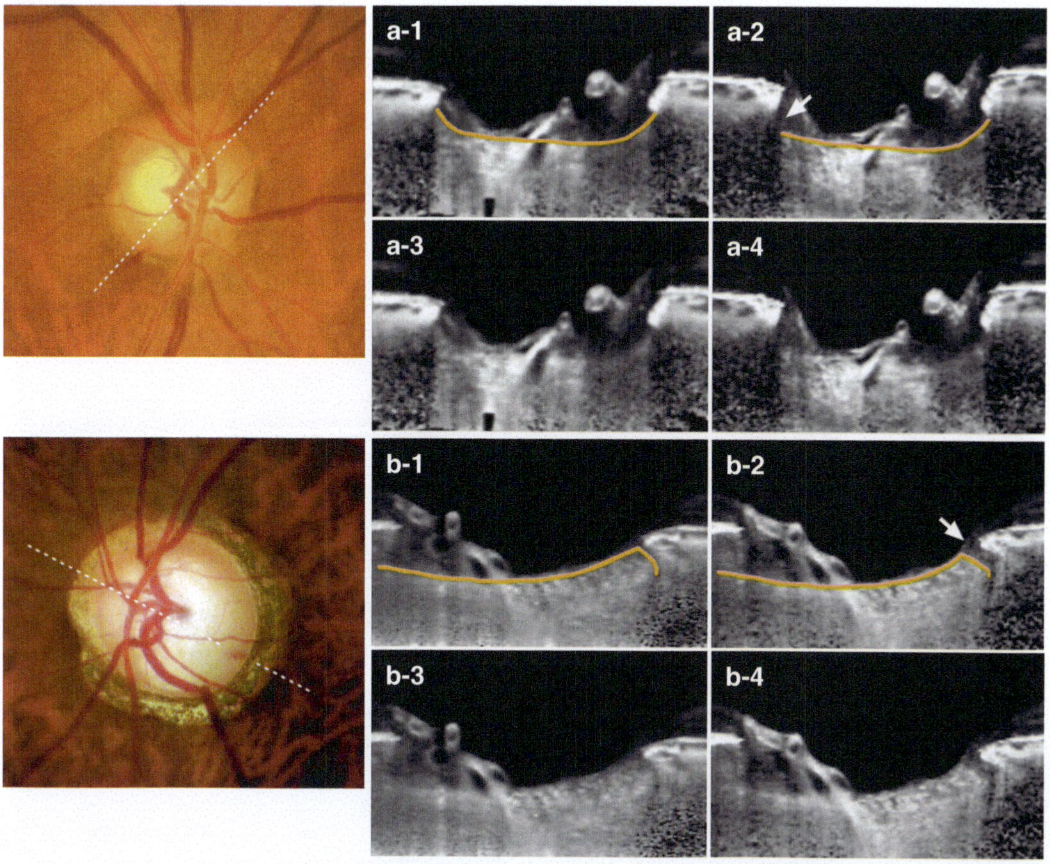

Fig. 9 Fundus photographs and SD-OCT B-scan images at the meridian (*dotted lines*) of disc hemorrhage. *Left images* (**a-1**, **a-3**, **b-1**, **b-3**) are the baseline B-scans and *right* (**a-2**, **a-4**, **b-2**, **b-4**) are the images obtained after detection of optic disc hemorrhage. *Orange lines* delineate the anterior surface of the lamina cribrosa (LC). (**a-3**, **a-4**) Same images as (**a-1**, **a-2**) without labels. (**b-3**, **b-4**) Same images as (**b-1**, **b-2**) without labels. (**a**) Structural alteration of the LC with outward deformation of the visible end of anterior LC surface. Note that the visible end of the anterior LC is more posteriorly located in the follow-up image (**a-2**, **b-2**) (*arrow*). The change in the curvature of the anterior LC surface also is noticeable (*orange lines*). (**b**) Recent structural alteration of the LC with radial disruption of the temporal LC. Note the enlarged cleft near the LC insertion in the follow-up image (*orange lines* and *arrow*). Adopted and modified from Lee et al. (2016b)

LCCI was associated with the rate of progressive RNFL thinning in glaucoma suspect eyes (Kim et al. 2018). This finding is consistent with experimental glaucoma model studies which demonstrated profoundly altered ONH connective tissues at the onset of detectable ONH surface change (Burgoyne et al. 2004). More recently, Lee et al. demonstrated that LCCI was the strongest prognostic factors for faster progressive RNFL thinning using regression tree model (Lee et al. 2019).

6 Applications of LC Imaging and Perspectives on Glaucoma Management

6.1 Differential Diagnosis from Other Optic Neuropathies

A characteristic feature of glaucoma is excavation of the optic nerve head (i.e., cupping). The excavation is composed of loss of neuronal tissue and posterior displacement/bowing of the lamina.

Mild degree of cupping is also noted in nonglaucomatous optic neuropathies, which often lead to misdiagnosis to glaucoma. Studies have shown that deep optic nerve head feature is different between glaucoma and other optic neuropathies. While deeply located or posteriorly curved LC together with loss of prelaminar tissue is the hallmark of glaucoma, those findings are not clearly seen in other optic neuropathies such as nonarteritic ischemic optic neuropathy and autosomal dominant optic neuropathy (Figs. 10 and 11) (Kim et al. 2020a; Fard et al. 2016; Lee et al. 2016b). This finding can be used to aid differential diagnosis in ambient cases with other differ-

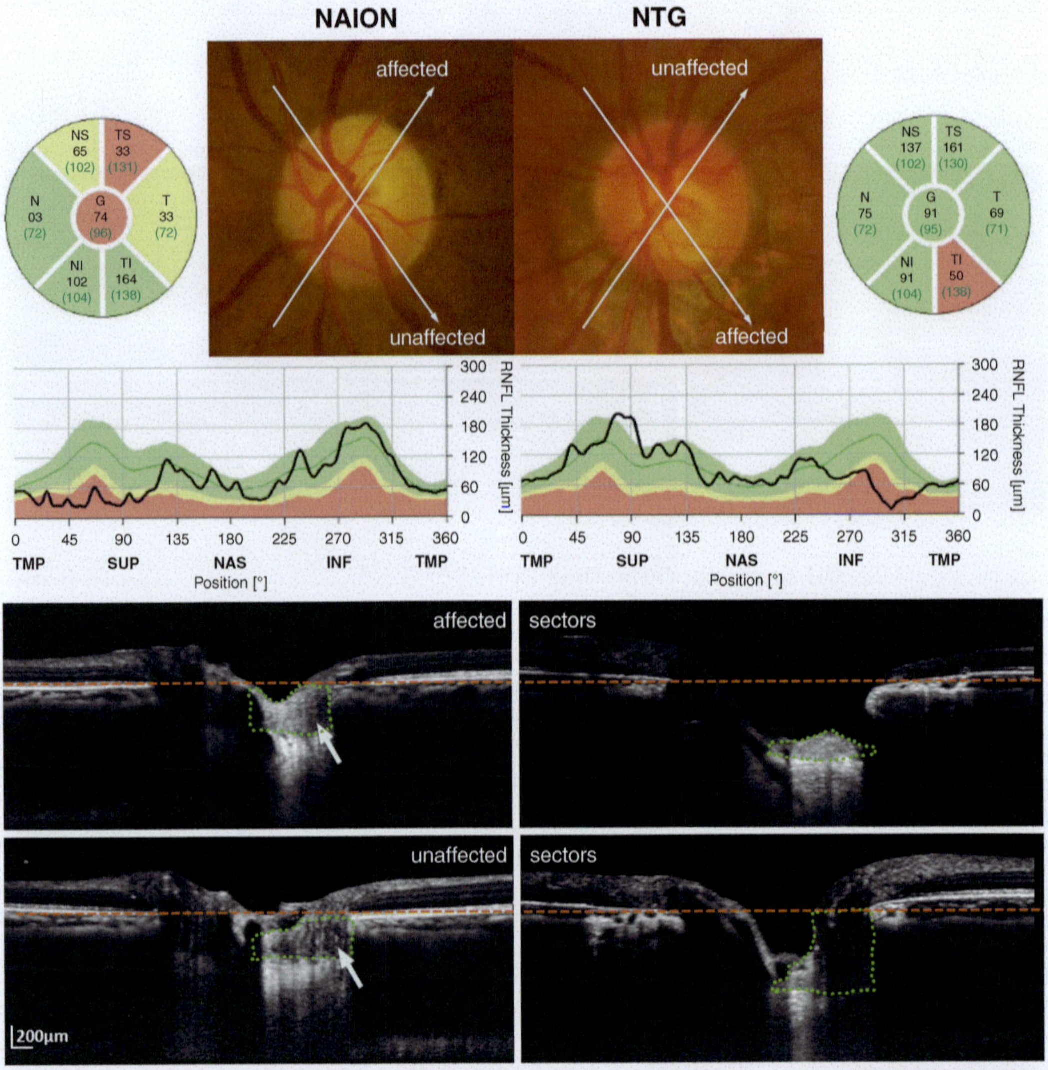

Fig. 10 Comparison of the prelaminar tissue thickness (PTT) between the affected and unaffected sectors in eyes with nonarteritic anterior ischemic optic neuropathy (NAION) (left) and normal tension glaucoma (NTG) (right). *Long arrows* in color disc photographs indicate the locations and directions of radial B-scans shown in the lower panels. *Orange dashed lines* indicate the level of the Bruch's membrane opening. *Green dotted lines* demarcate the area where the PTT was measured. Disc photographs in the top row show evident pallor (left) and notching (right) of the optic disc rims in the affected sectors in NAION and NTG eyes, respectively. Peripapillary OCT RNFL results show thinning of RNFL in the affected sectors in both NAION and NTG eyes. In NAION, the PT is thick in the affected sector, with the PTT being comparable to that in the unaffected sector (*arrows*). On the other hand, there is a remarkable difference in the PTT between the unaffected and the affected sectors in this NTG eye with an untreated IOP of 14 mmHg. Note that the anterior laminar surface is located deeper than in the affected sector than in the unaffected sector in NTG. Adopted and modified from Lee et al. (2016b)

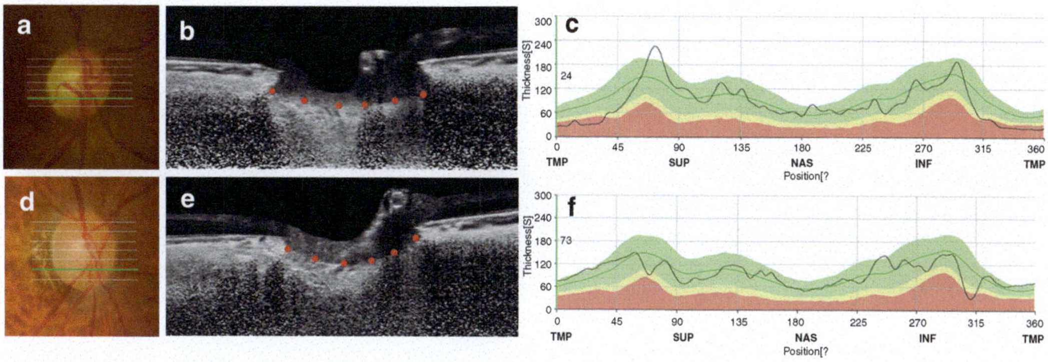

Fig. 11 Comparison of the anterior lamina cribrosa (red dots) curvature in an eye with autosomal dominant optic atrophy (ADOA) (**a–c**) in a 72-year-old woman, and an eye with normal tension glaucoma in a 77-year-old woman (**d–f**). (**b**, **e**) B-scan images at inferior midperipheral plane, indicated by the green lines in the optic disc photographs. (**c**) RNFL thinning is noted in the temporal region. (**f**) RNFL thinning is noted in the inferotemporal region. Adopted and modified from Kim et al. (2020b)

ential diagnosis point such more pronounced pallor than excavation, history of central vision loss and patter of visual field loss.

6.2 Predicting Rate of Future Glaucoma Progression

As describe earlier, several LC morphologic characteristics have been shown to be associated with rate of glaucoma progression as assessed by OCT or visual field in eyes with glaucoma. Those characteristics include thinner LC thickness, greater LCCI at baseline, presence of focal LC defects particularly with occurrence of disc hemorrhage (Ha et al. 2018; Faridi et al. 2014; Park et al. 2017b). The LC morphology can also be useful to predict development of glaucoma in suspect eyes (Fig. 12) (Kim et al. 2018). Characterization of high risk patients for disease progression will help clinicians to detect glaucoma progression early, so as to allow timely adjustment of the treatment.

6.3 Searching Mechanism of Optic Nerve Damage in Individual Patient

Glaucoma is a multifactorial disease. Although intraocular pressure induced stress is considered as the single most important risk factor, other factors including compromised circulation have been suggested as risk factors (Weinreb and Khaw 2004; Weinreb et al. 2014). Optic nerve damage often progresses despite substantial IOP lowering treatment. When a progression is noted despite maximum tolerable medical therapy, clinicians would consider other treatment options such as laser or surgical treatment for further IOP lowering. However, it is questionable whether such treatment approach is justified in every single glaucoma patient. This is due to the possibility that factors other than IOP related stress is the main cause of progression in certain patients.

There is no definite method to understand the mechanism of optic nerve damage in individual glaucoma patients. For better management of glaucoma, particularly for etiology targeted treatment approach, it is essential to develop method to identify specific etiology of optic nerve damage in individual patients. Theoretically, LC imaging can be a good candidate for such development because LC is a key structure in glaucoma biomechanics. The morphology of LC is variable among glaucoma patients, shedding light in this possibility. With further research and development of biomarkers, LC imaging might become a useful tool to help identify the specific mechanism of optic nerve damage in individual patients.

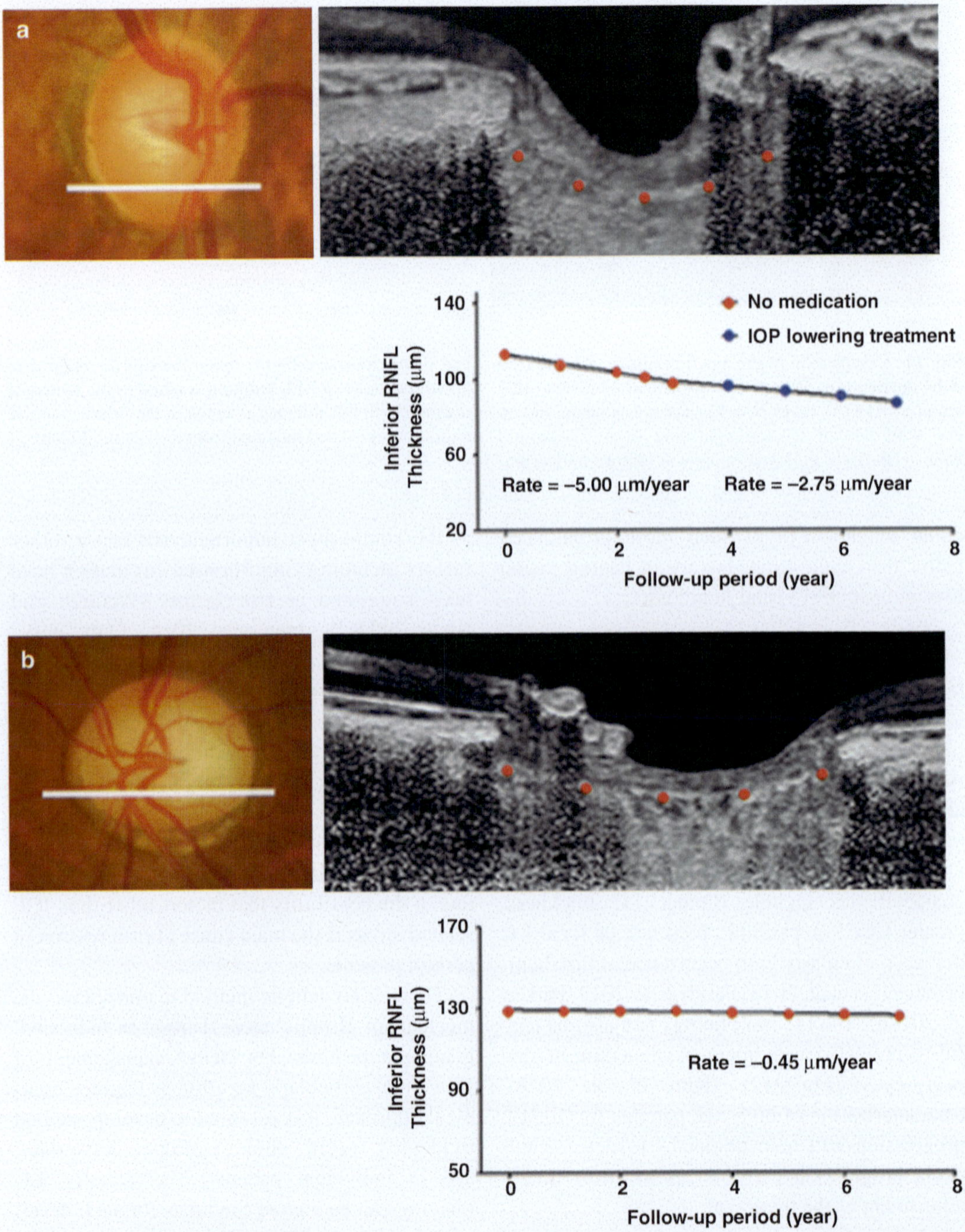

Fig. 12 Two cases of glaucoma suspect eyes. (**a**) A glaucoma suspect eye of a 61-year-old female with steeply curved lamina cribrosa (LC). The untreated intraocular pressure (IOP) and central corneal thickness were 16 mmHg and 537 μm, respectively. During the first 3 years following baseline examination, progressive retinal nerve fiber layer (RNFL) loss was observed in the inferior sector with the rate of −5.00 μm/year. After IOP lowering treatment, the rate of RNFL loss decreased to −2.75 μm/year. (**b**) A glaucoma-suspected eye of a 74-year-old female with a relatively fat LC. The untreated IOP and central corneal thickness were 16 mmHg and 545 μm, respectively. During 7 years of follow-up, the rate of RNFL loss in the inferior sector was −0.45 μm/year without any treatment. Adopted and modified from Kim et al. (2018)

6.4 Characterizing Optic Neuropathy in Myopic Eyes

Myopia is a risk factor for glaucoma (Mitchell et al. 1999; Liang et al. 2011; Suzuki et al. 2006). However, the rate of progression is often slower in myopic eyes with or even without IOP control (Lee et al. 2015; Araie et al. 2012). This finding suggests that mechanism of optic nerve damage may be different in myopic glaucomatous eyes. The LC configuration in myopic tilted disc eyes has some unique features. The LC is flatter and the pores are elongated to the direction of disc tilt/torsion (Fig. 13) (Sawada et al. 2018). This feature suggests that tensile stress to the LC arising from the axial elongation may play a role in the optic nerve damage.

If such stress is the main cause of optic nerve damage, the clinical course would be different from that of glaucoma derived from translaminar pressure gradient. Since axial elongation is not a lifelong process the tensile stress may be alleviated at some point. In addition, loss of axons may generate a room for remaining axons, thereby protecting them from the sustained tensile stress. If this is the case, the axonal loss can occur in the early life but the rate of loss can be slowed or halted in the late life (Kim et al. 2014). The treatment strategy should be different in those patients from the patients who have high risk of disease progression. Further study is needed to develop method to differentiate high risk and low risk patients for disease progression among myopic eyes. For those studies, LC imaging may play a central role.

7 Conclusions

Since LC is the primary site of axonal injury in glaucoma, imaging the LC provides an opportunity to enhance understanding on the pathogenesis of glaucomatous optic neuropathy. The LC imaging is not routinely used in the current clinical practice due to technical difficulty and lack of consensus in its utility. The devises for LC imaging and clinically useful biomarkers based on LC morphology are currently evolving. With further research and development, LC imaging may contribute to improvements in understanding biomechanics of glaucomatous optic neuropathy and specific mechanism of damage in individual patients, which will eventually facilitate development of patient-tailored treatment.

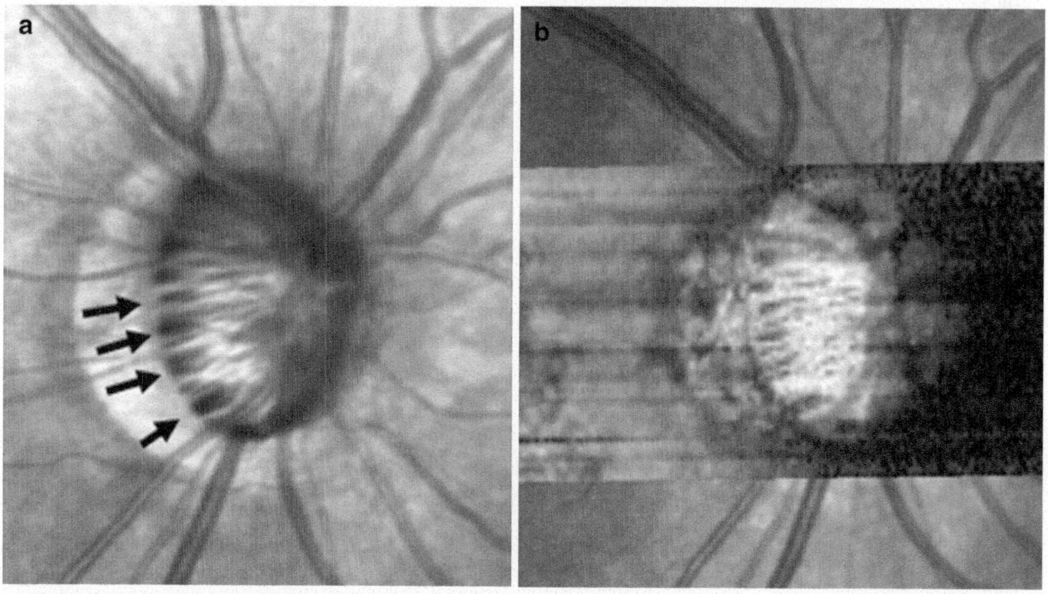

Fig. 13 Characteristic LC feature in myopic eyes shown in infrared fundus photo (**a**) and a coronal section of 3D reconstructed volume image (**b**). The laminar pores are large and elongated to the direction of disc tilt

References

Anderson DR, Hendrickson A. Effect of intraocular pressure on rapid axoplasmic transport in monkey optic nerve. Invest Ophthalmol. 1974;13(10):771–83.

Araie M, Shirato S, Yamazaki Y, Matsumoto C, Kitazawa Y, Ohashi Y, et al. Risk factors for progression of normal-tension glaucoma under beta-blocker monotherapy. Acta Ophthalmol. 2012;90(5):e337–43.

Barrancos C, Rebolleda G, Oblanca N, Cabarga C, Munoz-Negrete FJ. Changes in lamina cribrosa and prelaminar tissue after deep sclerectomy. Eye (Lond). 2014;28(1):58–65.

Burgoyne CF, Downs JC, Bellezza AJ, Hart RT. Three-dimensional reconstruction of normal and early glaucoma monkey optic nerve head connective tissues. Invest Ophthalmol Vis Sci. 2004;45(12):4388–99.

Burgoyne CF, Downs JC, Bellezza AJ, Suh JK, Hart RT. The optic nerve head as a biomechanical structure: a new paradigm for understanding the role of IOP-related stress and strain in the pathophysiology of glaucomatous optic nerve head damage. Prog Retin Eye Res. 2005;24(1):39–73.

Esfandiari H, Efatizadeh A, Hassanpour K, Doozandeh A, Yaseri M, Loewen NA. Factors associated with lamina cribrosa displacement after trabeculectomy measured by optical coherence tomography in advanced primary open-angle glaucoma. Graefes Arch Clin Exp Ophthalmol. 2018;256(12):2391–8.

Fard MA, Afzali M, Abdi P, Chen R, Yaseri M, Azaripour E, et al. Optic nerve head morphology in nonarteritic anterior ischemic optic neuropathy compared to open-angle glaucoma. Invest Ophthalmol Vis Sci. 2016;57(11):4632–40.

Faridi OS, Park SC, Kabadi R, Su D, De Moraes CG, Liebmann JM, et al. Effect of focal lamina cribrosa defect on glaucomatous visual field progression. Ophthalmology. 2014;121(8):1524–30.

Girard MJ, Tun TA, Husain R, Acharyya S, Haaland BA, Wei X, et al. Lamina cribrosa visibility using optical coherence tomography: comparison of devices and effects of image enhancement techniques. Invest Ophthal Vis Sci. 2015;56(2):865–74.

Goldbaum MH, Jeng SY, Logemann R, Weinreb RN. The extracellular matrix of the human optic nerve. Arch Ophthalmol. 1989;107(8):1225–31.

Ha A, Kim TJ, Girard MJA, Mari JM, Kim YK, Park KH, et al. Baseline lamina cribrosa curvature and subsequent visual field progression rate in primary open-angle glaucoma. Ophthalmology. 2018;125(12):1898–906.

Hernandez MR, Igoe F, Neufeld AH. Extracellular matrix of the human optic nerve head. Am J Ophthalmol. 1986;102(2):139–48.

Hernandez MR, Luo XX, Andrzejewska W, Neufeld AH. Age-related changes in the extracellular matrix of the human optic nerve head. Am J Ophthalmol. 1989;107(5):476–84.

Inoue R, Hangai M, Kotera Y, Nakanishi H, Mori S, Morishita S, et al. Three-dimensional high-speed optical coherence tomography imaging of lamina cribrosa in glaucoma. Ophthalmology. 2009;116(2):214–22.

Jonas JB, Berenshtein E, Holbach L. Lamina cribrosa thickness and spatial relationships between intraocular space and cerebrospinal fluid space in highly myopic eyes. Invest Ophthalmol Vis Sci. 2004;45(8):2660–5.

Kim YK, Park KH. Lamina cribrosa defects in eyes with glaucomatous disc haemorrhage. Acta Ophthalmol. 2016;94(6):e468–73.

Kim YW, Lee EJ, Kim TW, Kim M, Kim H. Microstructure of beta-zone parapapillary atrophy and rate of retinal nerve fiber layer thinning in primary open-angle glaucoma. Ophthalmology. 2014;121(7):1341–9.

Kim YW, Jeoung JW, Girard MJ, Mari JM, Park KH. Positional and curvature difference of lamina cribrosa according to the baseline intraocular pressure in primary open-angle glaucoma: a Swept-Source Optical Coherence Tomography (SS-OCT) study. PLoS One. 2016a;11(9):e0162182.

Kim YK, Jeoung JW, Park KH. Effect of focal lamina cribrosa defect on disc hemorrhage area in glaucoma. Invest Ophthalmol Vis Sci. 2016b;57(3):899–907.

Kim JA, Kim TW, Weinreb RN, Lee EJ, Girard MJA, Mari JM. Lamina cribrosa morphology predicts progressive retinal nerve fiber layer loss in eyes with suspected glaucoma. Sci Rep. 2018;8(1):738.

Kim JA, Kim TW, Lee EJ, Girard MJA, Mari JM. Lamina cribrosa morphology in glaucomatous eyes with hemifield defect in a Korean population. Ophthalmology. 2019a;126(5):692–701.

Kim JA, Kim TW, Lee EJ, Kim JM, Girard MJA, Mari JM. Intereye comparison of lamina cribrosa curvature in normal tension glaucoma patients with unilateral damage. Invest Ophthalmol Vis Sci. 2019b;60(7):2423–30.

Kim JA, Lee EJ, Kim TW, Kim H, Girard MJA, Mari JM, et al. Differentiation of nonarteritic anterior ischemic optic neuropathy from normal tension glaucoma by comparison of the lamina cribrosa. Invest Ophthalmol Vis Sci. 2020a;61(8):21.

Kim GN, Kim JA, Kim MJ, Lee EJ, Hwang JM, Kim TW. Comparison of lamina cribrosa morphology in normal tension glaucoma and autosomal-dominant optic atrophy. Invest Ophthalmol Vis Sci. 2020b;61(5):9.

Krzyzanowska-Berkowska P, Melinska A, Helemejko I, Robert Iskander D. Evaluating displacement of lamina cribrosa following glaucoma surgery. Graefes Arch Clin Exp Ophthalmol. 2018;256(4):791–800.

Lee EJ, Kim TW. Lamina cribrosa reversal after trabeculectomy and the rate of progressive retinal nerve fiber layer thinning. Ophthalmology. 2015;122(11):2234–42.

Lee EJ, Kim TW, Weinreb RN, Park KH, Kim SH, Kim DM. Visualization of the lamina cribrosa using enhanced depth imaging spectral-domain optical coherence tomography. Am J Ophthalmol. 2011;152(1):87–95. e1

Lee EJ, Kim TW, Weinreb RN. Reversal of lamina cribrosa displacement and thickness after trabeculectomy in glaucoma. Ophthalmology. 2012;119(7):1359–66.

Lee EJ, Kim TW, Weinreb RN. Variation of lamina cribrosa depth following trabeculectomy. Invest Ophthalmol Vis Sci. 2013a;54(8):5392–9.

Lee EJ, Kim TW, Weinreb RN, Kim H. Reversal of lamina cribrosa displacement after intraocular pressure reduction in open-angle glaucoma. Ophthalmology. 2013b;120(3):553–9.

Lee KM, Kim TW, Weinreb RN, Lee EJ, Girard MJ, Mari JM. Anterior lamina cribrosa insertion in primary open-angle glaucoma patients and healthy subjects. PLoS One. 2014a;9(12):e114935.

Lee EJ, Kim TW, Kim M, Girard MJ, Mari JM, Weinreb RN. Recent structural alteration of the peripheral lamina cribrosa near the location of disc hemorrhage in glaucoma. Invest Ophthalmol Vis Sci. 2014b;55(4):2805–15.

Lee JY, Sung KR, Han S, Na JH. Effect of myopia on the progression of primary open-angle glaucoma. Invest Ophthalmol Vis Sci. 2015;56(3):1775–81.

Lee SH, Yu DA, Kim TW, Lee EJ, Girard MJ, Mari JM. Reduction of the lamina cribrosa curvature after trabeculectomy in glaucoma. Invest Ophthalmol Vis Sci. 2016a;57(11):5006–14.

Lee EJ, Choi YJ, Kim TW, Hwang JM. Comparison of the deep optic nerve head structure between normal-tension glaucoma and nonarteritic anterior ischemic optic neuropathy. PLoS One. 2016b;11(4):e0150242.

Lee SH, Kim TW, Lee EJ, Girard MJ, Mari JM. Diagnostic power of lamina cribrosa depth and curvature in glaucoma. Invest Ophthalmol Vis Sci. 2017;58(2):755–62.

Lee EJ, Kim TW, Kim JA, Kim GN, Kim JM, Girard MJA, et al. Elucidation of the strongest factors influencing rapid retinal nerve fiber layer thinning in glaucoma. Invest Ophthalmol Vis Sci. 2019;60(10):3343–51.

Lee SH, Lee EJ, Kim JM, Girard MJA, Mari JM, Kim TW. Lamina cribrosa moves anteriorly after trabeculectomy in myopic eyes. Invest Ophthalmol Vis Sci. 2020;61(6):36.

Liang YB, Friedman DS, Zhou Q, Yang X, Sun LP, Guo LX, et al. Prevalence of primary open angle glaucoma in a rural adult Chinese population: the Handan eye study. Invest Ophthalmol Vis Sci. 2011;52(11):8250–7.

Mecham RP. Elastin synthesis and fiber assembly. Ann N Y Acad Sci. 1991;624:137–46.

Mitchell P, Hourihan F, Sandbach J, Wang JJ. The relationship between glaucoma and myopia: the Blue Mountains Eye Study. Ophthalmology. 1999;106(10):2010–5.

Morrison JC, L'Hernault NL, Jerdan JA, Quigley HA. Ultrastructural location of extracellular matrix components in the optic nerve head. Arch Ophthalmol. 1989;107(1):123–9.

Ogden TE, Duggan J, Danley K, Wilcox M, Minckler DS. Morphometry of nerve fiber bundle pores in the optic nerve head of the human. Exp Eye Res. 1988;46(4):559–68.

Park SC, Kiumehr S, Teng CC, Tello C, Liebmann JM, Ritch R. Horizontal central ridge of the lamina cribrosa and regional differences in laminar insertion in healthy subjects. Invest Ophthalmol Vis Sci. 2012a;53(3):1610–6.

Park HY, Jeon SH, Park CK. Enhanced depth imaging detects lamina cribrosa thickness differences in normal tension glaucoma and primary open-angle glaucoma. Ophthalmology. 2012b;119(1):10–20.

Park SC, Hsu AT, Su D, Simonson JL, Al-Jumayli M, Liu Y, et al. Factors associated with focal lamina cribrosa defects in glaucoma. Invest Ophthalmol Vis Sci. 2013;54(13):8401–7.

Park HY, Hwang YS, Park CK. Ocular characteristics associated with the location of focal lamina cribrosa defects in open-angle glaucoma patients. Eye (Lond). 2017a;31(4):578–87.

Park HL, Lee J, Jung Y, Park CK. Optic disc hemorrhage and lamina cribrosa defects in glaucoma progression. Sci Rep. 2017b;7(1):3489.

Park HL, Kim SI, Park CK. Influence of the lamina cribrosa on the rate of global and localized retinal nerve fiber layer thinning in open-angle glaucoma. Medicine (Baltimore). 2017c;96(14):e6295.

Quigley HA, Addicks EM. Regional differences in the structure of the lamina cribrosa and their relation to glaucomatous optic nerve damage. Arch Ophthalmol. 1981;99(1):137–43.

Quigley H, Anderson DR. The dynamics and location of axonal transport blockade by acute intraocular pressure elevation in primate optic nerve. Invest Ophthalmol. 1976;15(8):606–16.

Quigley HA, Hohman RM, Addicks EM, Massof RW, Green WR. Morphologic changes in the lamina cribrosa correlated with neural loss in open-angle glaucoma. Am J Ophthalmol. 1983;95(5):673–91.

Radius RL, Gonzales M. Anatomy of the lamina cribrosa in human eyes. Arch Ophthalmol. 1981;99(12):2159–62.

Rhodes LA, Huisingh C, Johnstone J, Fazio MA, Smith B, Wang L, et al. Peripapillary choroidal thickness variation with age and race in normal eyes. Invest Ophthalmol Vis Sci. 2015;56(3):1872–9.

Sawada Y, Araie M, Kasuga H, Ishikawa M, Iwata T, Murata K, et al. Focal lamina cribrosa defect in myopic eyes with nonprogressive glaucomatous visual field defect. Am J Ophthalmol. 2018;190:34–49.

Sigal IA, Yang H, Roberts MD, Grimm JL, Burgoyne CF, Demirel S, et al. IOP-induced lamina cribrosa deformation and scleral canal expansion: independent or related? Invest Ophthalmol Vis Sci. 2011;52(12):9023–32.

Suzuki Y, Iwase A, Araie M, Yamamoto T, Abe H, Shirato S, et al. Risk factors for open-angle glaucoma in a Japanese population: the Tajimi Study. Ophthalmology. 2006;113(9):1613–7.

Vianna JR, Lanoe VR, Quach J, Sharpe GP, Hutchison DM, Belliveau AC, et al. Serial changes in lamina cribrosa depth and neuroretinal parameters in glaucoma: impact of choroidal thickness. Ophthalmology. 2017;124(9):1392–402.

Weinreb RN, Khaw PT. Primary open-angle glaucoma. Lancet. 2004;363(9422):1711–20.

Weinreb RN, Aung T, Medeiros FA. The pathophysiology and treatment of glaucoma: a review. JAMA. 2014;311(18):1901–11.

You JY, Park SC, Su D, Teng CC, Liebmann JM, Ritch R. Focal lamina cribrosa defects associated with glaucomatous rim thinning and acquired pits. JAMA Ophthalmol. 2013;131(3):314–20.

OCT Angiography

Eun Ji Lee

Abstract

Optical coherence tomography angiography (OCTA) is a relatively new technology that enables noninvasive visualization of the microvasculature of ocular tissues. Altered ocular perfusion being understood as an important factor in the pathogenesis of glaucoma, OCTA has emerged as a promising tool to evaluate ocular blood flow in patients with glaucoma. OCTA may have the potential to provide new information about the pathophysiology of glaucoma, as well as to assist in its diagnosis and treatment. This chapter briefly describes the basic principles and interpretation of OCTA, and evaluates its clinical use in patients with glaucoma. This chapter also introduces recent research findings observed using OCTA in glaucoma, including microvascular changes in the optic nerve head, retina, and choroid, and discusses how they may be related to the pathophysiology of glaucoma.

Keywords

OCT angiography · Ocular perfusion Glaucoma · Microvasculature · Optic nerve head · Retina · Choroid

E. J. Lee (✉)
Seoul National University Bundang Hospital, Seongnam, Korea
e-mail: opticdisc@snubh.org

1 Introduction

Alterations in ocular perfusion have long been implicated in the pathogenesis of glaucoma. Compromised ocular blood flow (Huber et al. 2004; Findl et al. 2000; Shiga et al. 2016; Sehi et al. 2014) and reduced perfusion of the retina and choroid (Schwartz et al. 1977; Hitchings and Spaeth 1977; Yamazaki et al. 1996; Laatikainen 1971; O'Brart et al. 1997; Funaki et al. 1997) have been associated with glaucoma. Epidemiologic and clinical studies have demonstrated associations between glaucoma and low blood pressure (Tielsch et al. 1995; Bonomi et al. 2000; Leske et al. 1995) and nocturnal reductions in blood pressure (Graham and Drance 1999; Charlson et al. 2014). However, details of the role of ocular perfusion in glaucoma have remained elusive due to limitations in methods used to assess ocular blood flow.

Optical coherence tomography (OCT) angiography (OCTA) is a new imaging technique that enables visualization of the retinal and choroidal microvasculature, producing a three-dimensional (3D) reconstruction of vascular networks. OCTA providing structural and vascular maps in tandem, it is considered a promising tool to evaluate ocular perfusion in individual structural layers. Moreover, OCTA is noninvasive and does not require injection of dye, making it free from adverse effects and enabling repeated performance in busy clinics. Thus, OCTA imaging can

K. H. Park, T.-W. Kim (eds.), *OCT Imaging in Glaucoma*,
https://doi.org/10.1007/978-981-16-1178-0_6

not only help evaluate glaucoma patients in the clinic, but enables studies investigating the relationship of parapapillary microvascular compromise to the pathophysiologic features of glaucomatous optic neuropathy.

2 Basic Principles

Vascular imaging by OCTA is based on the OCT volume scan, which is auto-segmented and showed en-face to provide a view of the vasculature in individual segmented layers of the retina and choroid. The basic principle of OCTA is the taking of sequential B-scans at the same retinal location, followed by analysis to determine if there were any changes in the amplitude (intensity signal-based technique) (Jia et al. 2012a) and/or phase (phase signal-based technique) (Wang 2010) of the scan (Kashani et al. 2017). Changes signify movement of the retinal tissue at this location. This movement is thought to be due to the flow of red blood cells (RBCs) in the vasculature (i.e., functioning blood vessels Fig. 1). In contrast to traditional angiography (i.e., fluorescein or indocyanine green angiography), OCTA produces a static map of the vascular network without providing true information regarding blood flow or vascular leakage. Various systems are commercially available, with these systems using different acquisition, saving, and analytic processes (Li et al. 2018; Corvi et al. 2018).

3 Production of an En-Face Image from Segmented Tissue Layers

A two-dimensional (2D) en-face vascular map can be constructed from the 3D volume data obtained from any layer of interest. OCTA systems usually have preset layers of interest, with these layers segmented through an automated process. Although the preset layers vary slightly among systems, most systems provide images segmented in the radial peripapillary capillary plexus (RCP), superficial capillary plexus (SCP), deep capillary plexus (DCP), and choriocapillaris/choroidal layers (Fig. 2) (Spaide et al. 2015a). Manual segmentation can also be performed.

Most OCTA platforms generate en-face OCTA and B-scan OCT images with vascular signal overlay, enabling the in-tandem visualization of both the vasculature and structure (Fig. 2).

4 Strengths of OCTA

The outstanding feature of OCTA is that it does not require injection of a contrast dye, thus eliminating both systemic and local adverse effects. A single volume scan requires only a few seconds. OCTA has a high reproducibility and repeatability (Venugopal et al. 2018). Unlike conventional 2D angiography, OCTA is based on 3D images, allowing the depth-resolved en-face visualization

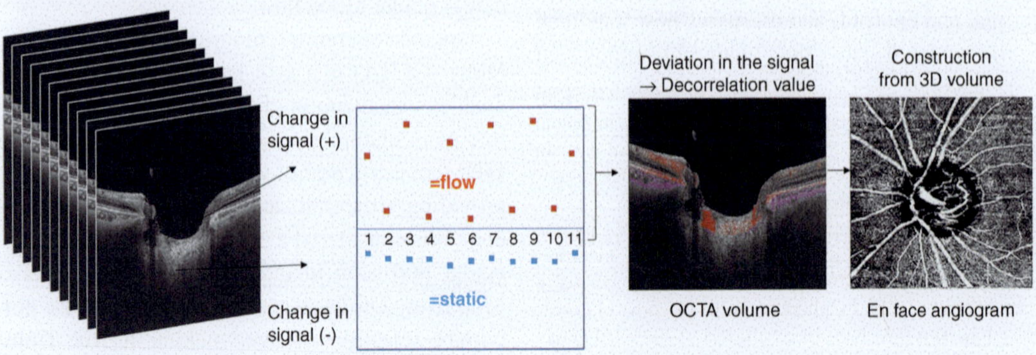

Fig. 1 Basic principle of OCTA. Sequential B-scans are taken at the same location, and compared to detect any changes in signal. A significant change in signal is thought to indicate blood flow. Alterations in signal are assessed mathematically to provide a decorrelation signal representing the amount of blood flow at that location. OCTA, optical coherence tomography angiography

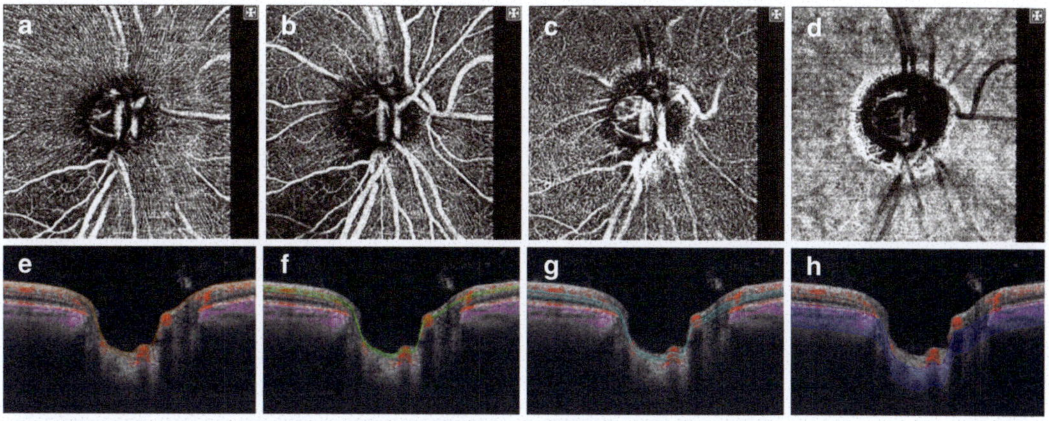

Fig. 2 Peripapillary OCTA images of a glaucomatous eye, obtained in the 4.5 × 4.5 mm area centered on the ONH using DRI OCT Triton (Topcon, Tokyo, Japan). The *upper panel* shows en-face OCTA images segmented in the (**a**) RCP, (**b**) SCP, (**c**) DCP, and (**d**) choroidal layers. The *lower panel* shows B-scan images (**e**–**h**) indicating the layers segmented to produce the en-face images in the *upper panel*. RCP, SCP, and DCP are segmented in the RNFL (**e**), GCL (**f**), and INL (**g**), respectively. OCTA, optical coherence tomography angiography; ONH, optic nerve head; RCP, radial peripapillary capillary plexus; SCP, superficial capillary plexus; DCP, deep capillary plexus; RNFL, retinal nerve fiber layer; GCL, ganglion cell layer; INL, inner nuclear layer

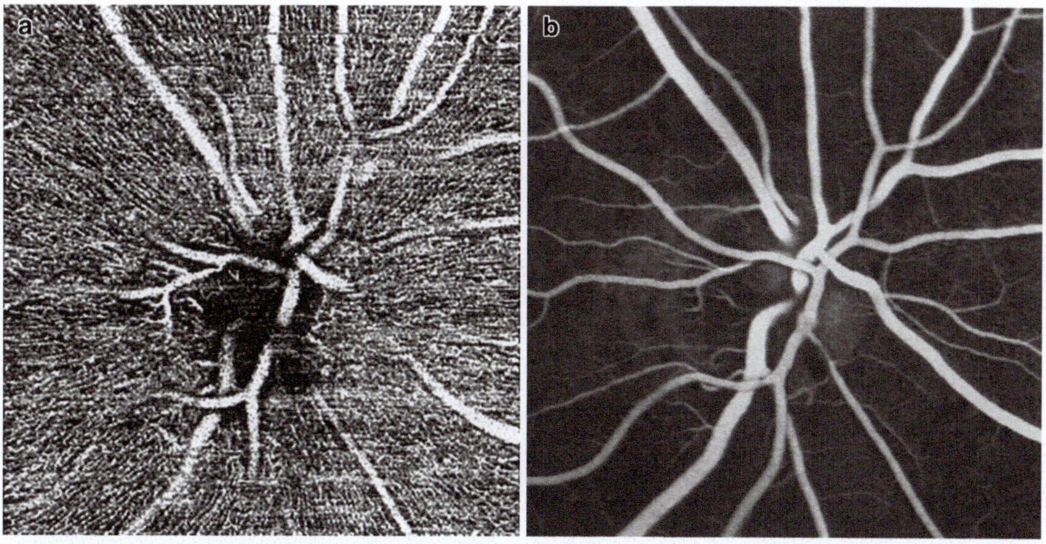

Fig. 3 (**a**) En-face OCTA image of the RCP and (**b**) an FA image of a healthy eye. The RCP is seen in exquisite detail on OCTA (**a**), whereas visualization on FA is poor (**b**). OCTA image was obtained using DRI OCT Triton (Topcon) and FA image was obtained Spectralis HRA + OCT (Heidelberg Engineering, Heidelberg, Germany). OCTA, optical coherence tomography angiography; RCP, radial peripapillary capillary plexus; FA, fluorescein angiography

of the different retinal capillary plexuses that cannot be distinguished by conventional fluorescein angiography (FA, Fig. 3). OCTA has been shown superior to traditional FA in imaging the RCP and DCP (Spaide et al. 2015a).

5 Limitations of OCTA

In contrast to traditional angiography (i.e., fluorescein or indocyanine green angiography), OCTA produces a static map of the vascular network and therefore does not provide true information regarding blood flow or vascular leakage. Quantitative assessment of flow speed using OCTA is currently unreliable.

OCTA is also prone to image artifacts resulting from patient motion, projection from superficial retinal vessels, and segmentation errors (Spaide et al. 2015b; Ghasemi Falavarjani et al. 2017). Because OCTA involves scans of the same area repeated multiple times, motion artifacts are likely to be caused by microsaccades, breathing, and cardiac cycle changes (Fig. 4). Blinking artifacts are caused by eye closure during image capture (Fig. 4). Fluctuating shadows from RBCs in superficial vessels can cast extra flow signals to deeper vascular networks, leading to projection artifacts (Fig. 4). Refracted, reflected, absorbed, or passing of the OCT beam through a vessel can generate false blood flow signals.

Various motion correction and eye-tracking technologies are applied to each OCTA system to reduce motion artifacts (Li et al. 2018). A recently developed projection resolved technique has been incorporated into OCTA (Takusagawa et al. 2017).

6 Evaluation of OCTA in Glaucoma

OCTA has been shown useful in distinguishing between glaucomatous and healthy eyes. As a diagnostic tool, OCTA can serve as an addition to conventional methods, or can substitute for the latter in eyes in which conventional tools are inconclusive, including eyes with high myopia (Shin et al. 2019; Lee et al. 2020a, b; Na et al. 2020) and advanced glaucoma (Kim et al. 2019a; Moghimi et al. 2019). OCTA may also be useful in the detection of glaucoma progression (Lee et al. 2019, c; Park et al. 2019; Hou et al. 2020).

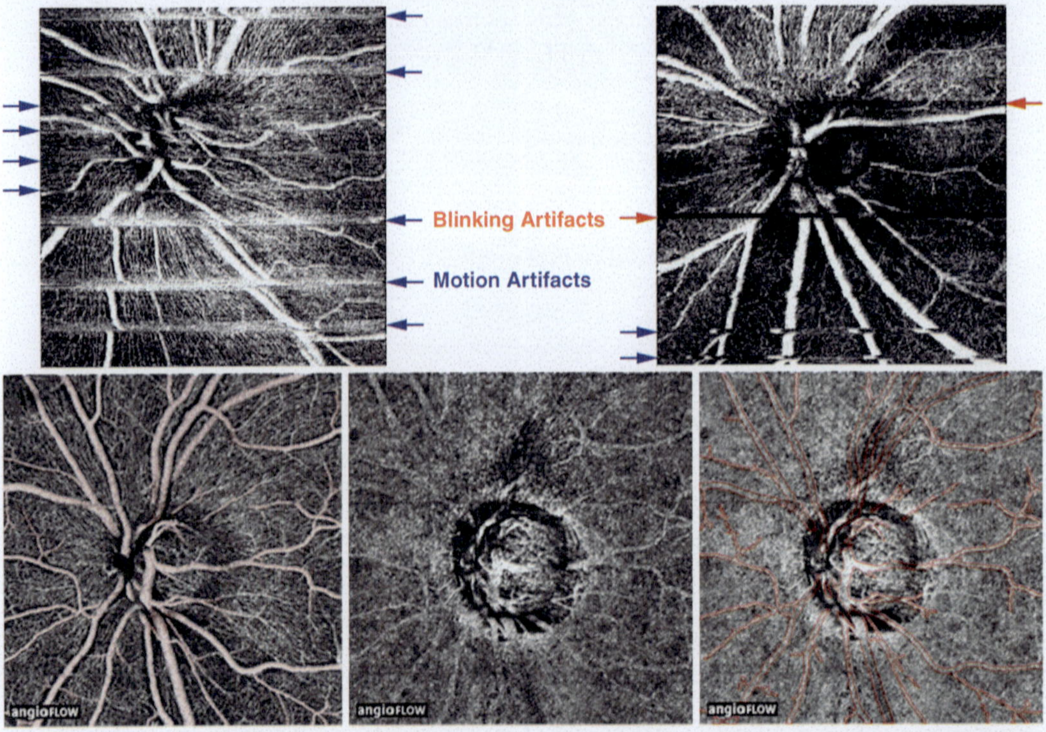

Fig. 4 Artifacts in OCTA. The *upper panel* shows en-face images of the SCP with motion (*blue arrows*) and blinking (*red arrows*) artifacts. The *lower panel* shows an example of a projection artifact. Signals of retinal vessels (colored in *light-red*) in the OCTA image of the SCP layer (**a**) are also observed (vessels demarcated with *red lines*) in the image of the choroidal layer (**b**, **c**). Images were obtained using DRI OCT Triton (Topcon) and RTVue XR Avanti (Optovue, Fremont Inc, California, USA), respectively. OCTA, optical coherence tomography angiography; SCP, superficial capillary plexus

6.1 Macular Imaging

OCTA imaging of the macula usually involves an area ranging from 3 × 3 to 9 × 9 mm^2 centered on the fovea. Vessel density (VD) in the segmented retinal layers and foveal avascular zone (FAZ) are the two most frequently used parameters in glaucoma evaluation.

6.1.1 FAZ

The FAZ is a region lacking capillaries at the center of the macula surrounded by interconnected capillary networks. FAZs are larger in area and have a more irregular shape in eyes with glaucoma than in healthy eyes (Zivkovic et al. 2017; Choi et al. 2017). These findings are topographically correlated with the location of visual field (VF) defects (Fig. 5)

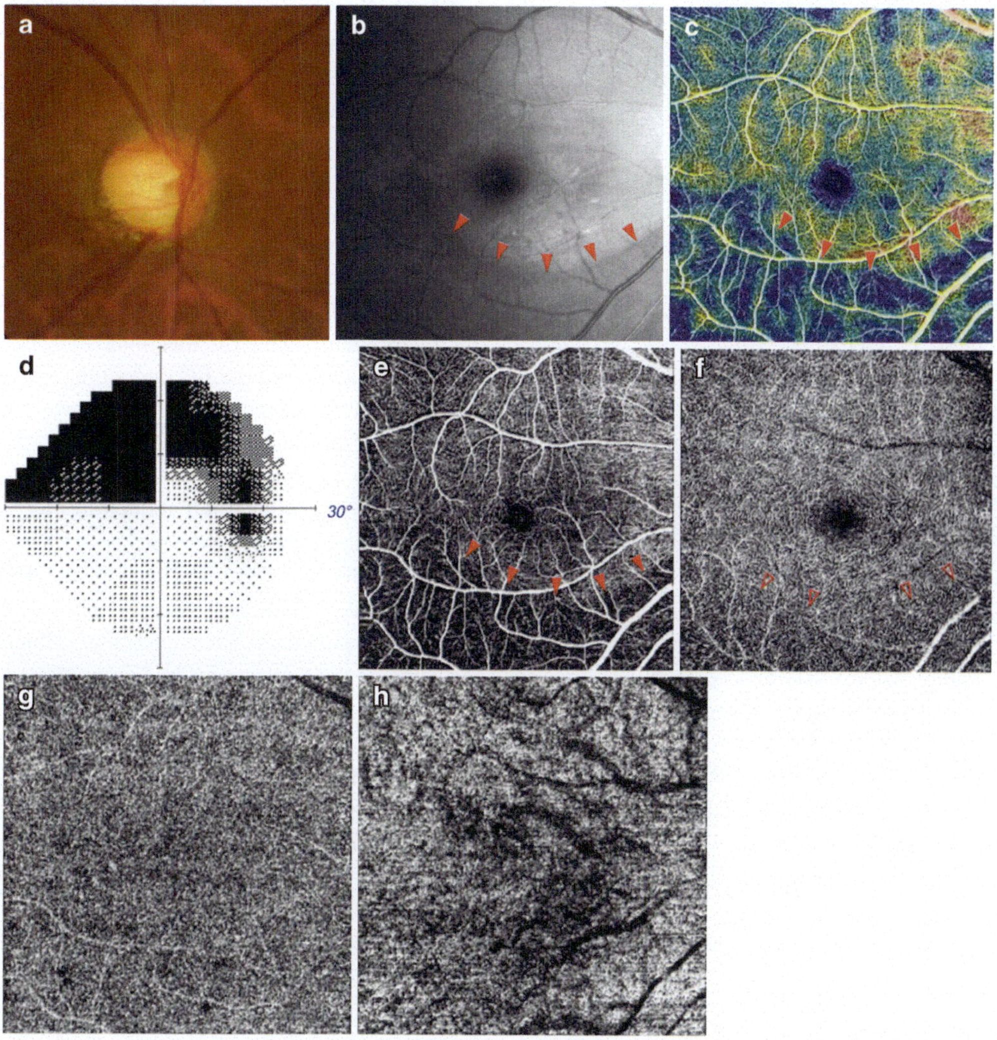

Fig. 5 Findings of macular OCTA (DRI OCT Triton, Topcon) in a glaucomatous eye with inferior ONH damage. The *upper panel* shows a color disc photograph (**a**), a red-free fundus photograph (**b**), an OCTA VD map (**c**), and a gray scale plot of VF examination (**d**). The *blue color* in the VD map (**c**, *arrowheads*) coincides with the localized RNFL defect shown in the red-free photograph (**b**, *arrowheads*). The *lower panel* shows en-face OCTA images of a 6.0 × 6.0 mm^2 area centered on the macula, segmented in the layers of SCP (**e**), DCP (**f**), choriocapillaris (**g**), and choroid (**h**). The localized reduction in macular VD is clearly visualized in the SCP (**e**, *arrowheads*), but less clearly in the DCP (**f**, *arrowheads*), and is not visible in the choriocapillaris (**g**) and choroidal (**h**) layers. Note that choroidal vessels are not clearly visible in the choroidal OCTA image (**h**), because of signal attenuation by the pigmented RPE and choriocapillaris. OCTA, optical coherence tomography angiography; ONH, optic nerve head; VD, vessel density; VF, visual field; RNFL, retinal nerve fiber layer; SCP, superficial capillary plexus; DCP, deep capillary plexus; RPE, retinal pigment epithelium

(Kwon et al. 2017a). FAZs are larger in eyes with pseudoexfoliative glaucoma than with open angle glaucoma (Philip et al. 2019). Moreover, FAZs are larger in women than in men, especially in older women (Gomez-Ulla et al. 2019), indicating that age and gender should be considered when assessing FAZs.

6.1.2 Macular Microvessel Density

Reduced macular VD has been observed in both the SCP and DCP of glaucomatous eyes (Choi et al. 2017; Wu et al. 2019; Kim et al. 2020a; Lommatzsch et al. 2018; Akil et al. 2017). These changes in macular microvessels were found to be well correlated with the degrees of structural (Wu et al. 2019; Kim et al. 2020a; Lommatzsch et al. 2018; Akil et al. 2017; Hou et al. 2019; Chung et al. 2017; Rao et al. 2017a; Lu et al. 2020) and functional (Lommatzsch et al. 2018; Lu et al. 2020) damage (Fig. 5) and were independent of age-related capillary loss (Wu et al. 2019). Choroidal imaging is limited in the macular area because the light is scattered or attenuated by the pigmented RPE and choriocapillaris with dense vascular structure (Fig. 5).

6.2 Peripapillary Imaging

Scanning of the ONH and peripapillary area is the most widely used OCTA imaging in glaucoma evaluation. Evaluation of the peripapillary microvasculature using OCTA helps to diagnose glaucoma (Moghimi et al. 2019; Liu et al. 2015; Enders et al. 2020; Rolle et al. 2019; Akagi et al. 2016; Yarmohammadi et al. 2018) and predict its progression (Jia et al. 2014; Cennamo et al. 2017). Abnormalities in the retinal and/or choroidal microvasculature may indicate reduced ocular perfusion, indicating that OCTA evaluation of the peripapillary microvasculature could shed a light on the vascular theory of glaucoma. However, it remains unclear whether the abnormal microvasculature in glaucomatous eyes is a causal factor in glaucoma pathogenesis or a secondary result of glaucomatous nerve fiber loss.

Peripapillary OCTA images are usually obtained from 3 × 3, 4.5 × 4.5 or 6 × 6 mm^2 areas centered on the ONH. The most common are those from peripapillary 4.5 × 4.5 mm^2 scans (Fig. 1), which have been shown to better detect glaucomatous changes than images from 6.0 × 6.0 mm^2 scans (Chang et al. 2019). However, one study reported that wider scans were superior in investigating capillary loss during early stages of glaucoma (Jia et al. 2017).

6.2.1 Optic Nerve Head

OCTA has been shown to detect abnormalities of ONH perfusion in glaucoma (Chung et al. 2017; Jia et al. 2012b, 2014). Imaging of the deeper ONH tissues (i.e., the lamina cribrosa [LC]) is limited by the shadowing or projection of large retinal vessels. However, there are studies where deep ONH tissues, including the LC and prelaminar tissues, have been imaged successfully (Numa et al. 2018; Kim et al. 2018, 2019b). The microvasculature in the LC was found to be negatively associated with the LC curvature, an indicator of mechanical stress derived from translaminar pressure difference (Fig. 6) (Kim et al. 2019b). In addition, reversal of the LC curvature following surgical IOP reduction was positively associated with the increased microvascular density in the LC (Fig. 6) (Kim et al. 2018). These findings indicate that LC deformation caused by mechanical stress can also influence perfusion of the ONH axons by compressing the laminar capillaries (Burgoyne et al. 2005).

6.2.2 Peripapillary Retina

Peripapillary retinal microvasculature can be assessed in the RCP, SCP, and DCP. In glaucoma, reduced VD is more prominent in the superficial than in the deeper layers (Liu et al. 2019). VD has been shown to correlate with both structural (Chung et al. 2017; Rao et al. 2017a; Enders et al. 2020; Lee et al. 2016a; Ichiyama et al. 2017) and functional (Liu et al. 2015; Akagi et al. 2016; Ichiyama et al. 2017; Shin et al. 2017a) damage, and is an excellent parameter for diagnosing glaucoma (Liu et al. 2015; Rolle et al. 2019; Bekkers et al. 2020). In patients with localized RNFL defects, reduced VD in the superficial retina was observed to coincide with wedge shaped RNFL defects (Fig. 7), suggesting that the

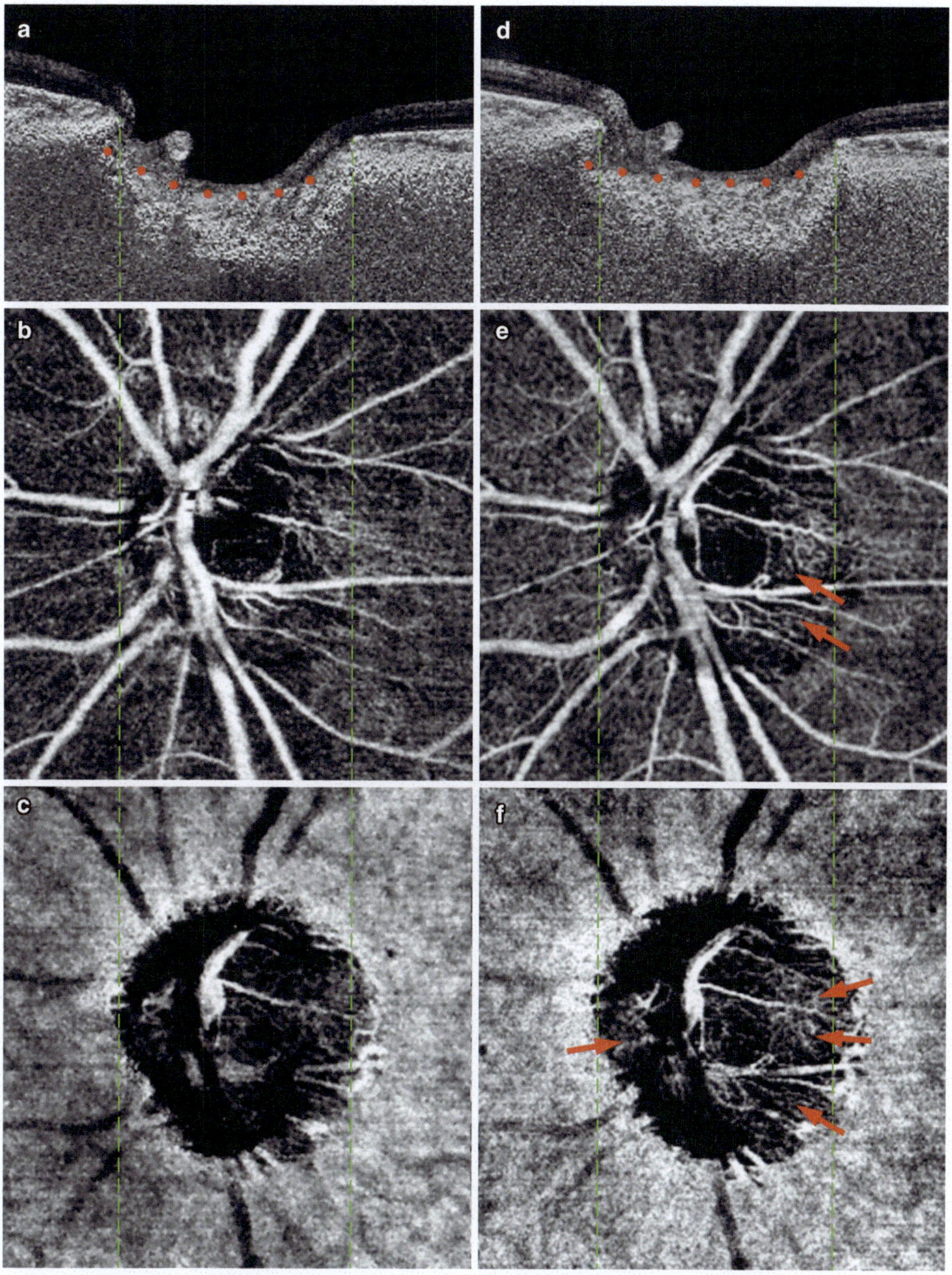

Fig. 6 A glaucomatous eye that underwent trabeculectomy, showing that reduction of the LC curvature (*red glyphs*) was associated with an increased microvascular density in ONH tissues (*arrows*). Images in the left column were obtained 1 day preoperatively (**a–c**), and images in the right column were obtained 3 months postoperatively (**d–f**). The top row (**a**, **d**) shows B-scan images of the central ONH, illustrating that the LC curvature was reduced after surgery (*red glyphs*). Note the increased microvasculature (*arrows*) in the prelaminar tissue (**e**) and in the LC (**f**). Images were obtained using DRI OCT Triton (Topcon). LC, lamina cribrosa; ONH, optic nerve head

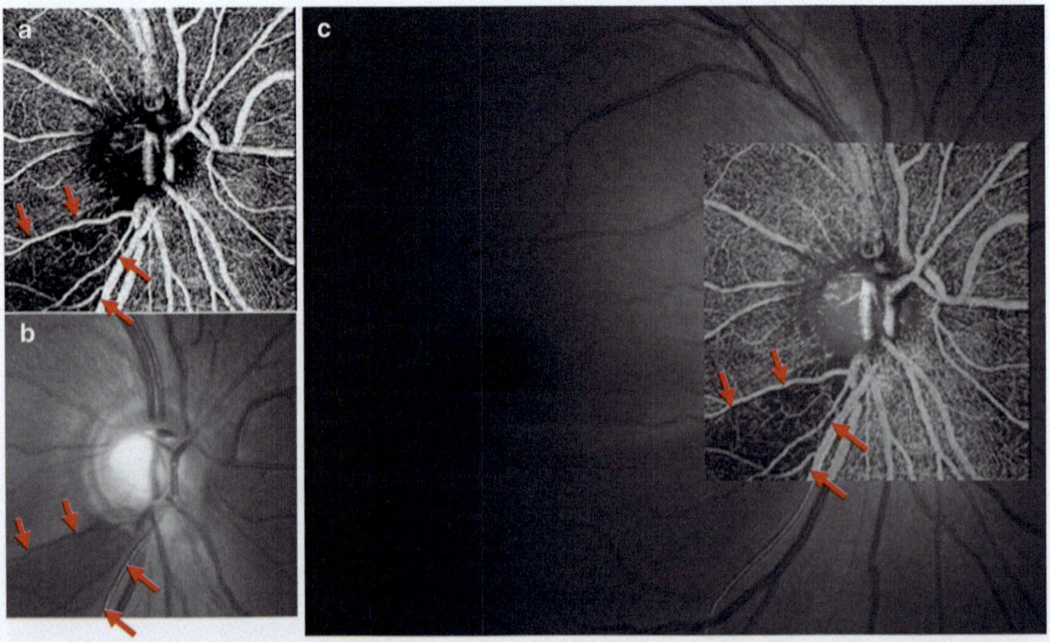

Fig. 7 En-face OCTA image of the superficial retina, including the RCP and SCP (**a**); a red-free fundus photograph (**b**); and the red-free fundus photograph superimposed on the en-face angiogram (**c**). The vascular impairment shown by OCTA appears to be identical to the RNFL defects evident in red-free photographs (*arrows*). OCTA Images were obtained using DRI OCT Triton (Topcon). OCTA, optical coherence tomography angiography; RCP, radial peripapillary capillary plexus; SCP, superficial capillary plexus; RNFL, retinal nerve fiber layer

decrease in retinal microvasculature is likely a secondary loss or closure of capillaries in areas of glaucomatous RNFL atrophy (Lee et al. 2016a).

6.2.3 Peripapillary Choroid

The peripapillary area, which is distinct from the macular area, frequently accompanies an area with atrophic RPE, thus allowing detailed OCTA imaging of the parapapillary choroidal microvasculature. Focal dropout of the juxtapapillary choroidal microvasculature has been observed in glaucomatous eyes (Suh et al. 2016), which had a good topographic correlation with glaucomatous RNFL (Lee et al. 2017a) and VF (Akagi et al. 2016; Suh et al. 2018) defects. Microvasculature dropout (MvD) in the peripapillary choroid has been shown to coincide with perfusion defects detected by indocyanine green angiography (ICGA, Fig. 8) (Lee et al. 2017b), indicating that MvD is likely indicative of a true perfusion defect in the choroid. Glaucoma progression was found to be faster in eyes with than without juxtapapillary choroidal MvD (Lee et al. 2019, 2020c).

6.3 Anterior Segment Imaging

Anterior segment OCTA has been utilized to image the vasculature in the conjunctiva and intrasclera. Hyperemia of the anterior segment, which has been associated with elevated IOP, as well as post-trabeculectomy avascular bleb could be imaged using the anterior segment OCTA (Akagi et al. 2019a, b). The clinical usefulness of anterior segment OCTA imaging in glaucoma remains to be determined. Experimental studies have attempted to image the aqueous humor outflow tract (Zhang et al. 2020; Gottschalk et al. 2019).

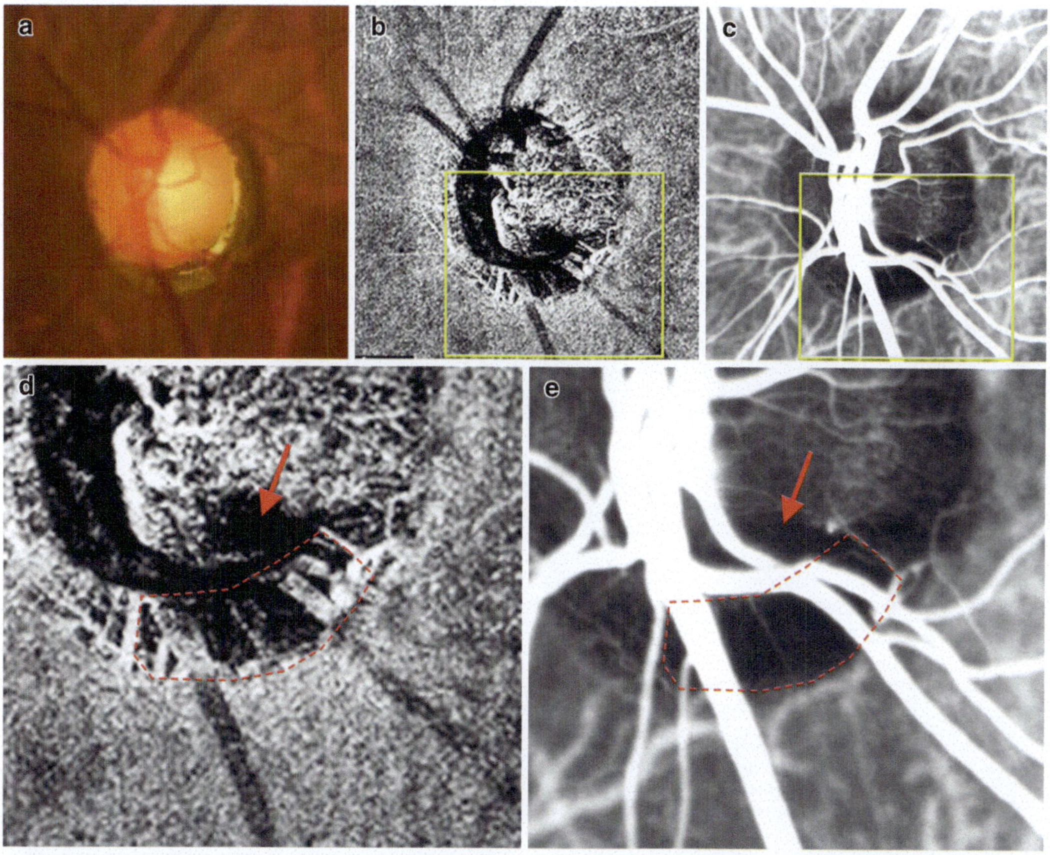

Fig. 8 Color disc photograph (**a**), en-face OCTA image of the choroid (**b**), and ICGA image at the peak phase (36 s, **c**) in a glaucomatous eye with an MvD. Images (**d**) and (**e**) are magnified images of (**b**) and (**c**), respectively. The parapapillary capillary dropout shown in the OCTA image exactly coincides with the perfusion defect shown in the ICGA image (areas demarcated by *dashed lines*). Focal dropout of intrapapillary microvessels is also observed in both the OCTA and ICGA images (*arrows*). OCTA and ICGA images were obtained using DRI OCT Triton (Topcon) and Spectralis HRA + OCT (Heidelberg Engineering), respectively. MvD, microvasculature dropout; OCTA, optical coherence tomography angiography; ICGA, indocyanine green angiography

7 Clinical Use of OCTA in Glaucoma Patients and OCTA in Glaucoma Research

7.1 Diagnosis of Glaucoma

Variable OCTA parameters can be useful in diagnosing glaucoma, with their diagnostic power being comparable to those of OCT (Yarmohammadi et al. 2018; Cennamo et al. 2017; Kumar et al. 2016) or VF examination (Kumar et al. 2016; Yarmohammadi et al. 2016). Sectors of the SCP and DCP with reduced microvessel density (Akagi et al. 2016; Lee et al. 2016a; Shin et al. 2017a) and the locations of MvD (Akagi et al. 2016; Lee et al. 2017a) and abnormal FAZ (Kwon et al. 2017a) were all well correlated with the locations of glaucomatous RNFL and VF loss. The magnitude of VD reduction (Cennamo et al. 2017; Shin et al. 2017a; Yarmohammadi et al. 2016) and MvD size (Lee et al. 2017a; Shin et al. 2018) and FAZ (Kwon et al. 2017a, b) also showed good correlations with the severity of glaucomatous damage.

The advantage of using OCTA in glaucoma assessment is that it is unaffected by the low reflectance of the RNFL or structural deformations of the optic nerve, such as optic disc tilt or PPA. Therefore, OCTA can be useful for evaluating glaucomatous damage in highly myopic eyes (Fig. 9) (Na et al. 2020).

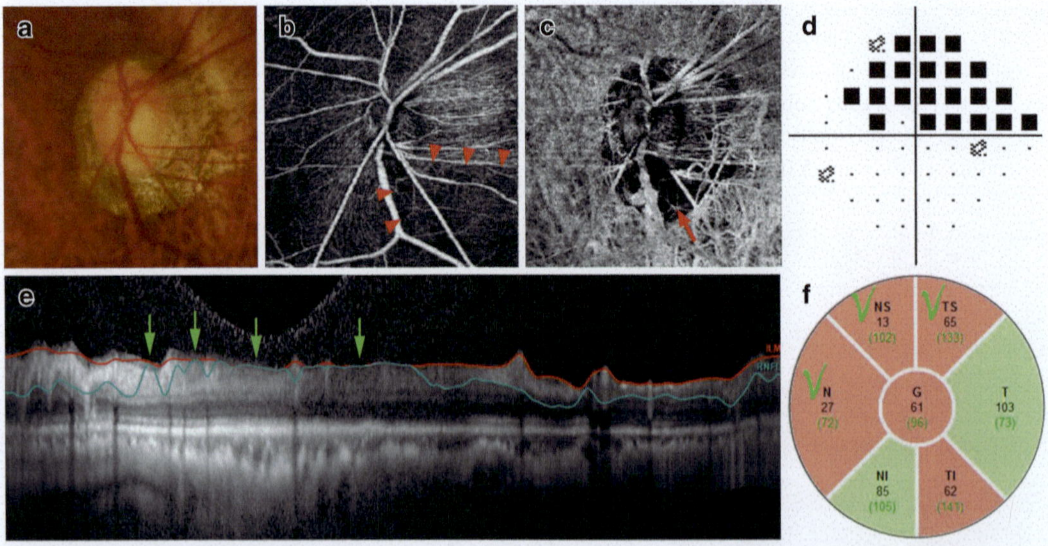

Fig. 9 A highly myopic glaucomatous eye with inferior ONH damage. Color disc photograph (**a**) shows inferior neuroretinal rim loss. En-face OCTA images (**b**, **c**) clearly show reduced retinal vessel density (*arrowheads*) and a choroidal MvD (*red arrow*) in the inferior hemisphere. The location of capillary loss corresponded well with the location of hemifield VF defect (**d**). In contrast, an OCT peripapillary scan (**e**) failed to demonstrate RNFL loss accurately, a failure that was due to segmentation error. The *light-green arrows* indicate the locations of segmentation errors resulting in false positive color codes in the N, NS, and TS sectors (**f**). OCTA images were obtained using DRI OCT Triton (Topcon). G, global; TS, temporal superior; T, temporal; TI, temporal inferior; NI, nasal inferior; N, nasal; NS, nasal superior; OCTA, optical coherence tomography angiography; MvD, microvasculature dropout; VF, visual field; OCT, optical coherence tomography; RNFL, retinal nerve fiber layer

In addition, OCTA measurements of microvessel density are less affected by the thickness of large vessels and are therefore unaffected by a floor effect. These advantages make OCTA particularly useful in evaluating glaucomatous damage in eyes with advanced damage (Kim et al. 2019a; Moghimi et al. 2019). OCTA can also be useful for monitoring disease progression in eyes with advanced glaucoma, with the rate of macular VD loss being more rapid than the rate of structural thinning (Hou et al. 2020).

The clinical usefulness of OCTA in patient diagnosis requires a technique to enhance image quality, a reliable algorithm to accurately quantify microvessel damage, and normative data based on a diverse population.

7.2 Study of Vascular Theory

The increased clinical availability of OCTA has led to an increase in the number of studies assessing the link between the OCTA vasculature and decreased ocular perfusion in the pathogenesis of glaucoma. Reductions in retinal microvasculature have been shown to precede VF damage in early preperimetric glaucoma (Lu et al. 2020; Kumar et al. 2016), with reduced retinal VD being more pronounced in glaucomatous eyes with lower than higher IOP (Xu et al. 2018). Lower baseline VD in the retina has been associated with a faster rate of RNFL thinning, suggesting that reduced ocular perfusion may have led to faster glaucomatous damage (Moghimi et al. 2018). Decreased VD on OCTA may represent dysfunctional retinal ganglion cells with lower metabolic demands. However, the findings of various studies have been inconsistent (Hou et al. 2019; Hirasawa et al. 2021; Kim et al. 2017; Mursch-Edlmayr et al. 2020; Bojikian et al. 2016), with results to date unable to determine whether reductions in retinal microvasculature are indicative of reduced ocular perfusion causing ischemic axonal damage. Based on our study, showing an exact overlap between localized RNFL defects and reduced retinal microvasculature (Lee et al. 2016a), this is more likely to be a secondary phenomenon resulting from glaucomatous atrophy of the RNFL and GCL (Fig. 7).

The retinal microvasculature consists of capillaries supplied by the central retinal artery system. However, the ONH is supplied with blood by the short posterior ciliary artery (SPCA). Layer segmentation in OCTA allows individual examination of the microvasculature supplied by the SPCA. The peripapillary choroidal microvasculature is of particular interest in understanding vascular theory, because this microvasculature is supplied by the SPCA, which also perfuses deep ONH tissues. OCTA has identified localized MvD in the peripapillary choroid of patients with glaucoma (Akagi et al. 2016). This localized MvD has been associated with both the location (Ichiyama et al. 2017; Lee et al. 2017a) and severity (Ichiyama et al. 2017; Suh et al. 2016) of glaucomatous damage. Areas of MvD were found to correspond to areas of perfusion defects on ICGA, indicating that MvD represents a true vascular compromise (Fig. 8) (Lee et al. 2017b). The presence of MvD was found to be associated with lower systemic blood pressure and lower ocular perfusion pressure (Suh et al. 2016; Lee et al. 2017b, 2018). In addition, MvD was a strong predictor of early parafoveal scotoma (Lee et al. 2018; Kwon et al. 2018), which is thought to represent systemic vascular risk factors (Park et al. 2011; Yoo et al. 2017). Taken together, these findings suggest that MvD may be a key to understanding vascular pathogenesis. MvD has been shown to be a strong predictor of glaucoma progression (Lee et al. 2019, 2020c; Kwon et al. 2019). A prospective study found that the occurrence of MvD was the second strongest predictor of glaucoma progression, with larger LC curvature, an indicator of mechanical stress, being the strongest predictor (Fig. 10) (Lee et al. 2019). Therefore, areas of MvD may represent the location of ischemia affecting the viability of axons and retinal ganglion cells, causing ischemic insult in addition to mechanical stress. Interestingly, areas of MvD could be identified in nonglaucomatous healthy eyes of patients with low systemic blood pressure profiles (Kim et al. 2020b). Further

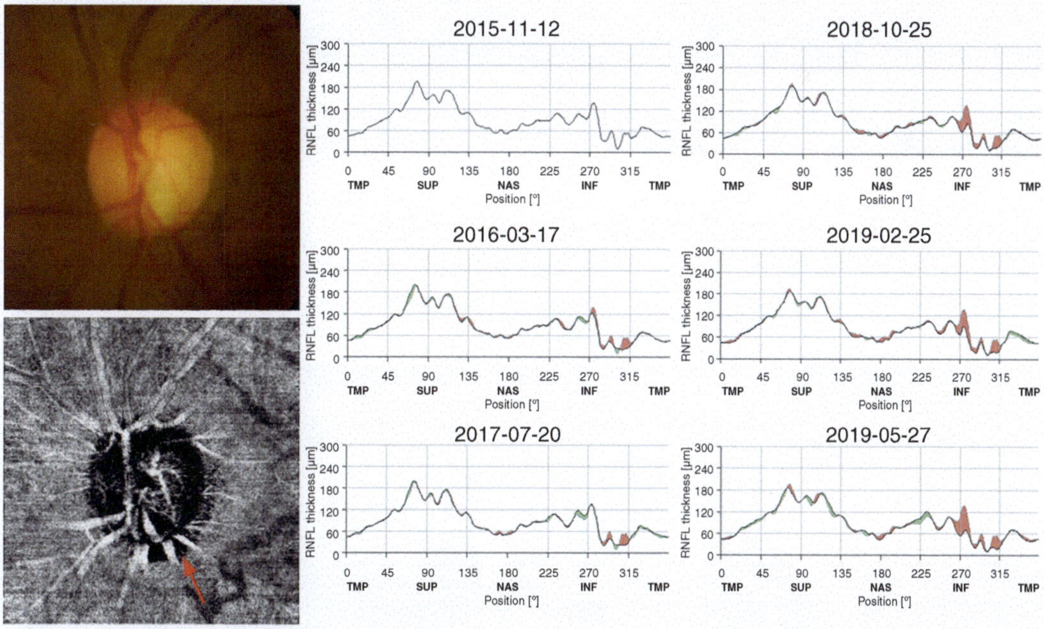

Fig. 10 Rapidly progressing glaucoma in an eye with an MvD in the inferior sector (*arrow*). The *right panel* shows progressive changes in RNFL thickness and rapid progressive thinning of the RNFL in the inferior sector (*red-colored area*). The diurnal IOP ranged from 15 to 17 mmHg before treatment and was maintained within a range of 10–12 mmHg during the entire treatment period. The OCTA image was obtained using DRI OCT Triton (Topcon). TMP, temporal; SUP, superior; NAS, nasal; INF, inferior; MvD, microvasculature dropout; RNFL, retinal nerve fiber layer; IOP, intraocular pressure

studies are warranted to determine whether such eyes would eventually undergo structural damage.

MvD has been frequently found in glaucomatous eyes with PPA β- and γ-zones associated with myopia. However, the β- and γ-zones have different pathomechanisms (Dai et al. 2013; Kim et al. 2013), and MvDs observed in these zones differ in their underlying microstructures, suggesting differences in the pathogenesis of parapapillary MvD in the β- and γ-zones (Fig. 11) (Lee et al. 2017c, d).

MvD-like structures have also been identified in nonglaucomatous eyes, including in highly myopic eyes without glaucoma (Fig. 12) (Kim et al. 2020c) and in eyes with compressive optic neuropathy (Fig. 13) (Lee et al. 2020d). However,

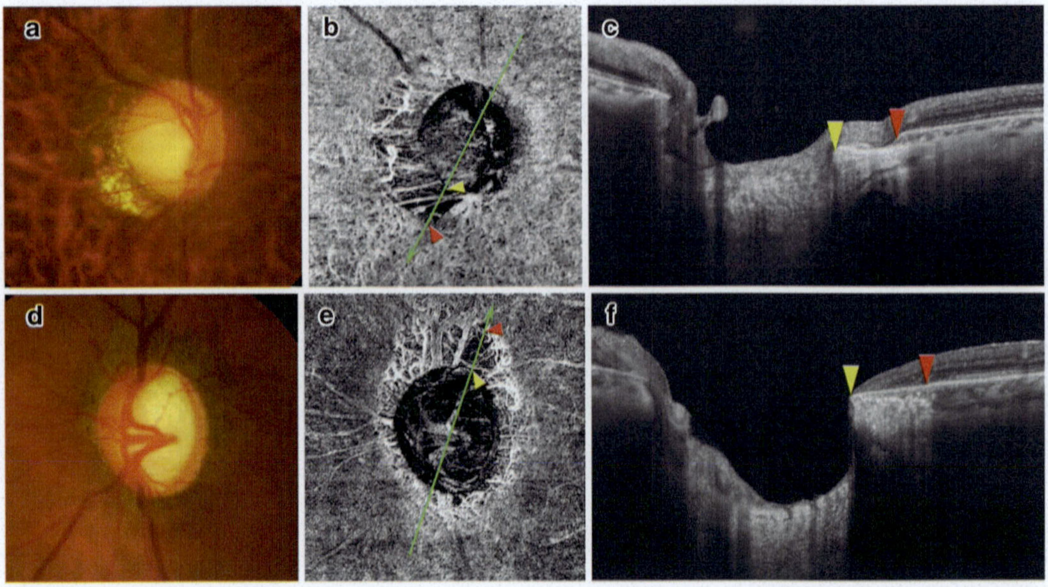

Fig. 11 Glaucomatous eyes having MvD in the γ-zone (*upper*) and β-zone (*lower*). Color disc photographs show PPA consisted of γ-zone (**a**) and β-zone (**d**) in each eye. *Light-green arrows* (**b**, **e**) indicate the locations of the B-scans in (**c**) and (**f**), respectively. *Yellow* and *red arrowheads* (**b**, **c**, **e**, **f**) indicate the points of the clinical disc margins (proximal MvD margins) and the distal margins of the MvD, respectively. Although choroidal tissue of noticeable thickness is present under the MvD in the β-zone (**f**), only the border tissue of Elschnig, which does not contain choroidal tissue, is present under the MvD in the γ-zone (**c**), suggesting differences in the pathogenesis of parapapillary MvD in the β- and γ-zones. OCTA images were obtained using DRI OCT Triton (Topcon). MvD, microvasculature dropout; PPA, parapapillary atrophy; OCTA, optical coherence tomography angiography

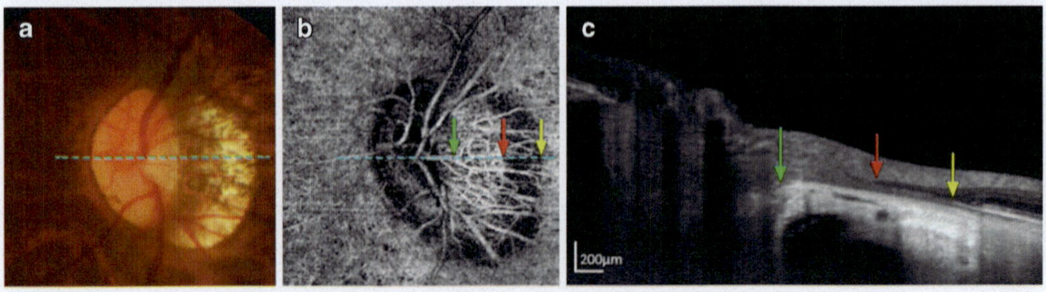

Fig. 12 A nonglaucomatous eye with high myopia. En-face choroidal OCTA image (**b**), showing an MvD-like structure in the non-juxtapapillary area (between the *red* and *yellow arrows*). The *light-green arrow* indicates the clinical optic disc margin. B-scan image (**c**), showing that the MvD-like structure did not consist of choroid, but mainly of border tissue and scleral flange. *Dashed lines* (**a**, **b**) indicate the location from which the B-scan image in (**c**) was obtained. OCTA image was obtained using DRI OCT Triton (Topcon). OCTA, optical coherence tomography angiography; MvD, microvasculature dropout

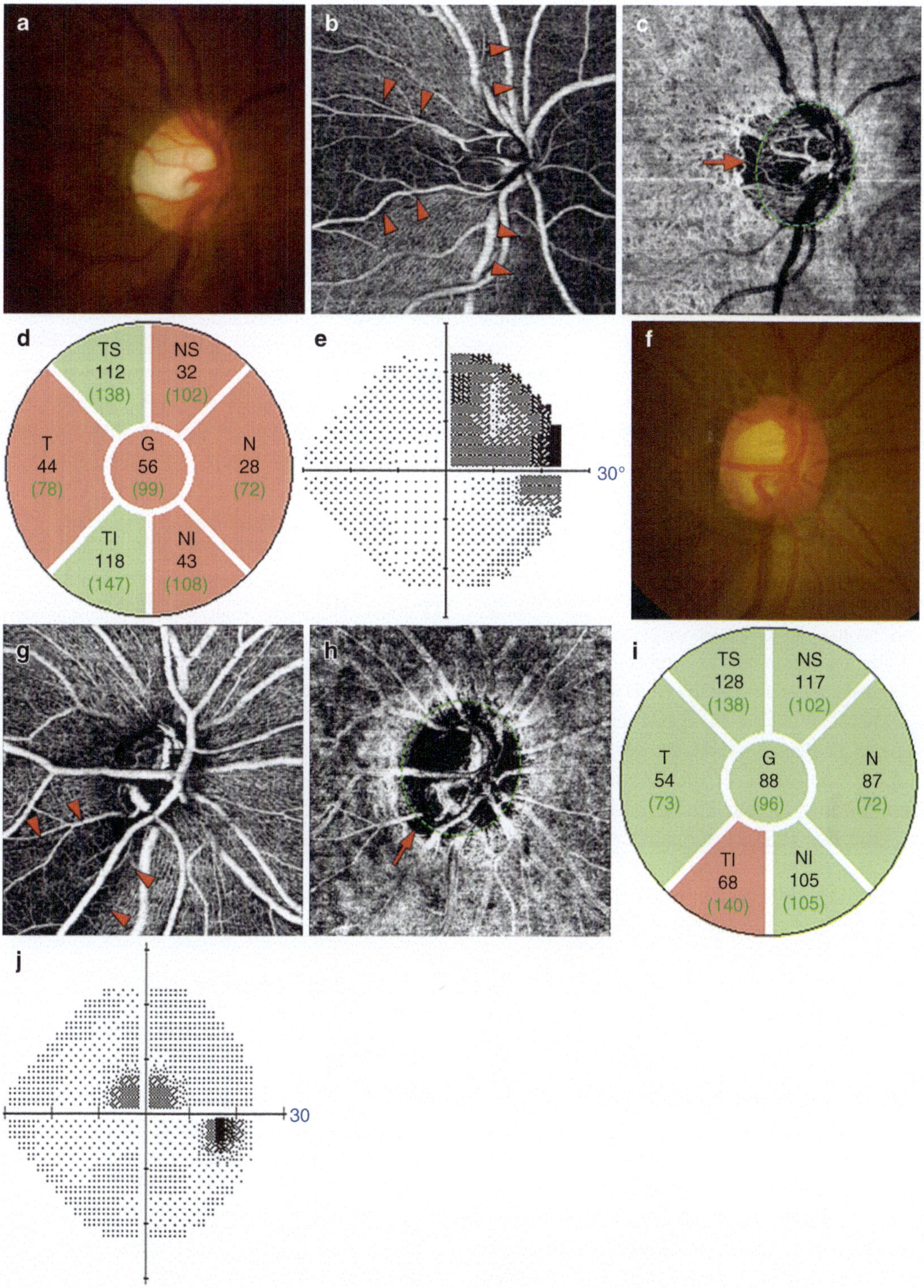

Fig. 13 Findings in a patient with compressive optic neuropathy associated with a pituitary adenoma (*upper panel*) and a patient with glaucomatous optic neuropathy (*lower panel*). The patterns and locations of reduced retinal VD (*arrowheads*) and choroidal capillary dropouts (*arrows*) in the en-face OCTA images clearly differed in these two eyes. OCTA images were obtained using DRI OCT Triton (Topcon). VD, vessel density; OCTA, optical coherence tomography angiography

the locations, structures, and accompanying clinical characteristics of these MvDs differed from the MvDs identified in glaucoma, suggesting that their pathogeneses and pathogenic meanings may differ from those of MvDs observed in glaucomatous eyes. These differences, however, remain to be determined.

7.3 Evaluation of Perfusion Recovery After Treatment

Reduced mechanical stress is thought to increase microvasculature in the peripapillary retina and in ONH tissues. IOP reduction following filtering surgery has been found to induce reversal of the deformed LC (Lee et al. 2012, 2016b). Studies using OCTA have shown that the increase in microvasculature was associated with the magnitude of LC reversal after IOP lowering surgery (Fig. 6) (Kim et al. 2018; Shin et al. 2017b), suggesting that this reversal of LC relieves compression on the capillaries within the LC trabeculae, potentially increasing blood flow to the ONH axons.

Microvasculature changes after application of topical medications have not yet been clarified. Topical application of the Rho-assisted coiled-coil forming protein kinase inhibitor ripasudil was found to enhance peripapillary VD, whereas topical application of the alpha-2 agonist brimonidine did not (Chihara et al. 2018). Because both medications reduce IOP to a similar extent, the increase in VD induced by ripasudil may not be caused by its reduction of mechanical stress but by its vasodilatory effect.

7.4 Differences Among Types of Glaucoma

OCTA does not seem to differentiate among different types of glaucoma. Studies have compared OCTA findings in eyes with normal-tension and high-tension glaucoma (Xu et al. 2018; Mursch-Edlmayr et al. 2020; Bojikian et al. 2016) and in eyes with primary angle-closure, primary open angle, and pseudoexfoliative glaucoma (Rao et al. 2017b; Jo et al. 2020; Simsek et al. 2020), but most of these studies failed to detect significant differences.

8 Conclusions

OCTA can provide reproducible information about the microvasculature in the ONH and retina, with an ability to diagnose glaucoma comparable to that of OCT and VF examinations. OCTA may therefore be a useful addition to these latter methods in diagnosing glaucoma, particularly when the findings from these conventional methods are inconclusive. The rapid, noninvasive, and reproducible nature of OCTA examinations may facilitate the evaluation of glaucoma patients in busy clinics.

En-face OCTA images show the microvascular structure in individual retinal layers and ONH tissues. These findings correspond to those of conventional angiography, and can even visualize vascular layers not evaluable by conventional methods. This capacity enables OCTA to assess individual microvasculature systems supplying the ONH and peripapillary area, resulting in increased understanding of vascular pathogenesis in glaucoma.

Current OCTA systems are limited by artifacts that affect image quality, by an inability to quantify blood flow, and by the lack of a reliable normative database. However, technologies are rapidly evolving, and it will not be long before these limitations are overcome.

References

Akagi T, Iida Y, Nakanishi H, et al. Microvascular density in glaucomatous eyes with hemifield visual field defects: an optical coherence tomography angiography study. Am J Ophthalmol. 2016;168:237–49.

Akagi T, Uji A, Okamoto Y, et al. Anterior segment optical coherence tomography angiography imaging of conjunctiva and intrasclera in treated primary open-angle glaucoma. Am J Ophthalmol. 2019a;208:313–22.

Akagi T, Okamoto Y, Tsujikawa A. Anterior segment OCT angiography images of avascular bleb after trabeculectomy. Ophthalmol Glaucoma. 2019b;2(2):102.

Akil H, Chopra V, Al-Sheikh M, et al. Swept-source OCT angiography imaging of the macular capillary network in glaucoma. Br J Ophthalmol. 2017. https://doi.org/10.1136/bjophthalmol-2016-309816.

Bekkers A, Borren N, Ederveen V, et al. Microvascular damage assessed by optical coherence tomography angiography for glaucoma diagnosis: a systematic review of the most discriminative regions. Acta Ophthalmol. 2020;98(6):537–58.

Bojikian KD, Chen CL, Wen JC, et al. Optic disc perfusion in primary open angle and normal tension glaucoma eyes using optical coherence tomography-based microangiography. PLoS One. 2016;11(5):e0154691.

Bonomi L, Marchini G, Marraffa M, Bernardi P, Morbio R, Varotto A. Vascular risk factors for primary open angle glaucoma: the Egna-Neumarkt Study. Ophthalmology. 2000;107(7):1287–93.

Burgoyne CF, Downs JC, Bellezza AJ, Suh JK, Hart RT. The optic nerve head as a biomechanical structure: a new paradigm for understanding the role of IOP-related stress and strain in the pathophysiology of glaucomatous optic nerve head damage. Prog Retin Eye Res. 2005;24(1):39–73.

Cennamo G, Montorio D, Velotti N, Sparnelli F, Reibaldi M, Cennamo G. Optical coherence tomography angiography in pre-perimetric open-angle glaucoma. Graefes Arch Clin Exp Ophthalmol. 2017;255(9):1787–93.

Chang R, Chu Z, Burkemper B, et al. Effect of scan size on glaucoma diagnostic performance using OCT angiography en face images of the radial peripapillary capillaries. J Glaucoma. 2019;28(5):465–72.

Charlson ME, de Moraes CG, Link A, et al. Nocturnal systemic hypotension increases the risk of glaucoma progression. Ophthalmology. 2014;121(10):2004–12.

Chihara E, Dimitrova G, Chihara T. Increase in the OCT angiographic peripapillary vessel density by ROCK inhibitor ripasudil instillation: a comparison with brimonidine. Graefes Arch Clin Exp Ophthalmol. 2018;256(7):1257–64.

Choi J, Kwon J, Shin JW, Lee J, Lee S, Kook MS. Quantitative optical coherence tomography angiography of macular vascular structure and foveal avascular zone in glaucoma. PLoS One. 2017;12(9):e0184948.

Chung JK, Hwang YH, Wi JM, Kim M, Jung JJ. Glaucoma diagnostic ability of the optical coherence tomography angiography vessel density parameters. Curr Eye Res. 2017;42(11):1458–67.

Corvi F, Pellegrini M, Erba S, Cozzi M, Staurenghi G, Giani A. Reproducibility of vessel density, fractal dimension, and foveal avascular zone using 7 different optical coherence tomography angiography devices. Am J Ophthalmol. 2018;186:25–31.

Dai Y, Jonas JB, Huang H, Wang M, Sun X. Microstructure of parapapillary atrophy: beta zone and gamma zone. Invest Ophthalmol Vis Sci. 2013;54(3):2013–8.

Enders P, Longo V, Adler W, et al. Analysis of peripapillary vessel density and Bruch's membrane opening-based neuroretinal rim parameters in glaucoma using OCT and OCT-angiography. Eye (Lond). 2020;34(6):1086–93.

Findl O, Rainer G, Dallinger S, et al. Assessment of optic disk blood flow in patients with open-angle glaucoma. Am J Ophthalmol. 2000;130(5):589–96.

Funaki S, Shirakashi M, Abe H. Parapapillary chorioretinal atrophy and parapapillary avascular area in glaucoma. Nippon Ganka Gakkai Zasshi. 1997;101(7):598–604.

Ghasemi Falavarjani K, Al-Sheikh M, Akil H, Sadda SR. Image artefacts in swept-source optical coherence tomography angiography. Br J Ophthalmol. 2017;101(5):564–8.

Gomez-Ulla F, Cutrin P, Santos P, et al. Age and gender influence on foveal avascular zone in healthy eyes. Exp Eye Res. 2019;189:107856.

Gottschalk HM, Wecker T, Khattab MH, et al. Lipid emulsion-based OCT angiography for ex vivo imaging of the aqueous outflow tract. Invest Ophthalmol Vis Sci. 2019;60(1):397–406.

Graham SL, Drance SM. Nocturnal hypotension: role in glaucoma progression. Surv Ophthalmol. 1999;43(Suppl 1):S10–6.

Hirasawa K, Smith CA, West ME, et al. Discrepancy in loss of macular perfusion density and ganglion cell layer thickness in early glaucoma. Am J Ophthalmol. 2021;221:39–47.

Hitchings RA, Spaeth GL. Fluorescein angiography in chronic simple and low-tension glaucoma. Br J Ophthalmol. 1977;61(2):126–32.

Hou H, Moghimi S, Zangwill LM, et al. Macula vessel density and thickness in early primary open-angle glaucoma. Am J Ophthalmol. 2019;199:120–32.

Hou H, Moghimi S, Proudfoot JA, et al. Ganglion cell complex thickness and macular vessel density loss in primary open-angle glaucoma. Ophthalmology. 2020;127(8):1043–52.

Huber K, Plange N, Remky A, Arend O. Comparison of colour Doppler imaging and retinal scanning laser fluorescein angiography in healthy volunteers and normal pressure glaucoma patients. Acta Ophthalmol Scand. 2004;82(4):426–31.

Ichiyama Y, Minamikawa T, Niwa Y, Ohji M. Capillary dropout at the retinal nerve fiber layer defect in glaucoma: an optical coherence tomography angiography study. J Glaucoma. 2017;26(4):e142–e5.

Jia Y, Tan O, Tokayer J, et al. Split-spectrum amplitude-decorrelation angiography with optical coherence tomography. Opt Express. 2012a;20(4):4710–25.

Jia Y, Morrison JC, Tokayer J, et al. Quantitative OCT angiography of optic nerve head blood flow. Biomed Opt Express. 2012b;3(12):3127–37.

Jia Y, Wei E, Wang X, et al. Optical coherence tomography angiography of optic disc perfusion in glaucoma. Ophthalmology. 2014;121(7):1322–32.

Jia Y, Simonett JM, Wang J, et al. Wide-field OCT angiography investigation of the relationship between radial peripapillary capillary plexus density and nerve fiber layer thickness. Invest Ophthalmol Vis Sci. 2017;58(12):5188–94.

Jo YH, Sung KR, Shin JW. Peripapillary and macular vessel density measurement by optical coherence tomography angiography in pseudoexfoliation and primary open-angle glaucoma. J Glaucoma. 2020;29(5):381–5.

Kashani AH, Chen CL, Gahm JK, et al. Optical coherence tomography angiography: A comprehensive review of current methods and clinical applications. Prog Retin Eye Res. 2017;60:66–100.

Kim M, Kim TW, Weinreb RN, Lee EJ. Differentiation of parapapillary atrophy using spectral-domain optical coherence tomography. Ophthalmology. 2013;120(9):1790–7.

Kim SB, Lee EJ, Han JC, Kee C. Comparison of peripapillary vessel density between preperimetric and perimetric glaucoma evaluated by OCT-angiography. PLoS One. 2017;12(8):e0184297.

Kim JA, Kim TW, Lee EJ, Girard MJA, Mari JM. Microvascular changes in peripapillary and optic nerve head tissues after trabeculectomy in primary open-angle glaucoma. Invest Ophthalmol Vis Sci. 2018;59(11):4614–21.

Kim GN, Lee EJ, Kim H, Kim TW. Dynamic range of the peripapillary retinal vessel density for detecting glaucomatous visual field damage. Ophthalmol Glaucoma. 2019a;2:103–10.

Kim JA, Kim TW, Lee EJ, Girard MJA, Mari JM. Relationship between lamina cribrosa curvature and the microvasculature in treatment-naive eyes. Br J Ophthalmol. 2019b. https://doi.org/10.1136/bjophthalmol-2019-313996.

Kim JS, Kim YK, Baek SU, et al. Topographic correlation between macular superficial microvessel density and ganglion cell-inner plexiform layer thickness in glaucoma-suspect and early normal-tension glaucoma. Br J Ophthalmol. 2020a;104(1):104–9.

Kim GN, Lee EJ, Kim TW. Parapapillary choroidal microvasculature dropout in nonglaucomatous healthy eyes. Acta Ophthalmol. 2020b;98(6):e754–e60.

Kim GN, Lee EJ, Kim TW. Microstructure of nonjuxtapapillary microvasculature dropout in healthy myopic eyes. Invest Ophthalmol Vis Sci. 2020c;61(2):36.

Kumar RS, Anegondi N, Chandapura RS, et al. Discriminant function of optical coherence tomography angiography to determine disease severity in glaucoma. Invest Ophthalmol Vis Sci. 2016;57(14):6079–88.

Kwon J, Choi J, Shin JW, Lee J, Kook MS. Glaucoma diagnostic capabilities of foveal avascular zone parameters using optical coherence tomography angiography according to visual field defect location. J Glaucoma. 2017a;26(12):1120–9.

Kwon J, Choi J, Shin JW, Lee J, Kook MS. Alterations of the foveal avascular zone measured by optical coherence tomography angiography in glaucoma patients with central visual field defects. Invest Ophthalmol Vis Sci. 2017b;58(3):1637–45.

Kwon J, Shin JW, Lee J, Kook MS. Choroidal microvasculature dropout Ii associated with parafoveal visual field defects in glaucoma. Am J Ophthalmol. 2018;188:141–54.

Kwon JM, Weinreb RN, Zangwill LM, Suh MH. Parapapillary deep-layer microvasculature dropout and visual field progression in glaucoma. Am J Ophthalmol. 2019;200:65–75.

Laatikainen L. Fluorescein angiographic studies of the peripapillary and perilimbal regions in simple, capsular and low-tension glaucoma. Acta Ophthalmol Suppl. 1971;111:3–83.

Lee EJ, Kim TW, Weinreb RN. Reversal of lamina cribrosa displacement and thickness after trabeculectomy in glaucoma. Ophthalmology. 2012;119(7):1359–66.

Lee EJ, Lee KM, Lee SH, Kim TW. OCT angiography of the peripapillary retina in primary open-angle glaucoma. Invest Ophthalmol Vis Sci. 2016a;57(14):6265–70.

Lee SH, Yu DA, Kim TW, Lee EJ, Girard MJ, Mari JM. Reduction of the lamina cribrosa curvature after trabeculectomy in glaucoma. Invest Ophthalmol Vis Sci. 2016b;57(11):5006–14.

Lee EJ, Lee SH, Kim JA, Kim TW. Parapapillary deep-layer microvasculature dropout in glaucoma: topographic association with glaucomatous damage. Invest Ophthalmol Vis Sci. 2017a;58(7):3004–10.

Lee EJ, Lee KM, Lee SH, Kim TW. Parapapillary choroidal microvasculature dropout in glaucoma: a comparison between optical coherence tomography angiography and indocyanine green angiography. Ophthalmology. 2017b;124(8):1209–17.

Lee EJ, Kim TW, Lee SH, Kim JA. Underlying microstructure of parapapillary deep-layer capillary dropout identified by optical coherence tomography angiography. Invest Ophthalmol Vis Sci. 2017c;58(3):1621–7.

Lee EJ, Kim TW, Kim JA, Kim JA. Parapapillary deep-layer microvasculature dropout in primary open-angle glaucoma eyes with a parapapillary gamma-zone. Invest Ophthalmol Vis Sci. 2017d;58(13):5673–80.

Lee EJ, Kim TW, Kim JA, Kim JA. Central visual field damage and parapapillary choroidal microvasculature dropout in primary open-angle glaucoma. Ophthalmology. 2018;125(4):588–96.

Lee EJ, Kim TW, Kim JA, et al. Elucidation of the strongest factors influencing rapid retinal nerve fiber layer thinning in glaucoma. Invest Ophthalmol Vis Sci. 2019;60(10):3343–51.

Lee SH, Lee EJ, Kim TW. Comparison of vascular-function and structure-function correlations in glaucomatous eyes with high myopia. Br J Ophthalmol. 2020a;104(6):807–12.

Lee K, Maeng KJ, Kim JY, et al. Diagnostic ability of vessel density measured by spectral-domain optical coherence tomography angiography for glaucoma in patients with high myopia. Sci Rep. 2020b;10(1):3027.

Lee EJ, Kim JA, Kim TW. Influence of choroidal microvasculature dropout on the rate of glaucomatous progression, a prospective study. Ophthalmol Glaucoma. 2020c;3(1):25–31.

Lee EJ, Kim JA, Kim TW, Kim H, Yang HK, Hwang JM. Glaucoma-like parapapillary choroidal microvasculature dropout in patients with compressive optic neuropathy. Ophthalmology. 2020d;127(12):1652–62.

Leske MC, Connell AM, Wu SY, Hyman LG, Schachat AP. Risk factors for open-angle glaucoma. The Barbados Eye Study. Arch Ophthalmol. 1995;113(7):918–24.

Li XX, Wu W, Zhou H, et al. A quantitative comparison of five optical coherence tomography angiography systems in clinical performance. Int J Ophthalmol. 2018;11(11):1784–95.

Liu L, Jia Y, Takusagawa HL, et al. Optical coherence tomography angiography of the peripapillary retina in glaucoma. JAMA Ophthalmol. 2015;133(9):1045–52.

Liu L, Edmunds B, Takusagawa HL, et al. Projection-resolved optical coherence tomography angiography of the peripapillary retina in glaucoma. Am J Ophthalmol. 2019;207:99–109.

Lommatzsch C, Rothaus K, Koch JM, Heinz C, Grisanti S. OCTA vessel density changes in the macular zone in glaucomatous eyes. Graefes Arch Clin Exp Ophthalmol. 2018;256(8):1499–508.

Lu P, Xiao H, Chen H, Ye D, Huang J. Asymmetry of macular vessel density in bilateral early open-angle glaucoma with unilateral central 10-2 visual field loss. J Glaucoma. 2020;29(10):926–31.

Moghimi S, Zangwill LM, Penteado RC, et al. Macular and optic nerve head vessel density and progressive retinal nerve fiber layer loss in glaucoma. Ophthalmology. 2018;125(11):1720–8.

Moghimi S, Bowd C, Zangwill LM, et al. Measurement floors and dynamic ranges of OCT and OCT angiography in glaucoma. Ophthalmology. 2019;126(7):980–8.

Mursch-Edlmayr AS, Waser K, Podkowinski D, Bolz M. Differences in swept-source OCT angiography of the macular capillary network in high tension and normal tension glaucoma. Curr Eye Res. 2020;45(9):1168–72.

Na HM, Lee EJ, Lee SH, Kim TW. Evaluation of peripapillary choroidal microvasculature to detect glaucomatous damage in eyes with high myopia. J Glaucoma. 2020;29(1):39–45.

Numa S, Akagi T, Uji A, et al. Visualization of the lamina cribrosa microvasculature in normal and glaucomatous eyes: a swept-source optical coherence tomography angiography study. J Glaucoma. 2018;27(11):1032–5.

O'Brart DP, de Souza LM, Bartsch DU, Freeman W, Weinreb RN. Indocyanine green angiography of the peripapillary region in glaucomatous eyes by confocal scanning laser ophthalmoscopy. Am J Ophthalmol. 1997;123(5):657–66.

Park SC, De Moraes CG, Teng CC, Tello C, Liebmann JM, Ritch R. Initial parafoveal versus peripheral scotomas in glaucoma: risk factors and visual field characteristics. Ophthalmology. 2011;118(9):1782–9.

Park HY, Shin DY, Jeon SJ, Park CK. Association between parapapillary choroidal vessel density measured with optical coherence tomography angiography and future visual field progression in patients with glaucoma. JAMA Ophthalmol. 2019;137(6):681–8.

Philip S, Najafi A, Tantraworasin A, Chui TYP, Rosen RB, Ritch R. Macula vessel density and foveal avascular zone parameters in exfoliation glaucoma compared to primary open-angle glaucoma. Invest Ophthalmol Vis Sci. 2019;60(4):1244–53.

Rao HL, Pradhan ZS, Weinreb RN, et al. A comparison of the diagnostic ability of vessel density and structural measurements of optical coherence tomography in primary open angle glaucoma. PLoS One. 2017a;12(3):e0173930.

Rao HL, Kadambi SV, Weinreb RN, et al. Diagnostic ability of peripapillary vessel density measurements of optical coherence tomography angiography in primary open-angle and angle-closure glaucoma. Br J Ophthalmol. 2017b;101(8):1066–70.

Rolle T, Dallorto L, Tavassoli M, Nuzzi R. Diagnostic ability and discriminant values of OCT-angiography parameters in early glaucoma diagnosis. Ophthalmic Res. 2019;61(3):143–52.

Schwartz B, Rieser JC, Fishbein SL. Fluorescein angiographic defects of the optic disc in glaucoma. Arch Ophthalmol. 1977;95(11):1961–74.

Sehi M, Goharian I, Konduru R, et al. Retinal blood flow in glaucomatous eyes with single-hemifield damage. Ophthalmology. 2014;121(3):750–8.

Shiga Y, Kunikata H, Aizawa N, et al. Optic nerve head blood flow, as measured by laser speckle flowgraphy, is significantly reduced in preperimetric glaucoma. Curr Eye Res. 2016;1–7.

Shin JW, Lee J, Kwon J, Choi J, Kook MS. Regional vascular density-visual field sensitivity relationship in glaucoma according to disease severity. Br J Ophthalmol. 2017a;101(12):1666–72.

Shin JW, Sung KR, Uhm KB, et al. Peripapillary microvascular improvement and lamina cribrosa depth reduction after trabeculectomy in primary open-angle glaucoma. Invest Ophthalmol Vis Sci. 2017b;58(13):5993–9.

Shin JW, Kwon J, Lee J, Kook MS. Choroidal microvasculature dropout is not associated with myopia, but is associated with glaucoma. J Glaucoma. 2018;27(2):189–96.

Shin JW, Kwon J, Lee J, Kook MS. Relationship between vessel density and visual field sensitivity in glaucomatous eyes with high myopia. Br J Ophthalmol. 2019;103:585–91.

Simsek M, Kocer AM, Cevik S, Sen E, Elgin U. Evaluation of the optic nerve head vessel density in the patients with asymmetric pseudoexfoliative glaucoma: an OCT angiography study. Graefes Arch Clin Exp Ophthalmol. 2020;258(7):1493–501.

Spaide RF, Klancnik JM Jr, Cooney MJ. Retinal vascular layers imaged by fluorescein angiography and optical coherence tomography angiography. JAMA Ophthalmol. 2015a;133(1):45–50.

Spaide RF, Fujimoto JG, Waheed NK. Image artifacts in optical coherence tomography angiography. Retina. 2015b;35(11):2163–80.

Suh MH, Zangwill LM, Manalastas PI, et al. Deep retinal layer microvasculature dropout detected by the optical coherence tomography angiography in glaucoma. Ophthalmology. 2016;123(12):2509–18.

Suh MH, Park JW, Kim HR. Association between the deep-layer microvasculature dropout and the visual field damage in glaucoma. J Glaucoma. 2018;27(6):543–51.

Takusagawa HL, Liu L, Ma KN, et al. Projection-resolved optical coherence tomography angiography of macular retinal circulation in glaucoma. Ophthalmology. 2017;124(11):1589–99.

Tielsch JM, Katz J, Sommer A, Quigley HA, Javitt JC. Hypertension, perfusion pressure, and primary open-angle glaucoma. A population-based assessment. Arch Ophthalmol. 1995;113(2):216–21.

Venugopal JP, Rao HL, Weinreb RN, et al. Repeatability of vessel density measurements of optical coherence tomography angiography in normal and glaucoma eyes. Br J Ophthalmol. 2018;102(3):352–7.

Wang RK. Optical microangiography: a label free 3D imaging technology to visualize and quantify blood circulations within tissue beds in vivo. IEEE J Sel Top Quantum Electron. 2010;16(3):545–54.

Wu J, Sebastian RT, Chu CJ, McGregor F, Dick AD, Liu L. Reduced macular vessel density and capillary perfusion in glaucoma detected using OCT angiography. Curr Eye Res. 2019;44(5):533–40.

Xu H, Zhai R, Zong Y, et al. Comparison of retinal microvascular changes in eyes with high-tension glaucoma or normal-tension glaucoma: a quantitative optic coherence tomography angiographic study. Graefes Arch Clin Exp Ophthalmol. 2018;256(6):1179–86.

Yamazaki S, Inoue Y, Yoshikawa K. Peripapillary fluorescein angiographic findings in primary open angle glaucoma. Br J Ophthalmol. 1996;80(9):812–7.

Yarmohammadi A, Zangwill LM, Diniz-Filho A, et al. Relationship between optical coherence tomography angiography vessel density and severity of visual field loss in glaucoma. Ophthalmology. 2016;123(12):2498–508.

Yarmohammadi A, Zangwill LM, Manalastas PIC, et al. Peripapillary and macular vessel density in patients with primary open-angle glaucoma and unilateral visual field loss. Ophthalmology. 2018;125(4):578–87.

Yoo E, Yoo C, Lee TE, Kim YY. Comparison of retinal vessel diameter between open-angle glaucoma patients with initial parafoveal scotoma and peripheral nasal step. Am J Ophthalmol. 2017;175:30–6.

Zhang X, Beckmann L, Miller DA, et al. In vivo imaging of Schlemm's canal and limbal vascular network in mouse using visible-light OCT. Invest Ophthalmol Vis Sci. 2020;61(2):23.

Zivkovic M, Dayanir V, Kocaturk T, et al. Foveal avascular zone in normal tension glaucoma measured by optical coherence tomography angiography. Biomed Res Int. 2017;2017:3079141.

Anterior Segment Imaging in Glaucoma

Young Kook Kim

Abstract

Anterior chamber (AC) angle visualization is essential for accurate glaucoma diagnosis, especially in angle-closure disease. The emergence of anterior segment imaging devices such as anterior segment optical coherence tomography (AS-OCT) has enabled objective quantitative analysis of the AC angle. AS-OCT is a noncontact and noninvasive, rapid *in vivo* imaging device that makes use of low-coherence interferometry to obtain cross-sectional anterior segment images. Over the years, technological improvements have increased capture speed and image resolution, thus accentuating AS-OCT imaging's impact on ocular-disease diagnosis and management. Also, image processing and software improvements have enhanced the ease and utility of AS-OCT image interpretation in everyday clinical practice. In this chapter, we summarize AS-OCT's historical development and update the research on its clinical applications in AC structural and aqueous outflow system imaging as well as postoperative assessment in glaucoma.

Y. K. Kim (✉)
Department of Medicine, Seoul National University College of Medicine, Seoul, Korea

Department of Ophthalmology, Seoul National University Hospital, Seoul, Korea

Keywords

Anterior segment optical coherence tomography · Anterior chamber angle · Glaucoma Angle-closure disease · Ultrasound biomicroscopy

1 Introduction

Anterior segment optical coherence tomography (AS-OCT) provides for noncontact and rapid *in vivo* imaging of ocular structures and has become a key tool for evaluation of the anterior segment of the eye. Over the years, technological improvements have increased capture speed and image resolution, thus leading to the increasing impact of AS-OCT imaging on clinical practice.

The current uses of AS-OCT for patients with established or suspected glaucoma are anterior chamber (AC) angle assessment as well as AC depth (ACD)-, lens position-, corneal thickness-, iris thickness-, and morphological analysis of filtering blebs or glaucoma implants. Anterior segment images can facilitate decision-making regarding laser treatment or the most appropriate surgical approach. Image processing and software improvements have enhanced the ease and utility of AS-OCT image interpretation in everyday clinical practice. Given the recent three-dimensional AS-OCT developments and the

K. H. Park, T.-W. Kim (eds.), *OCT Imaging in Glaucoma*,
https://doi.org/10.1007/978-981-16-1178-0_7

increasing speed of the scanning function, the future applications of this technology to glaucoma are promising.

In this chapter, we review AC-OCT's historical development and update the research on and clinical applications of AS-OCT in the field of glaucoma.

2 History and Technical Aspects of Anterior Segment Optical Coherence Tomography

Optical coherence tomography (OCT) is a modality utilizing low-coherence interferometry for noncontact *in vivo* imaging of ocular structures (Huang et al. 1991). In 1994, Izatt et al. used it, for the first time, to image the AC structures (Radhakrishnan et al. 2001). AS-OCT systems currently are classified according to their light source's wavelength. Dedicated systems use the 1310 nm wavelength, and include Zeiss Visante (Carl Zeiss Meditec Inc., Dublin, CA, USA), Heidelberg's SL-OCT (Heidelberg Engineering Inc., Heidelberg, Germany), and Tomey's CASIA (TOMEY Corp. Nagoya, Japan). Systems converted from a retinal scanner, meanwhile, use the 830 nm wavelength, and include Spectralis OCT (Heidelberg Engineering Inc., Heidelberg, Germany), Cirrus HD-OCT (Carl Zeiss Meditec Inc., Dublin, CA, USA), and Optovue's RTVue (Optovue iVue; Optovue Inc., Fremont, CA, USA). Shorter-wavelength systems provide higher axial resolution but limited imaging depth; longer-wavelength systems, on the other hand, allow for deeper penetration by reducing scattering caused by the sclera and limbus, thereby affording more detailed visualization of AC angle morphology. The axial resolutions of Fourier or spectral-domain AS-OCT systems range between 4 and 7 μm.

AS-OCT systems enable clinicians to visualize anterior segment anatomy in a cross-sectional view. Their measurements are semi-automated and have good reproducibility (Shabana et al. 2012; Sng et al. 2012). After acquisition, scanned images are processed by customized software that compensates for the transition of the index of refraction at the air–tear interface along with the different air, corneal and aqueous indices and accounts for the physical dimensions of images.

3 Imaging of Anterior Chamber Structures

3.1 Qualitative Assessment of AS-OCT

Evaluation of AC angle in the course of ophthalmic examination is crucial for determining the angle's susceptibility to closure (Nongpiur et al. 2011a). Although gonioscopy is the gold standard for AC angle assessment, its flaws include artifacts (caused by pressure on the cornea) and an excessive amount of light, and these factors can affect the results (Barkana et al. 2007). Also, gonioscopy findings are inherently subjective and semiquantitative (Maslin et al. 2015).

Qualitative and quantitative AC, AC angle, iris, and lens assessment can be accomplished using AS-OCT (Fig. 1). Angle closure in AC-OCT is determined by contact between the iris and the angle wall anterior to the scleral spur; with gonioscopy, however, the quadrant would be considered open in any cases other than those where the apposition reached the posterior trabecular meshwork. Thus, in AS-OCT, the scleral spur is an important landmark to be assessed. Sakata et al. have used Visante OCT to demonstrate the possibility of isolating the scleral spur location in cases where the AC angle is open (Sakata et al. 2008a). However, the difficulty of scleral spur identification as a reference point has been

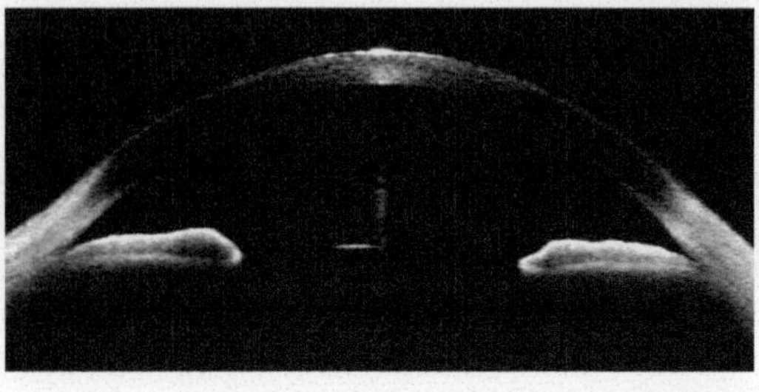

Fig. 1 Visante AS-OCT image of right eye showing normal anterior segment

reported in prior studies, where the rate of AS-OCT images in which such identification was impossible ranged from 15% to 28% (Sakata et al. 2008b; Wang et al. 2011).

In the literature, there is still no consensus on the relationships of AS-OCT-obtained measurements of aqueous humor outflow structures to each other. One study demonstrated that Spectralis OCT equipped with enhanced-depth imaging (EDI) could identify the Schwalbe's line and scleral spur in all nasal and temporal scans (Day et al. 2013). By modified Cirrus SD-OCT, Cheung et al. (2011) found that the Schwalbe's line was identifiable in 95% of scans and the scleral spur in 85%. By Casia OCT, the scleral spur was identifiable in all of the subjects; however, Schlemm's canal was identifiable in only 32% of those scans (McKee et al. 2013). Identification of scleral spur also has been reported to be subject to measurement error and variability (Sakata et al. 2008a; Li et al. 2007).

Variables such as eye quadrant (Sakata et al. 2008b), smaller ACD or a diagnosis of narrow angle, shorter axial length, or older age (Liu et al. 2010) can increase the difficulty of accurately identifying the scleral spur position. Such identification using AS-OCT is very important, and so several studies have sought to determine the best techniques for locating landmarks key to that goal. The three most common landmarks are as follows: (1) Schwalbe's line relative to scleral spur; (2) intersection of ciliary muscle (CM) and inner corneal margin; (3) bump-like structure in inner corneal-meshwork margin. A study by Seager et al. (2014) demonstrated that among these three approaches, locating the intersection of the CM and the inner corneal margin led to the highest rate of scleral spur identification with the lowest intra- and inter-observer variabilities.

3.2 Quantitative Assessment of AS-OCT

Automated algorithms for the provision of diagnostic and mechanistic classifications of angle closure based on AS-OCT images from Visante OCT, Casia SS-OCT, and Cirrus HD-OCT angle-to-angle scans have been developed (Fu et al. 2017; Niwas et al. 2016; Xu et al. 2013). The most important parameters in AC angle evaluation with AS-OCT are angle opening distance (AOD), angle recess area (ARA), trabecular-iris angle (TIA), and trabecular-iris space area (TISA) 500 or 750 μm from the scleral spur (Fig. 2). AOD is the distance from the cornea to the iris 500 or 750 μm from the scleral spur. The ARA is the area of the triangle bordered by the anterior iris surface, the corneal endothelium, and the line perpendicular to the corneal endothelium running from a point on the iris surface to a point 500 or 750 μm anterior to the scleral spur. The ARA is, theoretically, a better measurement parameter than the AOD, since it takes into account the entire iris surface contours rather than measuring a single point on the iris, as is the case with the AOD. The TIA is the angle formed from the angle recess to a point 500 or 750 μm

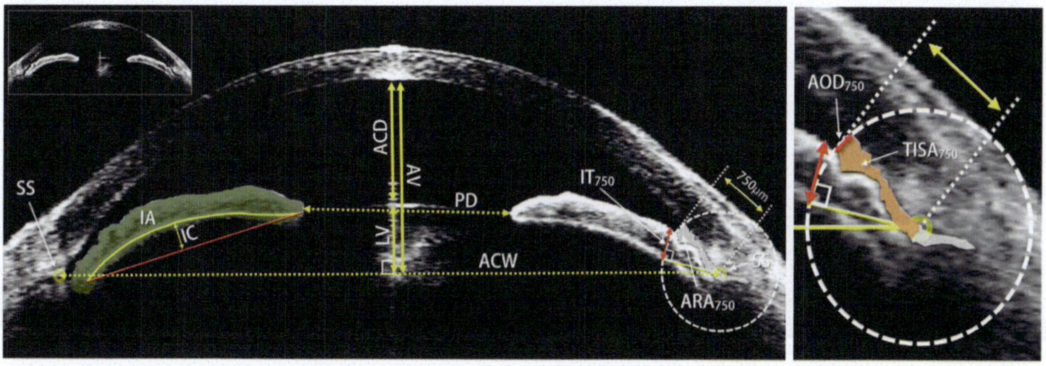

Fig. 2 AS-OCT's measured or calculated anterior segment parameters

from the scleral spur on the trabecular meshwork and perpendicular to the surface of the iris. The TISA is the trapezoid area between the iris and the cornea, as delimited by a line perpendicular to the scleral spur and a second line perpendicular to the cornea 500 or 750 μm from the scleral spur. Other biometric parameters measurable by AS-OCT are: Iris thickness (IT), iris curvature (IC), iris cross-sectional area (IA), ACD, AC width (ACW), trabecular meshwork ciliary process distance (TCPD), and lens vault (LV). Iris thickness (IT) usually is measured at a location where a line perpendicular to the cornea 500 μm from the scleral spur crosses the iris. Table 1 provides further descriptions of these and other parameters assessed by AS-OCT.

3.3 Comparisons with Gonioscopy or UBM

Although gonioscopy remains the gold standard for AC angle assessment, it has several limitations. It requires contact with the eye, which possibly leads to abrasions or the examiner's inadvertent pressure on the globe, which could change the angle's anatomic configuration. Additionally, gonioscopy's light source must be carefully controlled in order to prevent incident light from changing the diameter of the pupil and, thereby, the anatomic configuration of the angle. Finally, the skill required to perform the examination and interpret clinical findings is such as to require an adept, experi-

Table 1 Biometric parameters measured in AS-OCT

Parameter (abbreviation)	Description
Angle opening distance (AOD)	Linear distance between the point of the inner corneoscleral wall 500 or 750 μm from the scleral spur and the iris
Angle recess area (ARA)	The triangular area demarcated by the anterior iris surface, corneal endothelium, and a line perpendicular to the corneal endothelium drawn from a point 750 μm anterior to the scleral spur to the iris surface
Trabecular iris angle (TIA)	Angle formed from angle recess to points 500 μm from scleral spur on trabecular meshwork and perpendicular on the surface of the iris
Trabecular iris space area (TISA)	A trapezoidal area measuring the filtering area. The defining boundaries for this trapezoidal area are: anteriorly, the AOD; posteriorly, a line drawn from the scleral spur perpendicular to the plane of the inner scleral wall to the opposing iris; superiorly, the inner corneoscleral wall; and inferiorly, the iris surface
Iris thickness (IT)	Measured from a perpendicular point from the scleral spur
Iris curvature (IC)	The maximum perpendicular distance between iris pigment epithelium and the line connecting the most peripheral to most central point of the epithelium
Iris cross-sectional area (IA)	The average of the cross-sectional area of both nasal and temporal and nasal sides
Anterior chamber depth (ACD)	Distance from corneal endothelium to anterior surface of the lens
Anterior chamber width (ACW)	Distance of a horizontal line joining the two scleral spurs
Anterior chamber area (ACA)	The area whose boundaries are the corneo–scleral inner surface and the anterior iris and lens surfaces
Trabecular meshwork ciliary process distance (TCPD)	Measured from point on endothelium 500 μm from scleral spur through iris to ciliary process
Lens vault (LV)	Perpendicular distance between the anterior pole of the crystalline lens and the horizontal line joining the two scleral spurs
Anterior vault (AV)	Maximum distances between the horizontal line connecting the two scleral spurs and the posterior corneal surface
Relative lens vault (rVL)	Calculated by dividing the LV by the AV

AS-OCT anterior segment optical coherence tomography

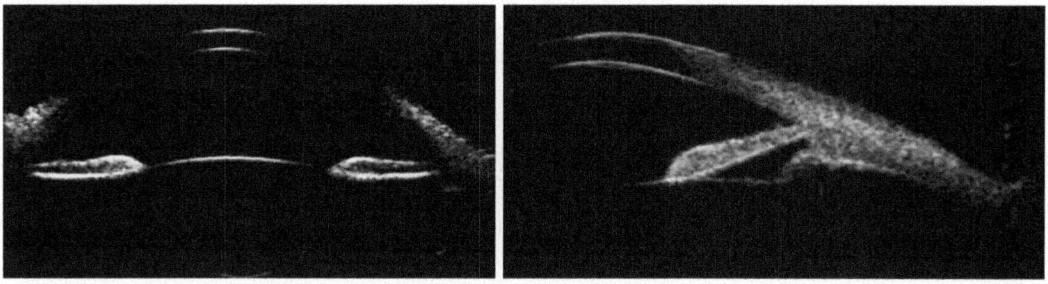

Fig. 3 UBM images of open-angle eye. UBM is better for visualization of the posterior chamber structures including the lens zonules and ciliary body

enced practitioner. Even when performed properly, gonioscopy provides only subjective and semiquantitative data.

AS-OCT is known to provide higher sensitivity than gonioscopy when detecting angle closure (Nolan et al. 2007). AS-OCT, with its ease of use, nonoperator dependence, and objective measurement of important quantitative parameters, allows for wider application in angle-closure glaucoma. AS-OCT can detect clinically important AC structural changes in patients under light-versus-dark conditions (Masoodi et al. 2014). It also is excellent for the measurement of iris parameters, which gonioscopy does not offer. Increased IC, IA, and thickness have been shown in previous studies to be independently associated with narrow angles (Wang et al. 2010, 2011).

Ultrasound biomicroscopy (UBM) utilizes high-frequency (50–100 MHz) ultrasound for anterior segment imaging. Then, a computer program converts these sound waves into a high-resolution B-scan image that can provide high-definition, reliable, and repeatable quantitative as well as qualitative data on the anterior segment. UBM previously has been shown to be in good agreement with gonioscopy in its utility for evaluation of angle closure as performed in a darkened room (Barkana et al. 2007). Also, because sound penetrates the pigment epithelium but light does not, UBM can visualize structures posterior to the iris pigment epithelium (Pavlin et al. 1990, 1991, 1992a, b; Wang et al. 1999; Foster et al. 2000). Thus, UBM is better for visualization of posterior chamber structures including the lens zonules, the ciliary body, and even the anterior choroid (Fig. 3). Furthermore, UBM, unlike AS-OCT, also can be performed with the subject lying down, and thus can be useful in the operating room when an examination is performed under general anesthesia. Compared with UBM, AS-OCT offers better resolution and does not require contact with the ocular surface (Li et al. 2007). It also provides a wider field of view than does UBM (Radhakrishnan et al. 2005; Dada et al. 2007; Memarzadeh et al. 2007; Ishikawa et al. 2000). Table 2 compares AS-OCT with UBM and highlights the main differences.

Table 2 Comparison of AS-OCT and UBM

AS-OCT	UBM
Optical	Ultrasound
Depth of penetration (~1 mm)	Depth of penetration (~6 mm)
Higher axial resolution	Lower axial resolution
Faster acquisition time	Slower acquisition time
Wider field of view (the entire anterior chamber in a single image)	Smaller field of view
Noncontact	Contact and requires a liquid coupling medium
Does not require a skilled operator	Requires skilled operator
Seated upright position	Seated upright or supine positions
Use for clear corneas	Can image through opaque media
Limited ability to visualize structures posterior to the iris pigment epithelium	Can visualize structures posterior to the iris pigment epithelium

AS-OCT anterior segment optical coherence tomography, *UBM* ultrasound biomicroscopy

4 Anterior Segment Optical Coherence Tomography Findings in Glaucoma

4.1 Pupillary Block

Aqueous humor flow resistance at the point of irido-lenticular contact increases pressure in the posterior chamber, widens its area, and produces anterior iris bowing leading to angle closure. In the pupillary block, the iris adopts a convex, forward-bowing appearance due to the AC/posterior chamber pressure gradient (Fig. 4).

Whereas shallow ACD and short axial length are the known risk factors for the development of primary angle-closure glaucoma, AS-OCT has shown that there are others as well. A number of AS-OCT parameters have been associated with angle-closure, including smaller ACW, AC area, and volume (Nongpiur et al. 2010; Wu et al. 2011); larger LV (Nongpiur et al. 2011b; Tan et al. 2012), along with greater IT, IC, and area (Wang et al. 2010). AC area and volume as well as LV have been demonstrated to be the most important determinants of angle width (Foo et al. 2012). An AS-OCT study by Cheung et al. (2010) determined iris bowing to be associated with angle width, independently of ACD.

AS-OCT has been employed to isolate the anatomic factors causing acute attacks of primary angle-closure glaucoma. A study by Sng investigated AS-OCT measurements in 31 unilateral acute angle-closure attack patients prior to therapeutic intervention (Sng et al. 2014). It was revealed that these patients tended to have shallower ACD and smaller IC (Sng et al. 2014). Also, another study revealed that eyes of this type had significantly greater LV relative to unaffected fellow eyes (Lee et al. 2014).

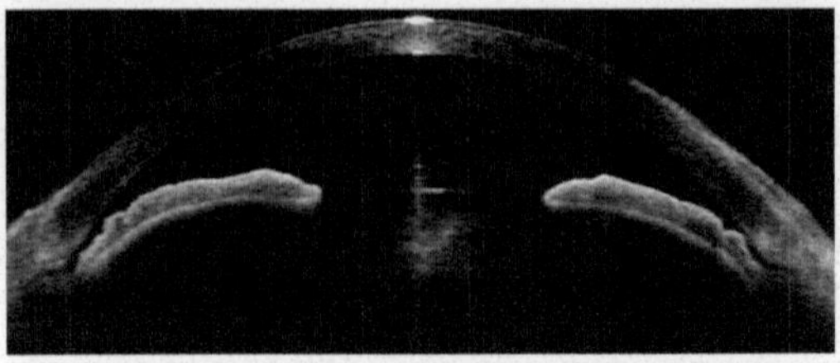

Fig. 4 AS-OCT imaging of primary angle-closure glaucoma case showing narrow angle and pupillary block

AS-OCT not only confirms diagnoses but also documents pressure balance restoration between anterior and posterior chambers after laser peripheral iridotomy (LPI) (Chalita et al. 2005). Anterior segment imaging can also explain why this procedure may be unsuccessful in angle-closure situations such as incomplete LPI, goniosynechiae, and plateau iris syndrome. A longitudinal AS-OCT study measuring angle structures 2 weeks and 6 months after LPI found that whereas significant angle widening was measured early after the procedure, this widening was significantly reduced at 6 months, which fact suggests that non-pupillary block mechanisms might contribute to primary angle-closure glaucoma (Jiang et al. 2014).

4.2 Plateau Iris

Plateau iris syndrome has been described in terms of persistent angle narrowing or occlusion with IOP elevation due to an abnormal plateau iris configuration following peripheral iridotomy (Mandell et al. 2003). Commonly it is caused by anteriorly positioned ciliary processes that push the peripheral iris forward, thus resulting in angle closure.

AS-OCT shows a generally thick, flat, slightly bowing iris that abruptly ascends after its insertion in the ciliary body's anterior surface, thereby assuming a "square root" appearance (Fig. 5). The most peripheral hump drapes over the rigid anteriorly positioned ciliary body, and the central hump rests on a long extension on the anterior lens surface. Anterior rotation of the ciliary body, which is associated with anterior positioning of the iris dilator's anchorage point, determines irido-ciliary sulcus narrowing, iris apposition to the trabecular meshwork, and angle closure (Pavlin et al. 1992c). The farther away the iris dilator joint is from the scleral spur, the lower is the probability of angle closure (Quigley 2009). It had been known that the AC has a relatively normal depth clinically (Quigley 2009; Ramakrishnan et al. 2016), until Mandell et al.

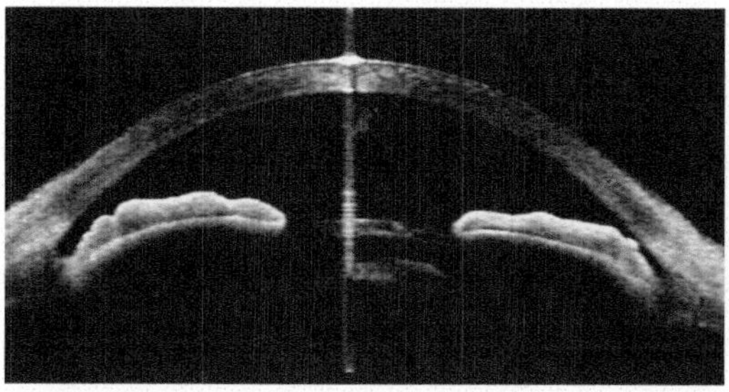

Fig. 5 Plateau iris. Despite the LPI, there remains a potential for a closing angle due to the iris root's steep angulation

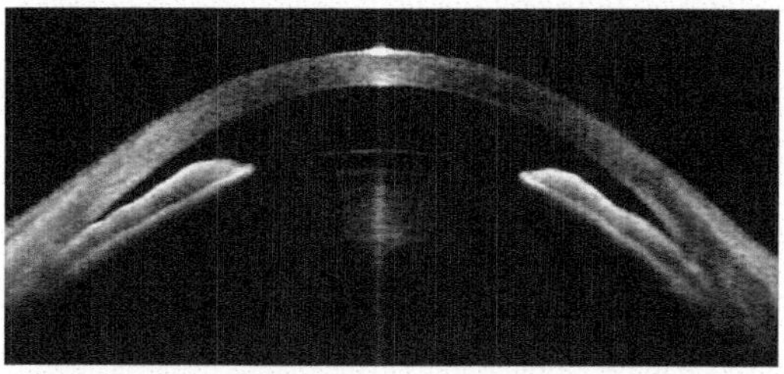

Fig. 6 Phacomorphic glaucoma. Note the shallow AC with high LV

found ACD measured by UBM to be shallower than that of both normal eyes and eyes with pupillary block (Mandell et al. 2003). Based on earlier-established UBM criteria, Verma et al. (2017) defined the plateau iris across three predefined AS-OCT patterns in 210 subjects. They could not differentiate the plateau iris based on any of the AS-OCT patterns, though increased peripheral IT in AS-OCT was associated with plateau iris likelihood. No ciliary-body-mediated posterior pushing of the peripheral iris (e.g., plateau iris or iris cysts) can be diagnosed with AS-OCT alone; rather, UBM also is necessary for ciliary process evaluation.

4.3 Phacomorphic Mechanism

AS-OCT can confirm the presence of a crystalline lens pushing the iris and ciliary body forward to cause iris-trabecular meshwork apposition (Fig. 6). An increased LV increases the probability of angle-closure glaucoma development, regardless of lens thickness or location (Nongpiur et al. 2011a). Nongpiur et al. (2011b) showed that higher LV, as representative of a greater portion of the lens being in the AC, determined angle crowding better than any other parameter for subjects of Chinese ethnicity. Several other parameters, for example, anterior LV and relative LV, also have been proposed to represent the lens contribution. Relative LV is the value of LV divided by the anterior vault (the sum of the LV and the ACD) to account for ACD differences (Kim et al. 2014). Kim et al. (2014) found that relative LV is more closely associated with primary angle-closure glaucoma than the absolute LV value is.

Subgrouping of AS-OCT images of angle closure identified two to four clusters, suggesting that the iris, lens, or both components may be predominant in the mechanism of angle closure (Niwas et al. 2016; Kwon et al. 2017; Baek et al. 2013; Nongpiur et al. 2013). Currently, there is a consensus that angle closure has multiple contributory factors and is not caused by a single mechanism. One of the most important of those factors might be pupillary block. However, other factors, namely the forward movement of the lens, increased iris volume, and plateau iris configuration, can be more important in some situations and can be evaluated in detail using AS-OCT.

4.4 Aqueous Misdirection

Classically, aqueous misdirection (i.e., malignant glaucoma) is characterized by a shallow AC associated with raised IOP in the presence of patent iridotomy (Ruben 1997). The mechanisms of the pathogenesis of this potentially devastating complication probably are related to abnormal anatomical relations among the lens, zonules, anterior vitreous face, and ciliary body. This can lead to misdirection of aqueous fluid, which flows into the vitreous cavity, subsequently increasing the vitreous volume, anteriorly displacing the central and peripheral anterior segment structures and, finally, increasing the IOP (Duy and Wollensak 1987; Byrnes et al. 1995).

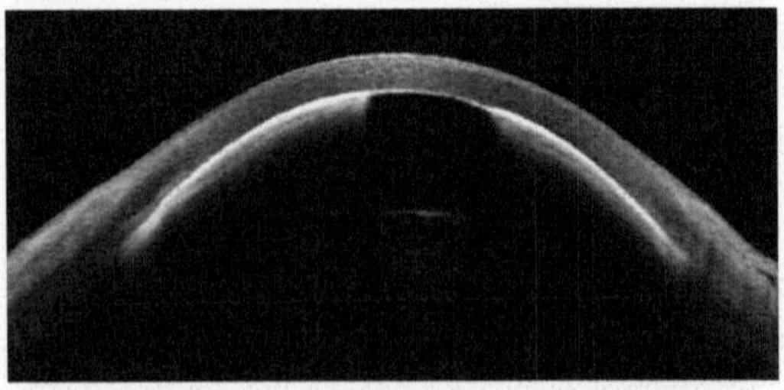

Fig. 7 Malignant glaucoma. The iris and lens directly contacting the corneal endothelium

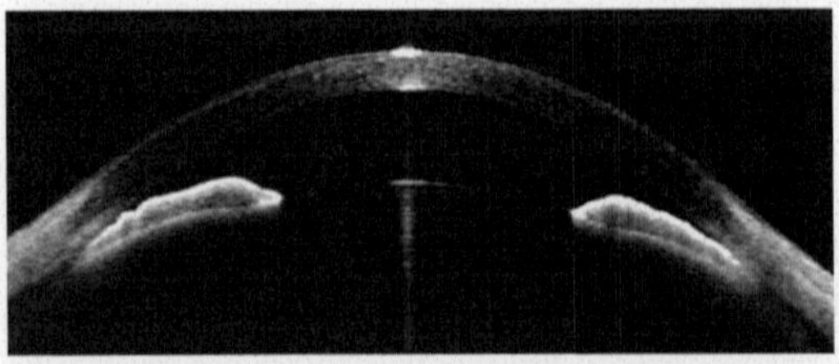

Fig. 8 Topiramate-induced angle closure. The AC is shallow, and the angles are narrowed. The lens-iris diaphragm is displaced forward. Note also the ciliochoroidal detachment accompanied by uveal effusion

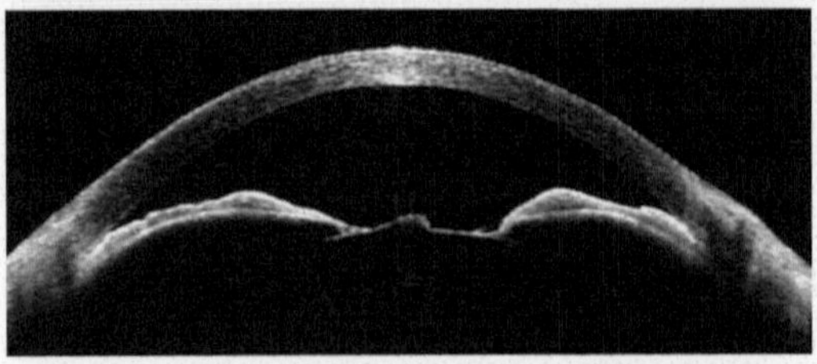

Fig. 9 Uveitis-associated secondary angle-closure case. The closed angles were caused by iris bombe due to absolute pupillary block (i.e., posterior synechiae)

AS-OCT has shown angle closure, forward movement of the crystalline lens or intraocular lens (IOL), and a flat AC (Fig. 7). Also, AS-OCT can document the absence of the posterior chamber and the presence of uveal effusion. Importantly too, it provides for objective assessment of medical and surgical therapeutic response, demonstrating, for example, increased AC angle after pars plana vitrectomy intervention (Jancevski and Foster 2010).

4.5 Other Causes of Angle Closure

Other disorders causing secondary angle closure, such as topiramate-induced acute-angle closure (Fig. 8), uveitis-related angle closure (Fig. 9), or iris cyst (Fig. 10), lead to discernible AS-OCT findings.

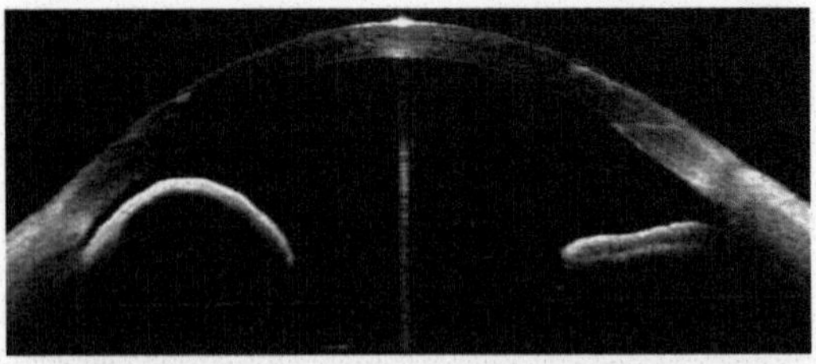

Fig. 10 Irido-ciliary cyst. Note the AS-OCT's indicated peripheral iris elevation. The typical UBM findings are a thin-walled structure with no internal reflectivity

5 Anterior Segment Optical Coherence Tomography Imaging in Glaucoma Surgery

5.1 Visualization of Filtering Blebs

Bleb morphology has been known as an important indicator of bleb function and potential future bleb failure (Wells et al. 2004). Bleb morphology in its external appearance can be assessed using slit-lamp biomicroscopy, but this modality cannot assess any of the bleb's internal structures. AS-OCT is useful in this regard, as it can show cross-sectional images of such structures. And, given its noncontact procedure, AS-OCT may be especially useful for fragile post-trabeculectomy blebs (Singh et al. 2009a).

Bleb types have been classified according to their characteristics on AS-OCT images (Leung et al. 2007). Four different patterns of intra-bleb morphology, namely diffuse filtering blebs, cystic blebs, encapsulated blebs, and flat blebs, were identified and closely related to slit-lamp appearance as well as bleb function. The scleral flap's thickness, height, and apposition to the scleral bed as well as the patency of the internal ostium can be assessed using properly sectioned AS-OCT images (Fig. 11). Tominaga et al. (2007) reported significantly lower mean IOP in eyes with a low-reflectivity bleb wall than in eyes with a more highly reflective wall. A study comparing *in vivo* confocal microscopy findings and AS-OCT filtering bleb reflectivity with filtering glaucoma surgery outcomes suggested that lower-reflective and heterogeneous suprascleral tissue is corre-

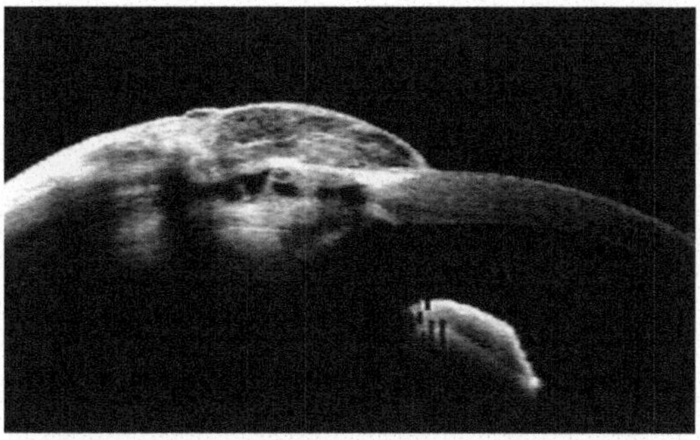

Fig. 11 Vertical AS-OCT section through conjunctival bleb after trabeculectomy and bleb revision. Note the open internal ostium, the filtration pathway guarded by the scleral flap, and the functioning elevated bleb

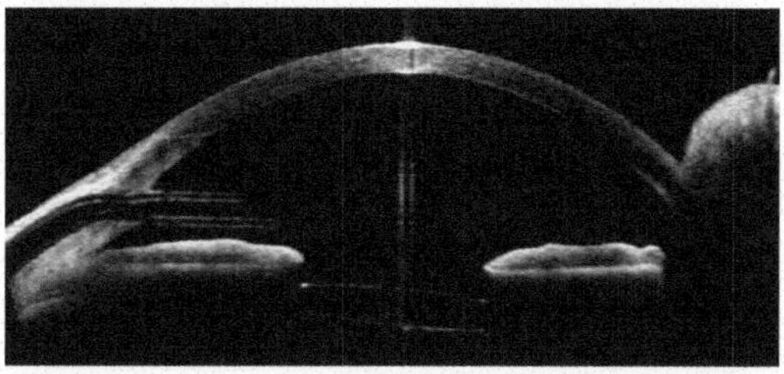

Fig. 12 Position, course, and patency of Ahmed glaucoma implant as successfully evaluated by AS-OCT

lated with loose connective tissue, where gaps and high fluid content abound, and where, correspondingly, functional blebs tend to arise (Messmer et al. 2006). Additionally, AS-OCT images potentially can be used for postoperative management purposes such as in suture lysis following filtration surgery (Singh et al. 2009b).

5.2 Imaging of Glaucoma Implants

AS-OCT can be employed to ascertain the position, course, and patency of aqueous drainage tubes (Koo et al. 2015; Park et al. 2012). Tube proximity to the corneal endothelium can be effectively visualized (Fig. 12). The thickness of tissue overlying the tube outside the AC and the presence of tube erosion can be assessed using properly obtained sections (Jung et al. 2013). Jung et al. (2013) found that the maximum bleb wall was significantly thinner in successful Ahmed glaucoma implant surgeries relative to unsuccessful ones. AS-OCT might also be helpful in assessments of tubes implanted into the ciliary sulcus.

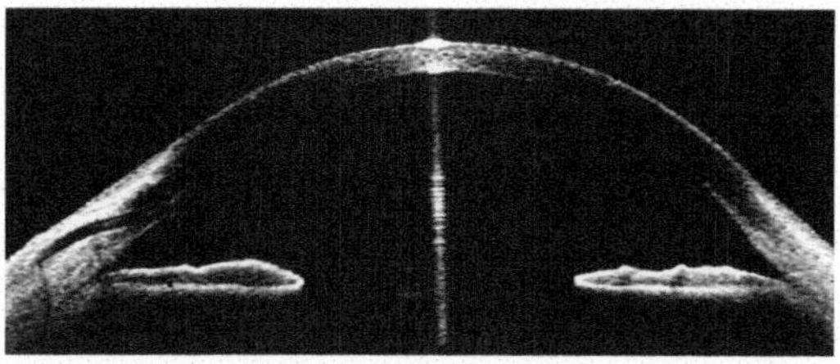

Fig. 13 AS-OCT image of Xen Gel stent. The implant is well positioned in the AC with an open ostium

As new glaucoma surgical techniques emerge, AS-OCT's role likely will continue to expand. Minimal Invasive Glaucoma Surgery (MIGS) has been evolving and is associated with several novel devices such as Glaukos iStent implant (Glaukos Corporation, Laguna Hills, CA, USA) and Xen Gel stent implant (AqueSys, CA, USA). The locations and patency of such implants can be evaluated by AS-OCT (Fig. 13). A study by Lenzhofer et al. evaluated longitudinal bleb morphologies after Xen Gel stent implantation surgery. They reported that the post-XEN bleb appearances seemed to differ from those after classic trabeculectomy (Lenzhofer et al. 2019). Also, the prevalence of small diffuse cysts is directly associated with lower IOP, while cystic encapsulation at 3 months predicts higher rates of surgical failure (Lenzhofer et al. 2019).

Compliance with Ethical Requirements

Conflict of interest: Young Kook Kim declares that he has no conflict of interest.

Informed consent: No human studies were carried out by the authors for this work.

Animal studies: No animal studies were carried out by the authors for this work.

References

Baek S, Sung KR, Sun JH, et al. A hierarchical cluster analysis of primary angle closure classification using anterior segment optical coherence tomography parameters. Invest Ophthalmol Vis Sci. 2013;54:848–53.

Barkana Y, Dorairaj SK, Gerber Y, Liebmann JM, Ritch R. Agreement between gonioscopy and ultrasound biomicroscopy in detecting iridotrabecular apposition. Arch Ophthalmol. 2007;125:1331–5.

Byrnes GA, Leen MM, Wong TP, Benson WE. Vitrectomy for ciliary block (malignant) glaucoma. Ophthalmology. 1995;102:1308–11.

Chalita MR, Li Y, Smith S, et al. High-speed optical coherence tomography of laser iridotomy. Am J Ophthalmol. 2005;140:1133–6.

Cheung CY, Liu S, Weinreb RN, et al. Dynamic analysis of iris configuration with anterior segment optical coherence tomography. Invest Ophthalmol Vis Sci. 2010;51:4040–6.

Cheung CY, Zheng C, Ho C-L, et al. Novel anterior-chamber angle measurements by high-definition optical coherence tomography using the Schwalbe line as the landmark. Br J Ophthalmol. 2011;95:955–9.

Dada T, Sihota R, Gadia R, Aggarwal A, Mandal S, Gupta V. Comparison of anterior segment optical coherence tomography and ultrasound biomicroscopy for assessment of the anterior segment. J Cataract Refract Surg. 2007;33:837–40.

Day AC, Garway-Heath DF, Broadway DC, et al. Spectral domain optical coherence tomography imaging of the aqueous outflow structures in normal participants of the EPIC-Norfolk Eye Study. Br J Ophthalmol. 2013;97:189–95.

Duy TP, Wollensak J. Ciliary block (malignant) glaucoma following posterior chamber lens implantation. Ophthalmic Surg Lasers Imaging Retina. 1987;18:741–4.

Foo L-L, Nongpiur ME, Allen JC, et al. Determinants of angle width in Chinese Singaporeans. Ophthalmology. 2012;119:278–82.

Foster FS, Pavlin CJ, Harasiewicz KA, Christopher DA, Turnbull DH. Advances in ultrasound biomicroscopy. Ultrasound Med Biol. 2000;26:1–27.

Fu H, Xu Y, Lin S, et al. Segmentation and quantification for angle-closure glaucoma assessment in anterior segment OCT. IEEE Trans Med Imaging. 2017;36:1930–8.

Huang D, Swanson EA, Lin CP, et al. Optical coherence tomography. Sience. 1991;254:1178–81.

Ishikawa H, Liebmann JM, Ritch R. Quantitative assessment of the anterior segment using ultrasound biomicroscopy. Curr Opin Ophthalmol. 2000;11:133–9.

Jancevski M, Foster CS, editors. Anterior segment optical coherence tomography. Semin Ophthalmol. 2010;25:317–23.

Jiang Y, Chang DS, Zhu H, et al. Longitudinal changes of angle configuration in primary angle-closure suspects: the Zhongshan Angle-Closure Prevention Trial. Ophthalmology. 2014;121:1699–705.

Jung KI, Lim SA, Park H-YL, Park CK. Visualization of blebs using anterior-segment optical coherence tomography after glaucoma drainage implant surgery. Ophthalmology. 2013;120:978–83.

Kim YK, Yoo BW, Kim HC, Aung T, Park KH. Relative lens vault in subjects with angle closure. BMC Ophthalmol. 2014;14:93.

Koo EB, Hou J, Han Y, Keenan JD, Stamper RL, Jeng BH. Effect of glaucoma tube shunt parameters on cornea endothelial cells in patients with Ahmed valve implants. Cornea. 2015;34:37–41.

Kwon J, Sung KR, Han S, Moon YJ, Shin JW. Subclassification of primary angle closure using anterior segment optical coherence tomography and ultrasound biomicroscopic parameters. Ophthalmology. 2017;124:1039–47.

Lee JR, Sung KR, Han S. Comparison of anterior segment parameters between the acute primary angle closure eye and the fellow eye. Invest Ophthalmol Vis Sci. 2014;55:3646–50.

Lenzhofer M, Strohmaier C, Hohensinn M, et al. Longitudinal bleb morphology in anterior segment OCT after minimally invasive transscleral ab interno Glaucoma Gel Microstent implantation. Acta Ophthalmol. 2019;97:e231–e7.

Leung CK, Yick DW, Kwong YY, et al. Analysis of bleb morphology after trabeculectomy with Visante anterior segment optical coherence tomography. Br J Ophthalmol. 2007;91:340–4.

Li H, Leung CKS, Cheung CYL, et al. Repeatability and reproducibility of anterior chamber angle measurement with anterior segment optical coherence tomography. Br J Ophthalmol. 2007;91:1490–2.

Liu S, Li H, Dorairaj S, et al. Assessment of scleral spur visibility with anterior segment optical coherence tomography. J Glaucoma. 2010;19:132–5.

Mandell MA, Pavlin CJ, Weisbrod DJ, Simpson ER. Anterior chamber depth in plateau iris syndrome and pupillary block as measured by ultrasound biomicroscopy. Am J Ophthalmol. 2003;136:900–3.

Maslin JS, Barkana Y, Dorairaj SK. Anterior segment imaging in glaucoma: an updated review. Indian J Ophthalmol. 2015;63:630.

Masoodi H, Jafarzadehpur E, Esmaeili A, Abolbashari F, Hosseini SMA. Evaluation of anterior chamber angle under dark and light conditions in angle closure glaucoma: an anterior segment OCT study. Cont Lens Anterior Eye. 2014;37:300–4.

McKee H, Ye C, Yu M, Liu S, Lam DS, Leung CK. Anterior chamber angle imaging with swept-source optical coherence tomography: detecting the scleral spur, Schwalbe's Line, and Schlemm's Canal. J Glaucoma. 2013;22:468–72.

Memarzadeh F, Li Y, Chopra V, Varma R, Francis BA, Huang D. Anterior segment optical coherence tomography for imaging the anterior chamber after laser peripheral iridotomy. Am J Ophthalmol. 2007;143:877–9.

Messmer EM, Zapp DM, Mackert MJ, Thiel M, Kampik A. In vivo confocal microscopy of filtering blebs after trabeculectomy. Arch Ophthalmol. 2006;124:1095–103.

Niwas SI, Lin W, Bai X, et al. Automated anterior segment OCT image analysis for Angle Closure Glaucoma mechanisms classification. Comput Methods Prog Biomed. 2016;130:65–75.

Nolan WP, See JL, Chew PT, et al. Detection of primary angle closure using anterior segment optical coherence tomography in Asian eyes. Ophthalmology. 2007;114:33–9.

Nongpiur ME, Sakata LM, Friedman DS, et al. Novel association of smaller anterior chamber width with angle closure in Singaporeans. Ophthalmology. 2010;117:1967–73.

Nongpiur ME, Ku JY, Aung T. Angle closure glaucoma: a mechanistic review. Curr Opin Ophthalmol. 2011a;22:96–101.

Nongpiur ME, He M, Amerasinghe N, et al. Lens vault, thickness, and position in Chinese subjects with angle closure. Ophthalmology. 2011b;118:474–9.

Nongpiur ME, Gong T, Lee HK, et al. Subgrouping of primary angle-closure suspects based on anterior segment optical coherence tomography parameters. Ophthalmology. 2013;120:2525–31.

Park HL, Jung K, Park C. Serial intracameral visualization of the Ahmed glaucoma valve tube by anterior segment optical coherence tomography. Eye. 2012;26:1256–62.

Pavlin CJ, Sherar MD, Foster FS. Subsurface ultrasound microscopic imaging of the intact eye. Ophthalmology. 1990;97:244–50.

Pavlin CJ, Harasiewicz K, Sherar MD, Foster FS. Clinical use of ultrasound biomicroscopy. Ophthalmology. 1991;98:287–95.

Pavlin CJ, Harasiewicz K, Foster FS. Ultrasound biomicroscopy of anterior segment structures in normal and glaucomatous eyes. Am J Ophthalmol. 1992a;113:381–9.

Pavlin CJ, McWhae JA, McGowan HD, Foster FS. Ultrasound biomicroscopy of anterior segment tumors. Ophthalmology. 1992b;99:1220–8.

Pavlin CJ, Ritch R, Foster FS. Ultrasound biomicroscopy in plateau iris syndrome. Am J Ophthalmol. 1992c;113:390–5.

Quigley HA. Angle-closure glaucoma–simpler answers to complex mechanisms: LXVI Edward Jackson memorial lecture. Am J Ophthalmol. 2009;148:657–69.

Radhakrishnan S, Rollins AM, Roth JE, et al. Real-time optical coherence tomography of the anterior segment at 1310 nm. Arch Ophthalmol. 2001;119:1179–85.

Radhakrishnan S, Goldsmith J, Huang D, et al. Comparison of optical coherence tomography and ultrasound biomicroscopy for detection of narrow anterior chamber angles. Arch Ophthalmol. 2005;123:1053–9.

Ramakrishnan R, Mitra A, Kader MA, Das S. To study the efficacy of laser peripheral iridoplasty in the treatment of eyes with primary angle closure and plateau iris syndrome, unresponsive to laser peripheral iridotomy, using anterior-segment OCT as a tool. J Glaucoma. 2016;25:440–6.

Ruben ST, Tsai J, Hitchings RA. Malignant glaucoma and its management. Br J Ophthalmol. 1997;81:163–7.

Sakata LM, Lavanya R, Friedman DS, et al. Comparison of gonioscopy and anterior segment ocular coherence tomography in detecting angle closure in different quadrants of the anterior chamber angle. Ophthalmology. 2008a;115:769–74.

Sakata LM, Lavanya R, Friedman DS, et al. Assessment of the scleral spur in anterior segment optical coherence tomography images. Arch Ophthalmol. 2008b;126:181–5.

Seager FE, Wang J, Arora KS, Quigley HA. The effect of scleral spur identification methods on structural measurements by anterior segment optical coherence tomography. J Glaucoma. 2014;23:e29–38.

Shabana N, Aquino MC, See J, et al. Quantitative evaluation of anterior chamber parameters using anterior segment optical coherence tomography in primary angle closure mechanisms. Clin Exp Ophthalmol. 2012;40:792–801.

Singh M, See JL, Aquino MC, Thean LS, Chew PT. High-definition imaging of trabeculectomy blebs using spectral domain optical coherence tomography adapted for the anterior segment. Clin Exp Ophthalmol. 2009a;37:345–51.

Singh M, Aung T, Aquino MC, Chew PT. Utility of bleb imaging with anterior segment optical coherence tomography in clinical decision-making after trabeculectomy. J Glaucoma. 2009b;18:492–5.

Sng CC, Foo L-L, Cheng C-Y, et al. Determinants of anterior chamber depth: the Singapore Chinese Eye Study. Ophthalmology. 2012;119:1143–50.

Sng CC, Aquino MCD, Liao J, et al. Pretreatment anterior segment imaging during acute primary angle closure: insights into angle closure mechanisms in the acute phase. Ophthalmology. 2014;121:119–25.

Tan GS, He M, Zhao W, et al. Determinants of lens vault and association with narrow angles in patients from Singapore. Am J Ophthalmol. 2012;154:39–46.

Tominaga A, Miki A, Yamazaki Y, Matsushita K, Otori Y. The assessment of the filtering bleb function with anterior segment optical coherence tomography. Br J Ophthalmol. 2007;91:340–4.

Verma S, Nongpiur ME, Oo HH, et al. Plateau Iris distribution across anterior segment optical coherence tomography defined subgroups of subjects with primary angle closure glaucoma. Invest Ophthalmol Vis Sci. 2017;58:5093–7.

Wang B, Sakata LM, Friedman DS, et al. Quantitative iris parameters and association with narrow angles. Ophthalmology. 2010;117:11–7.

Wang B, Narayanaswamy A, Amerasinghe N, et al. Increased iris thickness and association with primary angle closure glaucoma. Br J Ophthalmol. 2011;95:46–50.

Wang N, Ye T, Lai M, Ou Y, Zeng M, Yang C. Comparison of results of chamber angle examination by ultrasound biomicroscopy and gonioscopy. Chin J Ophthalmol. 1999;35:174–8, 10.

Wells A, Crowston J, Marks J, et al. A pilot study of a system for grading of drainage blebs after glaucoma surgery. J Glaucoma. 2004;13:454–60.

Wu R-Y, Nongpiur ME, He M-G, et al. Association of narrow angles with anterior chamber area and volume measured with anterior-segment optical coherence tomography. Arch Ophthalmol. 2011;129:569–74.

Xu Y, Liu J, Cheng J, et al. Automated anterior chamber angle localization and glaucoma type classification in OCT images. 2013 35th annual international conference of the IEEE Engineering in Medicine and Biology Society (EMBC); IEEE 2013:7380–7383.

Imaging in Myopic Glaucoma

Seok Hwan Kim

Abstract

Myopia is an important risk factor for glaucoma. The prevalence of myopia is increasing dramatically, and thus too, myopic glaucoma will be more often encountered. Recent advances in Spectral-Domain Optical Coherence Tomography (SD-OCT) technology enable fast, objective, and quantitative structural imaging of the optic nerve head (ONH), retinal nerve fiber layer (RNFL), and macula for facilitated and enhanced glaucoma diagnostics. However, myopic eyes have unique structural features, which might cause artifacts in OCT imaging or induce false positivity or negativity in interpreting OCT results. For correct diagnosis of glaucoma, it is essential to understand myopic eyes' structural features that might affect imaging and interpretation of OCT. The key OCT parameters in glaucoma diagnosis include peripapillary RNFL thickness, macular ganglion cell-inner plexiform layer (GCIPL) thickness, and neuroretinal rim thickness measurements. Here, I review the anatomical features of these structures in myopia, how they affect imaging and the diagnostic performance of OCT, how these structures and tests might be misinterpreted, and how to overcome pitfalls and to make correct diagnoses of myopic eyes with or without glaucoma.

Keywords

Optical coherence tomography · Myopia
Glaucoma · Retinal nerve fiber layer
Macular imaging · Optic nerve head imaging

1 RNFL Imaging in Myopia

1.1 Characteristics of RNFL Thickness in Myopia

Since the era of Stratus OCT, several studies have shown that myopic eyes have thinner-measured RNFL thickness (Choi and Lee 2006; Leung et al. 2006; Vernon et al. 2008; Budenz et al. 2007). Leung et al. (2006) reported that RNFL measurements were lower in highly myopic eyes than in low-to-moderate myopic eyes. Budenz et al. (2007) recruited 328 normal eyes with various refractive errors (−11.75 to +6.75 diopters) and reported that higher myopic eyes had a thinner-measured RNFL with a significant negative correlation between spherical equivalent/axial length and RNFL thickness. Studies utilizing SD-OCT have shown similar results (Kang et al. 2010; Wang et al. 2011; Mohammad Salih

S. H. Kim (✉)
Seoul National University, Boramae Medical Center, Seoul, Korea
e-mail: xcski1@snu.ac.kr

K. H. Park, T.-W. Kim (eds.), *OCT Imaging in Glaucoma*,
https://doi.org/10.1007/978-981-16-1178-0_8

2012). Although many studies have reported thinner RNFL thickness measurements in myopic eyes, it was uncertain if this finding resulted from an actual decrease of RNFL thickness in myopic eyes or if it was caused by factors affecting the accuracy of any OCT measurements.

Traditionally, peripapillary RNFL thickness has been measured along a circle scan of 1.73 mm radius. Because of the magnification effect, the actual scanning radius in a myopic eye could be longer than 1.73 mm. The relationship between the measurement obtained from the OCT image and the actual size of the fundus dimension can be expressed as $t = p * q * s$, where t is the actual fundus dimension, s is the measurement obtained using OCT, p is the magnification factor for the camera of the imaging system, and q is the magnification factor for the eye (Littmann 1982). The p is a constant in a telecentric system, which is 3.382 in the Cirrus and Stratus OCT systems (Carl Zeiss Meditec, California, USA). The ocular magnification factor q of the eye can be determined with the formula $q = 0.01306 * (\text{axial length} - 1.82)$ (Bennett et al. 1994). Therefore, the actual radius of the scan circle on the fundus (mm) equals $3.382 * 0.01306$ (axial length $- 1.82) * 1.73$ (mm). For example, in an eye of 28 mm axial length, the actual scanning radius will increase to 2.00 mm, and in an eye of 20 mm axial length, it will decrease to 1.39 mm (Savini et al. 2012). Thus, in myopic eyes with long axial length, the larger actual scanning circle in OCT might underestimate RNFL thickness.

Kang et al. (2010) first reported RNFL thickness measurement with Cirrus OCT after correction of the magnification effect in myopic eyes. Before adjusting the ocular magnification, the mean RNFL significantly decreased with spherical equivalent and increased with axial length. In contrast, after adjusting the ocular magnification, the mean RNFL thickness showed no correlation with spherical equivalent and only a weak positive correlation with axial length. Savini et al. (2012) also showed that RNFL thickness decreased with longer axial length, but this relationship disappeared with correction of axial-length-induced ocular magnification by the Littmann formula. These findings suggest that many previous studies reporting decreased mean RNFL thickness in myopia may, at least partly, have resulted from underestimation of thickness rather than from any true anatomical difference. Nevertheless, current OCT devices do not have any built-in function for correction of ocular magnification. Therefore, when evaluating OCT results for myopic eyes, it should be considered that even myopic eyes without glaucoma can show decreased peripapillary RNFL thickness.

1.2 Distribution Profile of RNFL Thickness in Myopia

Myopic eyes show different RNFL thickness profiles in OCT imaging. Kim et al. (2010) compared circumpapillary RNFL thickness profiles between a high-myopia group and a low-myopia group. Whereas the highly myopic eyes had significantly thinner RNFLs in the non-temporal sectors, they had significantly thicker RNFLs in the temporal quadrant compared with the low-myopia group. Hong et al. studied the angles of peaks in circumpapillary RNFL thickness profiles for young male adults and found a significant correlation between the angle and the degree of myopia (Hong et al. 2010). With increasing myopia, the peaks of RNFL thickness were closer to the temporal quadrant. Because the normative database of Stratus and Cirrus OCT devices largely comprises data from normal eyes with no or low myopia, both studies raised the possibility of misdiagnosis of glaucoma in myopic eyes without glaucoma. Leung et al. (2012) studied the RNFL distribution profile in myopic eyes using the RNFL thickness map of Cirrus OCT. They found that the RNFL distribution angle also diminished with increasing myopia and that this reduction could lead to false-positive classification of abnormal RNFL measurement on the RNFL thickness deviation map (Fig. 1).

Chung and Yoo (2011) raised the possibility of an inappropriate location of the OCT scan circle to explain the different RNFL thickness profiles in eyes with myopic tilted disc. After automated RNFL analysis by the Cirrus OCT built-in algorithm, the authors manually relocated the calcu-

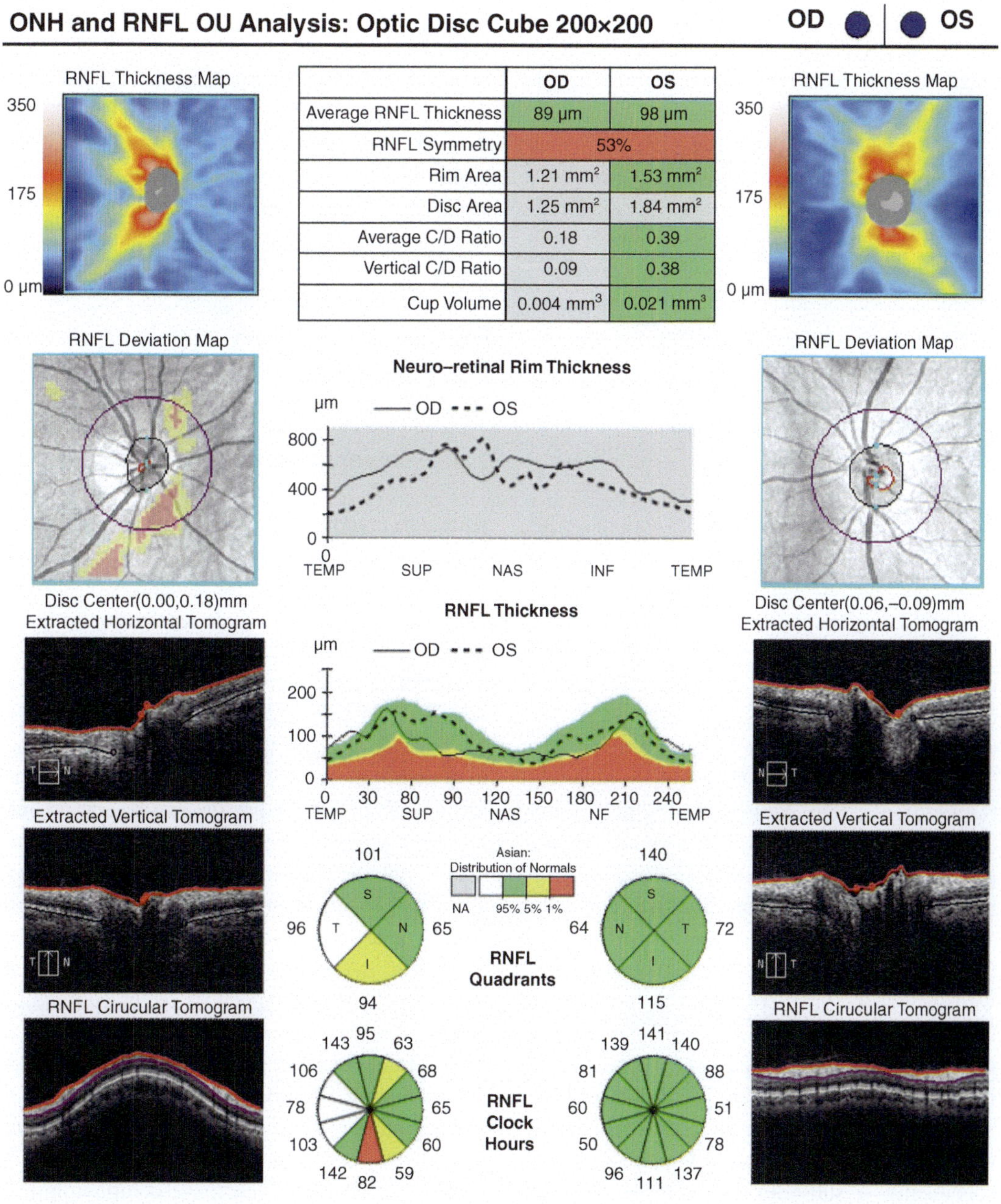

Fig. 1 The OCT RNFL image of a patient with unilateral myopia in the right eye. Despite normal disc, RNFL photo and visual field test, the OCT image of the right eye shows false-positives in the RNFL quadrants/clock hours analysis and deviation map due to the different profile of RNFL thickness

lation circle, centering it based on the contours of the neural canal opening (NCO). They found that in the new circle location, the mean number of abnormal clock-hour sectors as well as the proportion of eyes with abnormal clock-hour sectors at the 5% level of the built-in normative database was significantly lower. This result suggested that the NCO might be a suitable reference for peripapillary RNFL imaging. Lee et al. (2016) investigated circumpapillary RNFL thickness centered on the Bruch's membrane opening (BMO) with Spectralis OCT (Heidelberg

Engineering, Heidelberg, Germany), and showed that the new RNFL scanning algorithm had better diagnostic performance, particularly for myopic eyes with externally oblique border tissue.

In clinical practice, adjusting the circle scan location for every myopic eye might not be practical. However, clinicians, in order to minimize the probability of misdiagnosis, should always evaluate circumpapillary RNFL thickness or an RNFL thickness deviation map with caution considering the different RNFL profiles in myopic eyes.

1.3 High False Positivity in Myopia

The principal analysis of conventional OCT devices for diagnosis of glaucoma is based on measurement of RNFL thickness along the circle scan and comparison of the value to the built-in normative database. Due to the thinner RNFL thickness measurement and different distribution profiles in myopic eyes, high false-positivity rates for diagnostic performance of OCT have been reported from the era of Stratus OCT (Leung et al. 2006; Vernon et al. 2008). Leung et al. (2006) first reported that a significant proportion of myopic eyes were identified as abnormal based on the normative database provided in Stratus OCT. The most frequently abnormal sector was 2 o'clock, where 44.3% of myopic eyes were below the 95% confidence interval of the age-matched normative database. In addition, more eyes were classified as abnormal in the high-myopia group than in the low-to-moderate myopia group. Vernon et al. (2008) reported a similar finding with highly myopic Caucasians, specifically a substantial proportion of false-positivity errors. These studies both concluded that the normative database may not be entirely reliable for the evaluation of RNFL thickness in myopic eyes. Thus, the current in-machine normative database should be used with caution in the case of myopic eyes.

Studies with SD-OCT have shown similar findings (Leung et al. 2012; Aref et al. 2014; Qiu et al. 2011; Kim et al. 2011a). Leung et al. (2012) analyzed abnormal RNFL measurements on the RNFL thickness deviation map in Cirrus OCT and found that the reduction in the RNFL distribution angle with increasing myopia affected the false positivity. Qiu et al. (2011) reported that the frequency of false-positives was even higher in Cirrus OCT than in Stratus OCT. Kim et al. (2011a) studied the factors contributing to false-positive RNFL color-code results in Cirrus OCT. The overall false-positivity rate of 149 healthy eyes was as high as 26.2%, and eyes of longer axial length were more likely to show false-positive results.

1.4 Myopic Normative Database

Although myopic eyes have thinner RNFL thickness measurements and different thickness profiles in OCT, the normative databases of current OCT devices do not include moderate-to-highly myopic eyes. In the Cirrus OCT, the mean refractive error of 271 eyes in the normative database was −0.82D (SD 1.96D) (Knight et al. 2012). In order to decrease the frequency of false-positive errors in myopic eyes, the diagnostic performances of normative databases comprising myopic eyes have been studied. Biswas et al. (2016) obtained a normative database including 180 highly myopic eyes (spherical equivalent, −6.0D or less), and showed that the application of such a myopic normative database improved the specificity for detection of glaucomatous RNFL abnormalities in eyes with high myopia. This improvement in specificities did not tradeoff an overall sensitivity for detection of glaucoma; rather, improved sensitivity was observed in certain criteria. Similarly, Seol et al. (2017) obtained a normative database comprising 154 myopic eyes ranging from mild to severe myopia. They found that the myopic normative database showed a higher specificity than did the built-in normative database in quadrant RNFL thickness, clock-hour RNFL thickness, and GCIPL thickness, whereas the sensitivities of the OCT color probability codes after applying the built-in and myopic normative databases were not statistically different. Therefore, the authors of both studies suggested the importance of incorporating a myopic normative database in OCT instruments for the evaluation of RNFL measurements in myopic eyes. Unfortunately, none of the commercially available OCT devices has a built-in normative database of moderate-to-high myopia for RNFL thickness analysis. The retina scan–OCT (Nidek Co, Ltd) has a normative database including myopic eyes of long axial length (26–29 mm), but it is used only for macular map analysis (Nakanishi et al. 2015).

1.5 Imaging Artifacts in RNFL imaging

Proper segmentation of RNFL thickness is a fundamental step in the evaluation of OCT RNFL measurements. However, several studies have reported segmentation errors for myopic eyes. Nakano et al. (2013) reported that circumpapillary RNFL segmentation errors were more prevalent in patients with high myopia than in those without. The authors suggested that the error sources were related to myopic peripapillary changes that had crossed the circumpapillary RNFL circle scan and were of low signal intensity. Correspondingly, Suwan et al. (2018) found that 14% of normal myopic eyes and 44% of myopic glaucoma eyes had RNFL segmentation errors requiring manual correction in OCT. The authors also found that correction of the errors significantly improved the glaucoma-diagnostic capability. Kamal Salah et al. (2015) reported the effect of peripapillary neurosensory retinal detachment on RNFL measurement in high myopia. This study showed that eyes with peripapillary neurosensory retinal detachment had a significantly greater average RFNL thickness relative to those without peripapillary detachment, due to misidentification of the outer profile of the RFNL.

Retinal pathologies along the circle scan as well as segmentation errors of OCT software may affect RNFL thickness measurement of OCT. Thus, careful interpretation is required for the evaluation of OCT reports on myopic eyes. Because manual correction of segmentation errors is currently time-consuming and not provided for in all commercially available OCT devices, the development of a more accurate automated segmentation algorithm is necessary.

2 Macular Imaging in Myopia

2.1 Macular Imaging in Glaucoma

Glaucoma is characterized by selective loss of retinal ganglion cells (RGC). Since the macular area contains more than 50% of all RGCs and the RGC bodies are 10 to 20 times the diameter of their axons, the macular area is important in the detection of glaucomatous RGC damage (Hood et al. 2013). From the idea that macular thickness can reflect glaucomatous damage, the change of macular thickness as a measure of glaucoma had been studied prior to OCT's introduction (Zeimer et al. 1998). Later, with Stratus OCT, several studies tested whether assessment of macular thickness might outperform circumpapillary RNFL measurement. Initial research investigating total macular thickness showed that circumpapillary RNFL evaluation was superior to that of macular thickness, due probably to the retinal thickness other than the RGC layer masking glaucomatous change (Guedes et al. 2003; Wollstein et al. 2004). Customized segmentation of the inner retinal complex (RGC layer+inner plexiform and nuclear layers) by Stratus OCT showed comparable diagnostic performance to circumpapillary RNFL for glaucoma diagnosis, which served to raise the importance of segmentation analysis (Ishikawa et al. 2005).

Introduction of SD-OCT enabled segmented macular thickness measurements by a built-in segmentation algorithm. Several commercially available SD-OCTs provide different segmented macular thickness measurements. RTVue FD-OCT (Optovue, Fremont, California, USA) provides the macular ganglion cell complex (GCC), which is the sum of the macular RNFL, ganglion cell layer (GCL) and inner plexiform layer (IPL). Cirrus SD-OCT provides macular ganglion cell–inner plexiform layer (GCIPL) thickness via a macular ganglion cell analysis (GCA) algorithm. Topcon 3D-OCT (Topcon,

Tokyo, Japan) provides both GCC and GCIPL thickness. Spectralis OCT enables separate measurement of the entire retinal layers. Several studies have shown that the diagnostic ability of the macular thickness parameters is comparable to that of RNFL thickness for diagnosis of manifest glaucoma (Mwanza et al. 2012; Oddone et al. 2016).

Whereas circumpapillary RNFL thickness measurement is affected by several factors such as disc size (Savini et al. 2005), disc tilt (Hwang et al. 2012a), and axial length (Kang et al. 2010; Wang et al. 2011; Mohammad Salih 2012), macular GCIPL thickness is less influenced by them (Lee et al. 2014; Jeong et al. 2016). Therefore, the diagnostic benefit of macular thickness parameters in myopic glaucoma has been studied.

2.2 Diagnostic Ability of Macular Parameters in Myopia

Initial studies evaluating the ability of macular thickness to detect glaucoma in myopia have used RTVue OCT with GCC parameters. Kim et al. (2011b) compared the diagnostic ability to detect glaucoma between macular GCC and peripapillary RNFL thickness in highly myopic eyes using RTVue OCT. They found that the macular GCC thickness measurements had higher AUROC than did peripapillary RNFL thickness in highly myopic eyes for detection of glaucoma, but without statistical significance. Shoji et al. (2011) determined that the diagnostic power of GCC parameters was significantly higher than that of circumpapillary RNFL parameters in high myopia. Another paper by Shoji et al. studied the effects of high myopia on the glaucoma-diagnostic ability of OCT parameters. The ability of circumpapillary RNFL measurement to detect glaucoma in highly myopic eyes was inferior to that in emmetropic eyes, whereas macular GCC measurements showed a good ability to detect glaucoma in both groups. Based on the results of these studies, it can be concluded that macular GCC thickness has a glaucoma-diagnostic ability comparable or superior to that of circumpapillary RNFL thickness for highly myopic eyes.

GCC is the sum of three layers, the RNFL, GCL, and IPL, whereas GCIPL is the sum of the GCL and IPL. Thus, GCPIL is less influenced by RNFL thickness variation than GCC thickness is. Several studies have investigated its glaucoma detection ability for myopic eyes. Choi et al. (2013) compared the glaucoma-diagnostic ability of GCIPL with that of circumpapillary RNFL thickness in high myopia, finding them to be comparable. Seol et al. (2015) studied the glaucoma detection ability of GCIPL in myopic preperimetric glaucoma and determined the inferotemporal macular GCIPL thickness parameter to be the best for detection of PPG in myopic eyes, superior to the RNFL thickness parameters.

Besides measuring GCIPL thickness and comparing the values with a normative database, other approaches to the improvement of glaucoma-diagnostic ability have been reported as well. Kim et al. introduced a MATLAB-based GCIPL hemifield test for detection of GCIPL thickness difference across the temporal horizontal raphe and evaluated its glaucoma-diagnostic ability in highly myopic eyes (Kim et al. 2015a, 2016). They found that the AUC value for the GCIPL hemifield test, as compared with the RNFL and GCIPL thickness parameters, was the best (Kim et al. 2016). Baek et al. (2018) proposed a new scoring system combining the topographic signs of both RNFL and GCIPL analysis. The system had a higher diagnostic ability than the RNFL or GCIPL thickness parameters for myopic eyes and even for highly myopic eyes. The recently introduced swept-source OCT (SS-OCT) provides a wide 12- $*$ 9-mm^2 area in a single scan showing the macular and peripapillary structures simultaneously. Kim et al. determined that SS-OCT wide-field imaging, as compared with conventional SD-OCT, had greater diagnostic power for glaucoma with myopia (Kim et al. 2020).

Although the macular parameters in myopic eyes have shown similar or better diagnostic ability relative to the RNFL thickness parameters, GCA maps can miss abnormal findings if the angular distance between the fovea and an RNFL defect is great (Hwang et al. 2014; Kim et al. 2014). In addition, several factors (see below) affect macular thickness in myopia. Therefore, macular thickness parameters cannot substitute for RNFL thickness evaluation by OCT but rather should be considered as complementary to it.

2.3 Imaging Artifacts in Macular Imaging

Several studies have reported that segmentation errors in OCT total retinal thickness measurements could be found in various macular diseases including age-related macular degeneration, epiretinal membrane (ERM), diabetic retinopathy, and retinal vein occlusion (Ray et al. 2005; Ho et al. 2009; Giani et al. 2010; Han and Jaffe 2010). Abnormal segmentations in GCIPL also have been reported in eyes with macular degeneration and ERM (Hwang 2014). Even in eyes without macular disorders, segmentation errors in macular GCA can be found in some cases. Hwang et al. (2016) reported that 9.7% of glaucoma or healthy eyes without macular disorder had segmentation errors and that only higher-degree myopia was associated with the presence of segmentation errors. Therefore, the possibility of segmentation errors as well as accompanying macular pathologies should be considered when evaluating macular analysis in myopic eyes, especially in eyes with high myopia.

False-positive classification is frequently observed in the case of the color-code GCA map. Kim et al. (2015b) reported that 40.4% of 104 healthy eyes showed abnormal classifications on any of the GCA maps. Abnormal classification was associated with longer axial length and larger fovea-disc angle. Due to the higher frequency of false-positive GCA classification, macular thickness analyses should be carefully evaluated, especially in myopic eyes (Fig. 2).

3 Disc Imaging in Myopia

3.1 Disc Imaging with OCT

Stratus OCT provides various ONH parameters including disc area, cup area, rim area, cup/disc area ratio, cup/disc horizontal ratio, cup/disc vertical ratio, vertical integrated rim area (volume), and horizontal integrated rim width (area). However, owing to the low reproducibility of ONH scans, frequent inappropriate recognition of optic disc margin, and imaging artifacts, ONH analysis has not been widely used in glaucoma diagnostics using Stratus OCT (Iliev et al. 2006; Ortega Jde et al. 2009; Marsh et al. 2010).

SD-OCT provides excellent reproducibility and a low rate of incorrect optic disc margin detection ranging from 0.5 to 2.6% (Mwanza et al. 2010; Cheung et al. 2011; Sung et al. 2012). In addition, studies using Cirrus-OCT have reported that ONH parameters are comparable to RNFL thickness measurements in terms of differentiating normal eyes from glaucoma (Mwanza et al. 2011; Hwang and Kim 2012). In myopic eyes, however, errors in neuroretinal rim measurement by Cirrus HD-OCT were found in 17.6% of myopic eyes, especially eyes with PPA, higher myopia, greater axial length, vitreous opacity, or acute cup slope angle (Hwang et al. 2012b).

3.2 BMO-MRW

Studies comparing the clinical disc margin and structures in SD-OCT have found that the clinical disc margin is neither a single anatomic entity nor a clinical construct that underlies a consistent anatomical structure within or between eyes (Reis et al. 2012a, b). Because RGC axons exit the eye through the BMO from the inner retinal layer, and because axons cannot pass through an intact Bruch's membrane, neuroretinal rim measurements using the BMO as a reference plane have been proposed (Chauhan and Burgoyne 2013; Chauhan et al. 2013). The BMO-minimum rim width (BMO-MRW), defined as the minimum distance between the BMO and the internal limiting membrane, has shown a higher sensitivity compared with peripapillary RNFL thickness measurements for diagnosis of early glaucoma (Chauhan et al. 2013).

In myopic eyes, evaluation of glaucomatous optic disc changes has been challenging due to the unique optic disc morphology, including large peripapillary atrophy, varying degrees of disc tilt

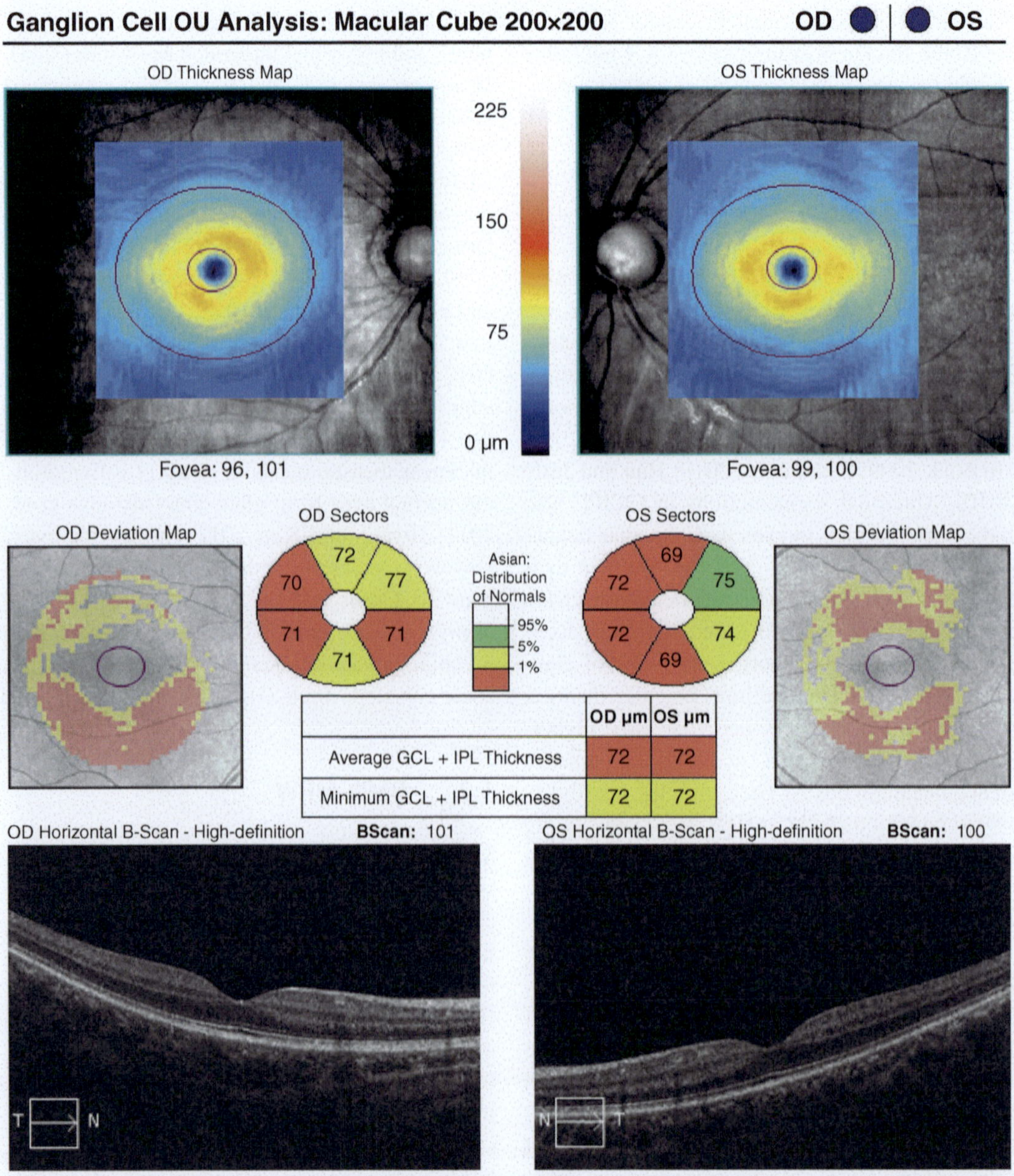

Fig. 2 The OCT macular GCIPL image of a patient with bilateral myopia. Despite normal disc, RNFL photo, and visual field test, the OCT image of both eyes shows false-positives in the deviation map and the average/minimum GCIPL thickness parameters

or torsion, and abnormally large or small optic disc size. Therefore, several studies have evaluated the usefulness of BMO-MRW for myopic eyes. Malik et al. (2016) reported that the sensitivity of BMO-MRW was comparable to that of RNFL thickness; however, the sensitivity of both parameters was only 71.4% at 90% specificity. Recent studies have reported that for healthy myopic eyes, the BMO-MRW parameter shows a lower rate of false-positives than does RNFL thickness (Rebolleda et al. 2016; Sastre-Ibañez et al. 2018). Kim et al. studied the diagnostic accuracy of three-dimensional neuroretinal rim (3D-NRR) thickness, which is defined as the distance between the BMO and the vitreoretinal interface, in myopic eyes (Kim and Park 2018). They found that the false-positivity rate was significantly lower for 3D-NRR thickness than for RNFL thickness and that its diagnostic accuracy for glaucoma outperformed RNFL thickness. However, Zheng et al. (2018) demonstrated that in high myopia, 32% of eyes had indiscernible BMO in at least one meridian. Furthermore, the BMO was indistinct most frequently at the temporal, inferotemporal, and superotemporal meridians where glaucomatous neuroretinal rim loss is most common. Therefore, utilization of BMO-MRW might be compromised in highly myopic eyes. Based on these results, it can be concluded that rim evaluation referencing the BMO as an anatomic landmark can be a complementary tool to RNFL thickness measurements for the diagnosis of glaucoma in myopic eyes (Fig. 3).

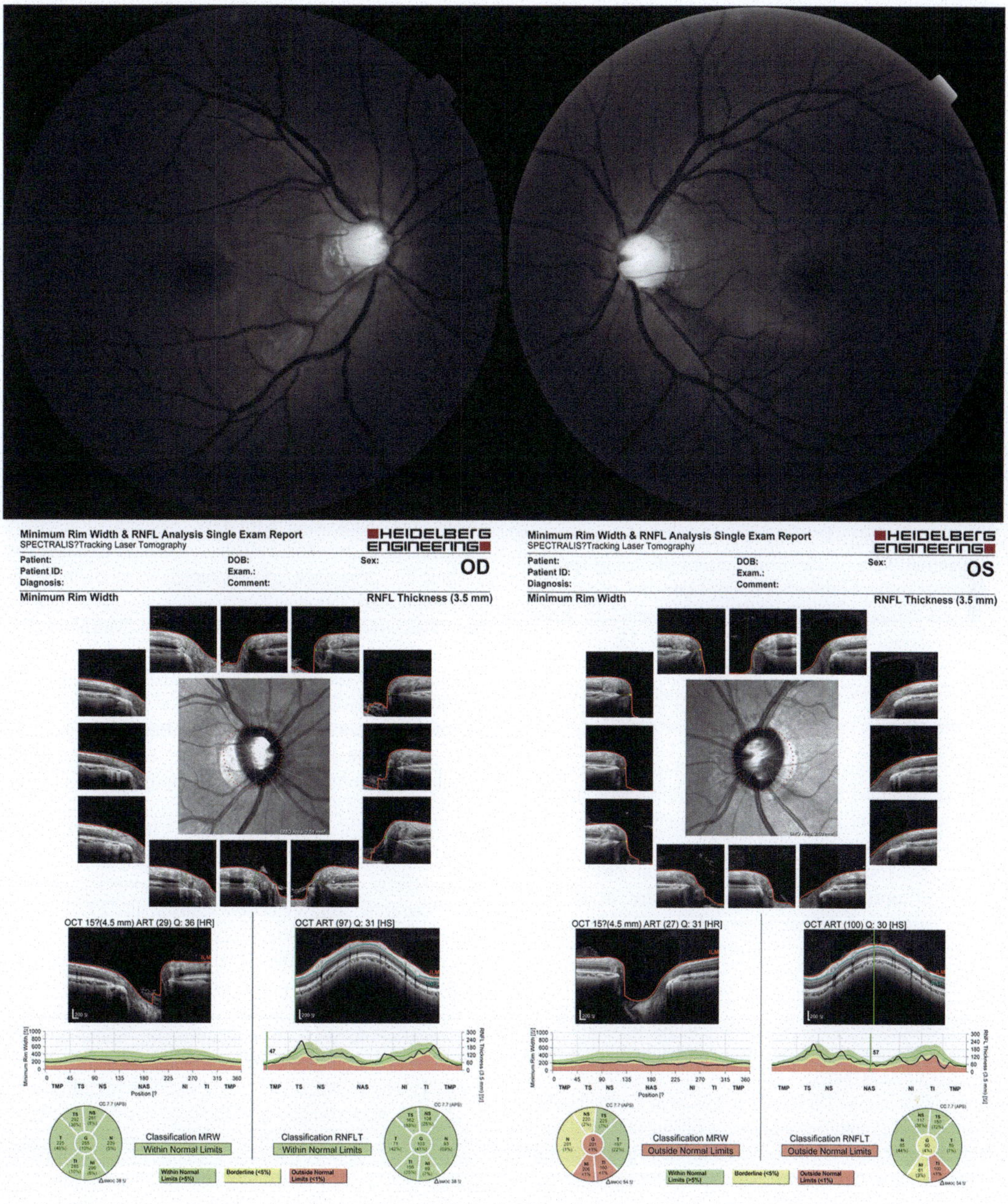

Fig. 3 The RNFL photographs and the OCT BMO-MRW/RNFL analysis of a patient with unilateral myopic glaucoma in the left eye. The BMO-MRW and RNFL analysis indicate abnormalities in the inferior sectors of the left eye

References

Aref AA, Sayyad FE, Mwanza JC, Feuer WJ, Budenz DL. Diagnostic specificities of retinal nerve fiber layer, optic nerve head, and macular ganglion cell-inner plexiform layer measurements in myopic eyes. J Glaucoma. 2014;23(8):487–93.

Baek SU, Kim KE, Kim YK, Park KH, Jeoung JW. Development of topographic scoring system for identifying glaucoma in myopic eyes: a spectral-domain OCT study. Ophthalmology. 2018;125(11):1710–9.

Bennett AG, Rudnicka AR, Edgar DF. Improvements on Littmann's method of determining the size of retinal features by fundus photography. Graefes Arch Clin Exp Ophthalmol. 1994;232(6):361–7.

Biswas S, Lin C, Leung CK. Evaluation of a myopic normative database for analysis of retinal nerve fiber layer thickness. JAMA Ophthalmol. 2016;134(9):1032–9.

Budenz DL, Anderson DR, Varma R, et al. Determinants of normal retinal nerve fiber layer thickness measured by Stratus OCT. Ophthalmology. 2007;114(6):1046–52.

Chauhan BC, Burgoyne CF. From clinical examination of the optic disc to clinical assessment of the optic nerve head: a paradigm change. Am J Ophthalmol. 2013;156(2):218–27.e2.

Chauhan BC, O'Leary N, AlMobarak FA, et al. Enhanced detection of open-angle glaucoma with an anatomically accurate optical coherence tomography-derived neuroretinal rim parameter. Ophthalmology. 2013;120(3):535–43.

Cheung CY, Chen D, Wong TY, et al. Determinants of quantitative optic nerve measurements using spectral domain optical coherence tomography in a population-based sample of non-glaucomatous subjects. Invest Ophthalmol Vis Sci. 2011;52(13):9629–35.

Choi SW, Lee SJ. Thickness changes in the fovea and peripapillary retinal nerve fiber layer depend on the degree of myopia. Korean J Ophthalmol. 2006;20(4):215–9.

Choi YJ, Jeoung JW, Park KH, Kim DM. Glaucoma detection ability of ganglion cell-inner plexiform layer thickness by spectral-domain optical coherence tomography in high myopia. Invest Ophthalmol Vis Sci. 2013;54(3):2296–304.

Chung JK, Yoo YC. Correct calculation circle location of optical coherence tomography in measuring retinal nerve fiber layer thickness in eyes with myopic tilted discs. Invest Ophthalmol Vis Sci. 2011;52(11):7894–900.

Giani A, Cigada M, Esmaili DD, et al. Artifacts in automatic retinal segmentation using different optical coherence tomography instruments. Retina. 2010;30(4):607–16.

Guedes V, Schuman JS, Hertzmark E, et al. Optical coherence tomography measurement of macular and nerve fiber layer thickness in normal and glaucomatous human eyes. Ophthalmology. 2003;110(1):177–89.

Han IC, Jaffe GJ. Evaluation of artifacts associated with macular spectral-domain optical coherence tomography. Ophthalmology. 2010;117(6):1177–89.e4.

Ho J, Sull AC, Vuong LN, et al. Assessment of artifacts and reproducibility across spectral- and time-domain optical coherence tomography devices. Ophthalmology. 2009;116(10):1960–70.

Hong SW, Ahn MD, Kang SH, Im SK. Analysis of peripapillary retinal nerve fiber distribution in normal young adults. Invest Ophthalmol Vis Sci. 2010;51(7):3515–23.

Hood DC, Raza AS, de Moraes CG, Liebmann JM, Ritch R. Glaucomatous damage of the macula. Prog Retin Eye Res. 2013;32:1–21.

Hwang YH. Patterns of macular ganglion cell abnormalities in various ocular conditions. Invest Ophthalmol Vis Sci. 2014;55(6):3995–6.

Hwang YH, Kim YY. Glaucoma diagnostic ability of quadrant and clock-hour neuroretinal rim assessment using cirrus HD optical coherence tomography. Invest Ophthalmol Vis Sci. 2012;53(4):2226–34.

Hwang YH, Yoo C, Kim YY. Myopic optic disc tilt and the characteristics of peripapillary retinal nerve fiber layer thickness measured by spectral-domain optical coherence tomography. J Glaucoma. 2012a;21(4):260–5.

Hwang YH, Kim YY, Jin S, Na JH, Kim HK, Sohn YH. Errors in neuroretinal rim measurement by Cirrus high-definition optical coherence tomography in myopic eyes. Br J Ophthalmol. 2012b;96(11):1386–90.

Hwang YH, Jeong YC, Kim HK, Sohn YH. Macular ganglion cell analysis for early detection of glaucoma. Ophthalmology. 2014;121(8):1508–15.

Hwang YH, Kim MK, Kim DW. Segmentation errors in macular ganglion cell analysis as determined by optical coherence tomography. Ophthalmology. 2016;123(5):950–8.

Iliev ME, Meyenberg A, Garweg JG. Morphometric assessment of normal, suspect and glaucomatous optic discs with Stratus OCT and HRT II. Eye (Lond). 2006;20(11):1288–99.

Ishikawa H, Stein DM, Wollstein G, Beaton S, Fujimoto JG, Schuman JS. Macular segmentation with optical coherence tomography. Invest Ophthalmol Vis Sci. 2005;46(6):2012–7.

Jeoung JH, Choi YJ, Park KH, Kim DM, Jeoung JW. Macular ganglion cell imaging study: covariate effects on the spectral domain optical coherence tomography for glaucoma diagnosis. PLoS One. 2016;11(8):e0160448.

Kamal Salah R, Morillo-Sánchez MJ, García-Ben A, et al. The effect of peripapillary detachment on retinal nerve fiber layer measurement by spectral domain optical coherence tomography in high myopia. Ophthalmologica. 2015;233(3–4):209–15.

Kang SH, Hong SW, Im SK, Lee SH, Ahn MD. Effect of myopia on the thickness of the retinal nerve fiber layer measured by Cirrus HD optical coherence tomography. Invest Ophthalmol Vis Sci. 2010;51(8):4075–83.

Kim KE, Jeoung JW, Park KH, Kim DM, Kim SH. Diagnostic classification of macular ganglion cell and retinal nerve fiber layer analysis: differentiation of false-positives from glaucoma. Ophthalmology. 2015b;122(3):502–10.

Kim MJ, Lee EJ, Kim TW. Peripapillary retinal nerve fibre layer thickness profile in subjects with myopia measured using the Stratus optical coherence tomography. Br J Ophthalmol. 2010;94(1):115–20.

Kim MJ, Jeoung JW, Park KH, Choi YJ, Kim DM. Topographic profiles of retinal nerve fiber layer defects affect the diagnostic performance of macular scans in preperimetric glaucoma. Invest Ophthalmol Vis Sci. 2014;55(4):2079–87.

Kim NR, Lim H, Kim JH, Rho SS, Seong GJ, Kim CY. Factors associated with false positives in retinal nerve fiber layer color codes from spectral-domain optical coherence tomography. Ophthalmology. 2011a;118(9):1774–81.

Kim NR, Lee ES, Seong GJ, et al. Comparing the ganglion cell complex and retinal nerve fibre layer measurements by Fourier domain OCT to detect glaucoma in high myopia. Br J Ophthalmol. 2011b;95(8):1115–21.

Kim YK, Yoo BW, Kim HC, Park KH. Automated detection of hemifield difference across horizontal raphe on ganglion cell-inner plexiform layer thickness map. Ophthalmology. 2015a;122(11):2252–60.

Kim YK, Yoo BW, Jeoung JW, Kim HC, Kim HJ, Park KH. Glaucoma-diagnostic ability of ganglion cell-inner plexiform layer thickness difference across temporal raphe in highly myopic eyes. Invest Ophthalmol Vis Sci. 2016;57(14):5856–63.

Kim YW, Park KH. Diagnostic accuracy of three-dimensional neuroretinal rim thickness for differentiation of myopic glaucoma from myopia. Invest Ophthalmol Vis Sci. 2018;59(8):3655–66.

Kim YW, Lee J, Kim JS, Park KH. Diagnostic accuracy of wide-field map from swept-source optical coherence tomography for primary open-angle glaucoma in myopic eyes. Am J Ophthalmol. 2020;218:182–91.

Knight OJ, Girkin CA, Budenz DL, Durbin MK, Feuer WJ. Effect of race, age, and axial length on optic nerve head parameters and retinal nerve fiber layer thickness measured by Cirrus HD-OCT. Arch Ophthalmol. 2012;130(3):312–8.

Lee EJ, Lee KM, Kim H, Kim TW. Glaucoma diagnostic ability of the new circumpapillary retinal nerve fiber layer thickness analysis based on Bruch's membrane opening. Invest Ophthalmol Vis Sci. 2016;57(10):4194–204.

Lee KH, Kim CY, Kim NR. Variations of retinal nerve fiber layer thickness and ganglion cell-inner plexiform layer thickness according to the torsion direction of optic disc. Invest Ophthalmol Vis Sci. 2014;55(2):1048–55.

Leung CK, Mohamed S, Leung KS, et al. Retinal nerve fiber layer measurements in myopia: an optical coherence tomography study. Invest Ophthalmol Vis Sci. 2006;47(12):5171–6.

Leung CK, Yu M, Weinreb RN, et al. Retinal nerve fiber layer imaging with spectral-domain optical coherence tomography: interpreting the RNFL maps in healthy myopic eyes. Invest Ophthalmol Vis Sci. 2012;53(11):7194–200.

Littmann H. Determination of the real size of an object on the fundus of the living eye. Klin Monatsbl Augenheilkd. 1982;180(4):286–9.

Malik R, Belliveau AC, Sharpe GP, Shuba LM, Chauhan BC, Nicolela MT. Diagnostic accuracy of optical coherence tomography and scanning laser tomography for identifying glaucoma in myopic eyes. Ophthalmology. 2016;123(6):1181–9.

Marsh BC, Cantor LB, WuDunn D, et al. Optic nerve head (ONH) topographic analysis by stratus OCT in normal subjects: correlation to disc size, age, and ethnicity. J Glaucoma. 2010;19(5):310–8.

Mohammad Salih PA. Evaluation of peripapillary retinal nerve fiber layer thickness in myopic eyes by spectral-domain optical coherence tomography. J Glaucoma. 2012;21(1):41–4.

Mwanza JC, Chang RT, Budenz DL, et al. Reproducibility of peripapillary retinal nerve fiber layer thickness and optic nerve head parameters measured with cirrus HD-OCT in glaucomatous eyes. Invest Ophthalmol Vis Sci. 2010;51(11):5724–30.

Mwanza JC, Oakley JD, Budenz DL, Anderson DR. Ability of cirrus HD-OCT optic nerve head parameters to discriminate normal from glaucomatous eyes. Ophthalmology. 2011;118(2):241–8.e1.

Mwanza JC, Durbin MK, Budenz DL, et al. Glaucoma diagnostic accuracy of ganglion cell-inner plexiform layer thickness: comparison with nerve fiber layer and optic nerve head. Ophthalmology. 2012;119(6):1151–8.

Nakanishi H, Akagi T, Hangai M, et al. Sensitivity and specificity for detecting early glaucoma in eyes with high myopia from normative database of macular ganglion cell complex thickness obtained from normal non-myopic or highly myopic Asian eyes. Graefes Arch Clin Exp Ophthalmol. 2015;253(7):1143–52.

Nakano N, Hangai M, Noma H, et al. Macular imaging in highly myopic eyes with and without glaucoma. Am J Ophthalmol. 2013;156(3):511–23.e6.

Oddone F, Lucenteforte E, Michelessi M, et al. Macular versus retinal nerve fiber layer parameters for diagnosing manifest glaucoma: a systematic review of diagnostic accuracy studies. Ophthalmology. 2016;123(5):939–49.

Ortega Jde L, Kakati B, Girkin CA. Artifacts on the optic nerve head analysis of the optical coherence tomography in glaucomatous and nonglaucomatous eyes. J Glaucoma. 2009;18(3):186–91.

Qiu KL, Zhang MZ, Leung CK, et al. Diagnostic classification of retinal nerve fiber layer measurement in myopic eyes: a comparison between time-domain and spectral-domain optical coherence tomography. Am J Ophthalmol. 2011;152(4):646–53.e2.

Ray R, Stinnett SS, Jaffe GJ. Evaluation of image artifact produced by optical coherence tomography of retinal pathology. Am J Ophthalmol. 2005;139(1):18–29.

Rebolleda G, Casado A, Oblanca N, Muñoz-Negrete FJ. The new Bruch's membrane opening – minimum rim width classification improves optical coherence tomography specificity in tilted discs. Clin Ophthalmol. 2016;10:2417–25.

Reis AS, Sharpe GP, Yang H, Nicolela MT, Burgoyne CF, Chauhan BC. Optic disc margin anatomy in patients with glaucoma and normal controls with spectral domain optical coherence tomography. Ophthalmology. 2012a;119(4):738–47.

Reis AS, O'Leary N, Yang H, et al. Influence of clinically invisible, but optical coherence tomography detected, optic disc margin anatomy on neuroretinal rim evaluation. Invest Ophthalmol Vis Sci. 2012b;53(4): 1852–60.

Sastre-Ibañez M, Martinez-de-la-Casa JM, Rebolleda G, et al. Utility of Bruch membrane opening-based optic nerve head parameters in myopic subjects. Eur J Ophthalmol. 2018;28(1):42–6.

Savini G, Zanini M, Carelli V, Sadun AA, Ross-Cisneros FN, Barboni P. Correlation between retinal nerve fibre layer thickness and optic nerve head size: an optical coherence tomography study. Br J Ophthalmol. 2005;89(4):489–92.

Savini G, Barboni P, Parisi V, Carbonelli M. The influence of axial length on retinal nerve fibre layer thickness and optic-disc size measurements by spectral-domain OCT. Br J Ophthalmol. 2012;96(1):57–61.

Seol BR, Jeoung JW, Park KH. Glaucoma detection ability of macular ganglion cell-inner plexiform layer thickness in myopic preperimetric glaucoma. Invest Ophthalmol Vis Sci. 2015;56(13):8306–13.

Seol BR, Kim DM, Park KH, Jeoung JW. Assessment of optical coherence tomography color probability codes in myopic glaucoma eyes after applying a myopic normative database. Am J Ophthalmol. 2017;183:147–55.

Shoji T, Sato H, Ishida M, Takeuchi M, Chihara E. Assessment of glaucomatous changes in subjects with high myopia using spectral domain optical coherence tomography. Invest Ophthalmol Vis Sci. 2011;52(2):1098–102.

Sung KR, Na JH, Lee Y. Glaucoma diagnostic capabilities of optic nerve head parameters as determined by Cirrus HD optical coherence tomography. J Glaucoma. 2012;21(7):498–504.

Suwan Y, Rettig S, Park SC, et al. Effects of circumpapillary retinal nerve fiber layer segmentation error correction on glaucoma diagnosis in myopic eyes. J Glaucoma. 2018;27(11):971–5.

Vernon SA, Rotchford AP, Negi A, Ryatt S, Tattersal C. Peripapillary retinal nerve fibre layer thickness in highly myopic Caucasians as measured by Stratus optical coherence tomography. Br J Ophthalmol. 2008;92(8):1076–80.

Wang G, Qiu KL, Lu XH, et al. The effect of myopia on retinal nerve fibre layer measurement: a comparative study of spectral-domain optical coherence tomography and scanning laser polarimetry. Br J Ophthalmol. 2011;95(2):255–60.

Wollstein G, Schuman JS, Price LL, et al. Optical coherence tomography (OCT) macular and peripapillary retinal nerve fiber layer measurements and automated visual fields. Am J Ophthalmol. 2004;138(2):218–25.

Zeimer R, Asrani S, Zou S, Quigley H, Jampel H. Quantitative detection of glaucomatous damage at the posterior pole by retinal thickness mapping. A pilot study. Ophthalmology. 1998;105(2):224–31.

Zheng F, Wu Z, Leung CKS. Detection of Bruch's membrane opening in healthy individuals and glaucoma patients with and without high myopia. Ophthalmology. 2018;125(10):1537–46.

Pitfalls in OCT Imaging

Eunoo Bak

Abstract

Optical coherence tomography (OCT)-based imaging of the optic nerve head, retinal nerve fiber layer, and the ganglion cell complex has become a key tool in the diagnosis and evaluation of glaucoma. The structural details available from OCT continue to improve with advances in technology. However, artifacts and misinterpretation of OCT still can lead to clinical misdiagnosis of glaucoma. Owing to the "floor effect" of retinal imaging, red and green disease may lead to erroneous results. Common OCT artifacts are classified as (1) patient-related factors (e.g., myopia, media opacities, vitreoretinal interface problems, optic nerve head pathologies, motion artifact, blink artifact); (2) instrument factors (e.g., poor image quality or device performance, inaccurate optic disc margin delineation, segmentation errors); and (3) operator factors (e.g., incorrect scan-circle placement, incorrect axial alignment). Understanding the potential limitations and pitfalls of each instrument is imperative in patient care.

Keywords

Glaucoma · Optical coherence tomography Artifact · Segmentation error · Red disease Green disease

1 Introduction

Optical coherence tomography (OCT) is a noninvasive imaging modality that has become a useful ancillary tool for diagnosis and monitoring of glaucoma. It is widely used by ophthalmologists worldwide in daily practice, and they are now basing their treatment plans on OCT results for early glaucoma patients and glaucoma suspects (Stein et al. 2012; Gabriele et al. 2011; Dong et al. 2016). Despite the improvements in OCT technology, the user must be able to accurately interpret the data and be aware of potential artifacts and limitations that can lead to a false-positive or false-negative diagnosis.

Previous studies with various Spectral-domain OCT (SD-OCT) instruments have reported that over a quarter of patients may have artifacts of the retinal nerve fiber layer (RNFL) and/or ganglion cell-inner plexiform layer (GCIPL) complex analysis (Giani et al. 2010; Sull et al. 2010). Errors either in data acquisition or software analysis may result in artifacts of RNFL measurements, which may lead to inaccurate clinical

E. Bak (✉)
Department of Ophthalmology, Seoul National University College of Medicine, Seoul, Korea

Department of Ophthalmology, Seoul National University Hospital, Seoul, Korea
e-mail: eunoobak@snu.ac.kr

K. H. Park, T.-W. Kim (eds.), *OCT Imaging in Glaucoma*,
https://doi.org/10.1007/978-981-16-1178-0_9

assessment. It takes time for users to understand the potential limitations and pitfalls of OCT. Regardless, understanding these limitations and being able to distinguish artifacts from true disease are imperative in patient care and can prevent further unnecessary, expensive investigations.

This chapter is devoted to the common artifacts affecting OCT that can lead to diagnostic errors.

2 Causes and Classification of OCT Artifacts

2.1 Floor Effect

In retinal imaging, the "floor effect" is defined as the point at which no further structural damage can be detected. Given this effect, OCT measurements are less useful for measuring tissue thickness in cases of advanced disease (Mwanza et al. 2015), possibly due to the presence of residual tissue (e.g., glial cells, blood vessels, nonfunctioning ganglion cell axons) or failure of tissue segmentation algorithms (i.e., artifactual floor) (Asrani et al. 2014). Thus, even though an advanced disease may be progressing, it is often challenging to detect identifiable changes with OCT. Disease monitoring in these eyes should not depend solely on optical imaging but must rely on standard automated perimetry or other visual function tests.

2.2 Red and Green Disease

Red and green are the main colors used in the OCT platforms to indicate that the results are within normal limits (within the 5–95% prediction interval) or abnormal (less than 1% prediction interval) when compared with the normative database. "Red disease" is a false-positive diagnosis, where the software mistakenly identifies an eye as abnormal even though there is no glaucomatous damage (Asrani et al. 2014; Chong and Lee 2012). In contrast, "green disease" is a false-negative diagnosis, when the software interprets actual glaucomatous damage as normal (Sayed et al. 2017). Green disease artifacts can present as the result of the averaging of sectors that include a subtle notch in the RNFL, or an RNFL defect in an eye that started with a high value of RNFL thickness. In addition, RNFL can become thicker in eyes with RNFL edema, which can mask RNFL thinning (Moore et al. 2015). Clinicians therefore should not rely solely on the color scheme to interpret an OCT report. Also, they are encouraged to keep in mind that the red and green colors in OCT evaluations depend on the normative database of the manufacturer, which commonly includes only 300–500 patients. Depending on the manufacturer, these normative databases mostly do not include children, high refractive error, diverse races, or corrections for such variations. This may lead to erroneous results for some patient groups.

2.3 Classification of OCT Artifacts in Optic Disc Scan Analysis

The rates, types, and causes of OCT artifacts can vary according to the methods used for their definition and classification. OCT artifacts are classified as follows: (1) patient-related factors, (2) instrument factors, and (3) operator factors (Asrani et al. 2014; Han and Jaffe 2010). If no definite patient-related artifact is identified and the artifacts did not show any association with the operator, the cause of the artifact can be classified as an instrument error. However, there is a large overlap among these categories (i.e., scan artifacts often result from a combination of patient-related, instrument, and operator factors).

3 Patient-Related Factors

These are the most common causes and most confusing artifacts. It is common to see red areas in the results of a reliable good-quality OCT scan in a routine eye exam performed on a healthy person with no ocular disease. Some of these patients are diagnosed with glaucoma and start on medical therapy. The person diagnosed requires lifelong treatment and follow-up, which leads to a psychological burden both to the patient and the family. In order to avoid misinforming patients, ophthalmologists must be able to differentiate among the common artifacts and anatomical variants that can lead to errors on OCT reports.

3.1 Split Bundle

In the majority of individuals, the superior and inferior poles of the optic nerve head receive the largest number of retinal ganglion cell axons in the form of two thick bundles. This configuration is the basis for the color-coded normative database comparisons of temporal–superior–nasal–inferior–temporal (TSNIT) profiles. In some individuals, the superior and/or inferior RNFL bundles are divided in two and enter the optic disc in the form of a pair of separate bundles each, thus masquerading as a local RNFL defect. This is called a split RNFL, which is an anatomical variant rather than an imaging artifact (Kaliner et al. 2007; Colen and Lemij 2001) (Fig. 1). This finding is one of the most common reasons for red disease in younger patients with good-quality OCT scans. A careful evaluation of the RNFL TSNIT profiles, lack of optic nerve head parameter abnormalities, normal macular ganglion cell analysis, and typical split RNFL images on RNFL thickness maps are important clues for correct diagnosis.

3.2 Myopia

Myopic eyes with longer axial length are associated with a higher percentage of abnormal diagnostic classifications, because the RNFL normative databases are typically adjusted only by age and not by axial length or refractive error (Qiu et al. 2011; Yoo et al. 2012). The normal population database used by the manufacturer specifically excludes subjects with high refractive error, which usually encompasses spherical equivalents between −5.00 and +5.00.

The overall RNFL thickness in high-myopic refractive error, typically with longer axial length, is thinner compared with the normal population (Budenz et al. 2007; Kang et al. 2010; Leung et al. 2006; Savini et al. 2012; Wang et al. 2011). In addition, hyperopia and shorter axial eye lengths show increases in RNFL thickness (Savini et al. 2012). These findings are attributed to the ocular magnification effects of axial eye length. When adjusting for ocular magnification, the negative correlation between these OCT measurements and both axial eye length and refractive error is removed (Savini et al. 2012; Leung et al. 2007). Moreover, the effects of axial-length magnification remain in patients who have undergone refractive surgery and cataract operation. When their axial eye length is unknown and their preoperative status is unrecognized, incorrect interpretation of OCT may result. Because most current OCT machines do not account for ocular magnification, patients with long or short axial eye lengths will have artificially low or high OCT measurements, respectively, when compared with the normative database. If the axial eye length is known, the OCT measurements can be corrected with the modified Littmann formula, as described by Bennet et al. (1994). However, in pathological myopia, true retinal thinning, such as myopic retinal schisis affecting the peripapillary RNFL thickness, may be present.

In addition to the changes of overall RNFL thickness, the peaks on the TSNIT RNFL thickness plot are shifted temporally toward the fovea in myopes relative to the general population (Kang et al. 2010; Hong et al. 2010; Hwang et al. 2012; Yamashita et al. 2014) (Fig. 2). Due to the more temporal shift of the RNFL peaks in myopia, the temporal RNFL thickness may be elevated, and the superior and inferior RNFL thicknesses may be reported as decreased (Wang et al. 2011; Yamashita et al. 2013). In other words, the thickness of RNFL bundles is normal, but with an abnormal topographic position. Hong et al. stated that RNFL peaks may deviate in normal individuals, leading to red disease artifacts, which have been associated with myopia and increased axial length (Hong et al. 2010). Hood

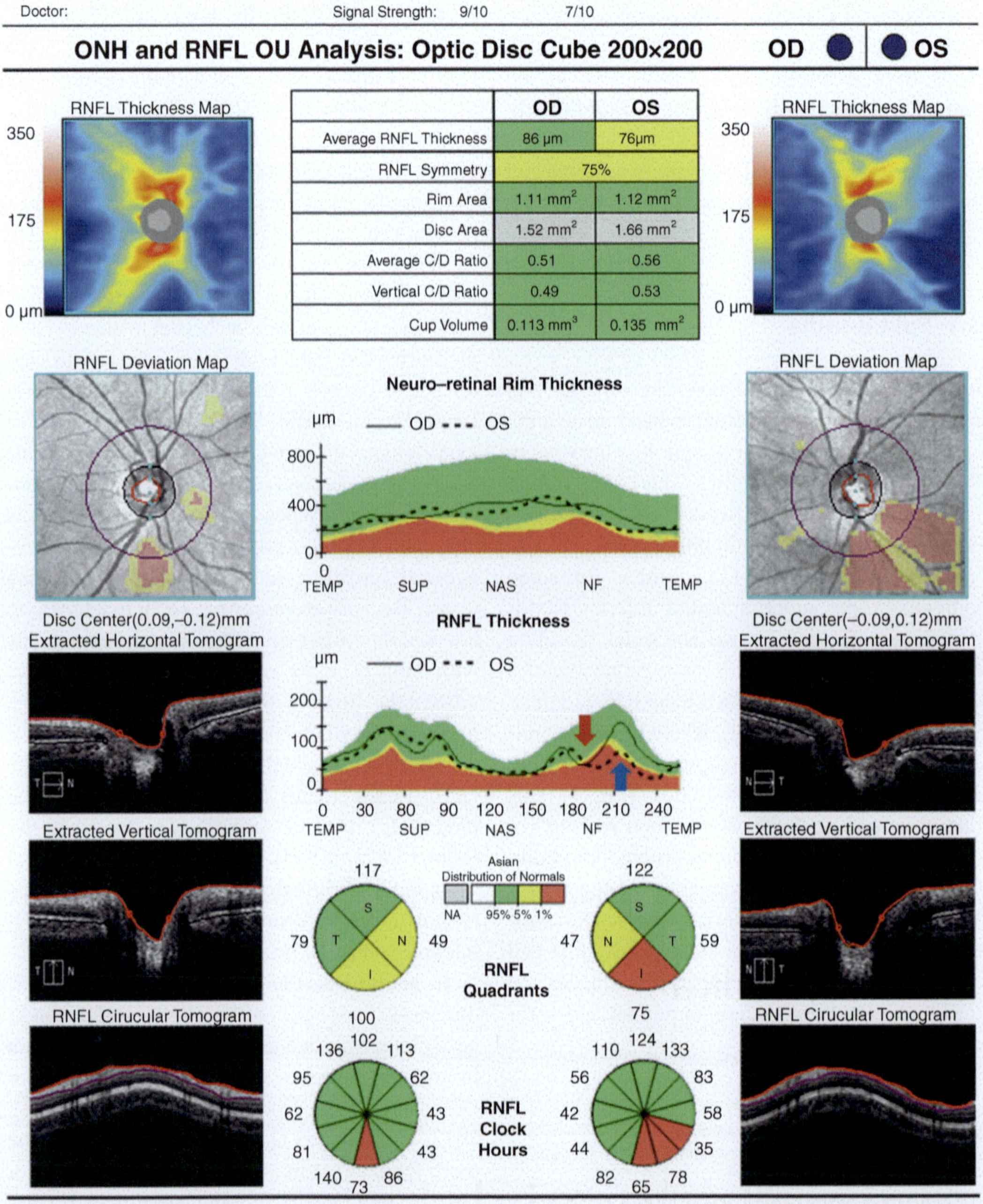

Fig. 1 Inferior RNFL bundle of right eye showing split RNFL defect. On the TSNIT profile, the inferior vertex is split into two peaks separated by a valley (red arrow). The left eye shows a glaucomatous RNFL defect in the infero-temporal area (blue arrow)

et al. (2010) stated that the positions of RNFL peaks on TSNIT graphs are in the same regions as major retinal vessels. Careful examination of the RNFL TSNIT profile and major retinal vessels, as combined with the optic nerve head parameters and macular scan results, is important for the recognition of these anomalies.

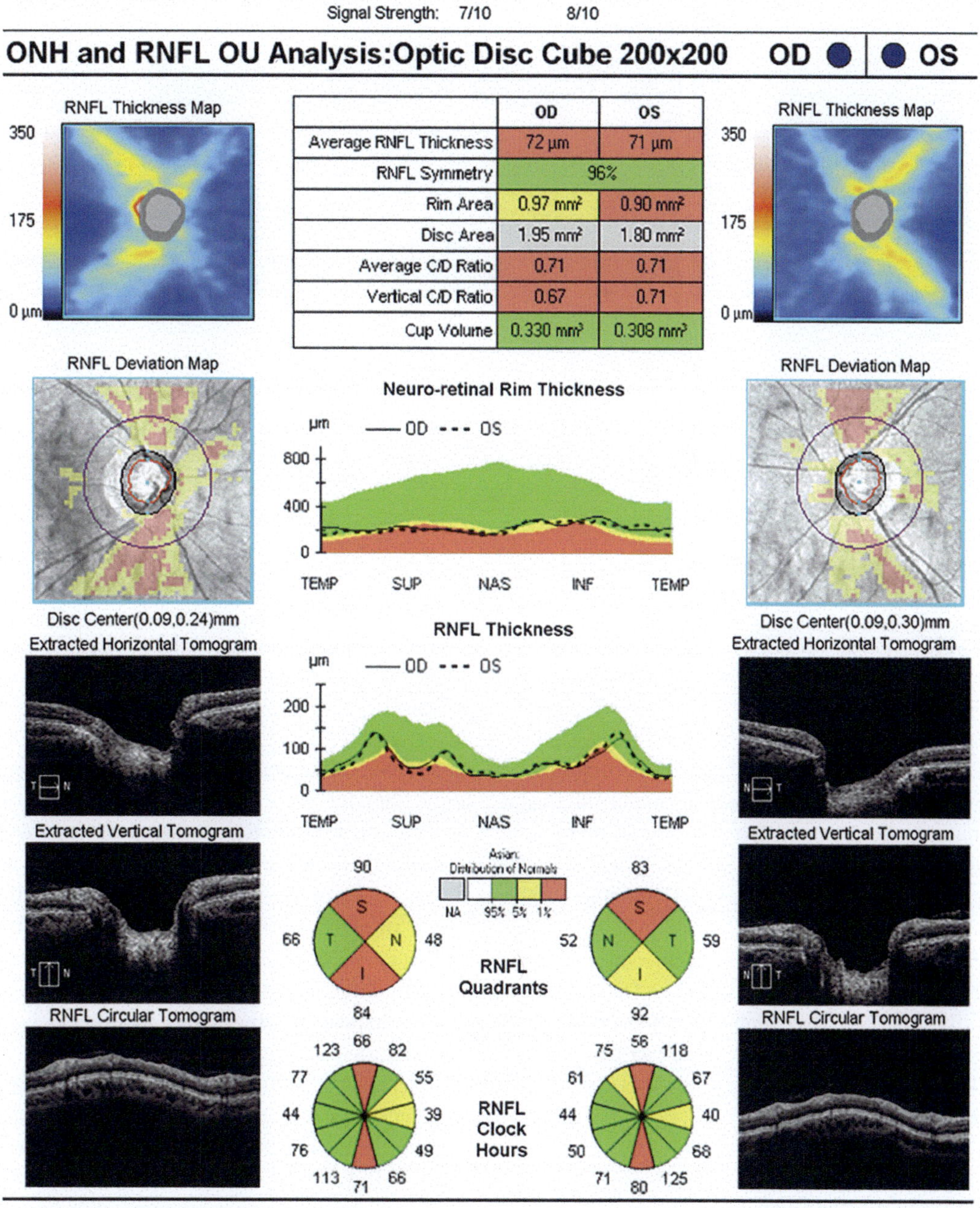

Fig. 2 Low values of RNFL thickness in nasal sectors on TSNIT profile of myopic patient due to temporal displacement of RNFL peaks. This occurred because the peaks did not align with the expected positions in the TSNIT graphs based on the normative database

3.3 Peripapillary Atrophy

Peripapillary atrophy, which frequently accompanies myopia, is another cause of OCT segmentation error (Fig. 3). This is clinically important, because peripapillary atrophy is found commonly in glaucoma patients (Jonas et al. 1989). Peripapillary atrophy occurs mostly with time-

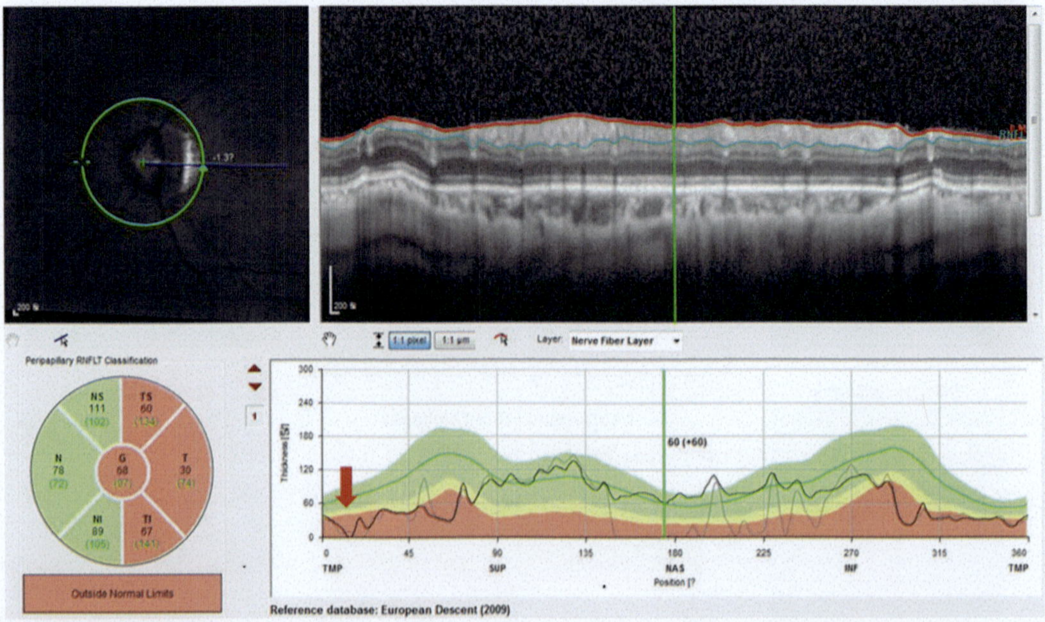

Fig. 3 Section seen to be passing through the area of peripapillary atrophy on careful examination of regions covered by peripapillary scanning ring (normally 3.46 mm in diameter). The segmentation error resulted from the passage of the scanning ring over an atrophic area in the temporal quadrant. The values on the TSNIT profile are zero in that area (red arrow)

domain OCT (TD-OCT), due to the inability of the segmentation software to accurately align and register the A scans along the retinal pigmented epithelial border, which adversely affects segmentation of the retinal layers (Kim et al. 2012). Fortunately, with the advent of the newer SD-OCT, the inaccuracy of segmentation caused by peripapillary atrophy with TD-OCT is markedly reduced. Also, along with the presence of peripapillary staphyloma, there can be localized RNFL thinning depending on the size of the lesion (Fig. 4).

3.4 Media Opacity

Media opacities (e.g., dry eye, corneal opacity, cataract, and vitreous opacity) are the most common cause of artifacts in elderly patients (Fig. 5). They reduce signal strength and compromise retinal layer segmentation (Cheung et al. 2008; Vizzeri et al. 2009). In healthy patients analyzed with Stratus OCT, a positive linear relationship between signal strength and mean RNFL thickness has been reported. It was found that for each unit of decrease in signal strength, the average RNFL thickness had a corresponding decrease of 2 mm (Vizzeri et al. 2009). Also, in the Cirrus platform, once the signal strength drops below a value of 7, the segmentation algorithm can sometimes fail and produce large regional errors in the derived RNFL thickness. Other OCT platforms have similar signal strength measurements.

The presence of vitreous opacities in the scanning area can cause imaging artifacts, often leading to red disease and sometimes to green disease. It can also cause the device to incorrectly detect the disc center, resulting in scanning of the wrong area. Focal media opacities, such as posterior vitreous detachment and hemorrhage, can cause a focal loss of signal strength, giving a false appearance of local areas of RNFL drop out that can lower the average RNFL thickness or artificially create segmental areas of thinning. Careful inspection of the RNFL thickness map, the deviation map, and the TSNIT graph can help clinicians identify this type of artifact.

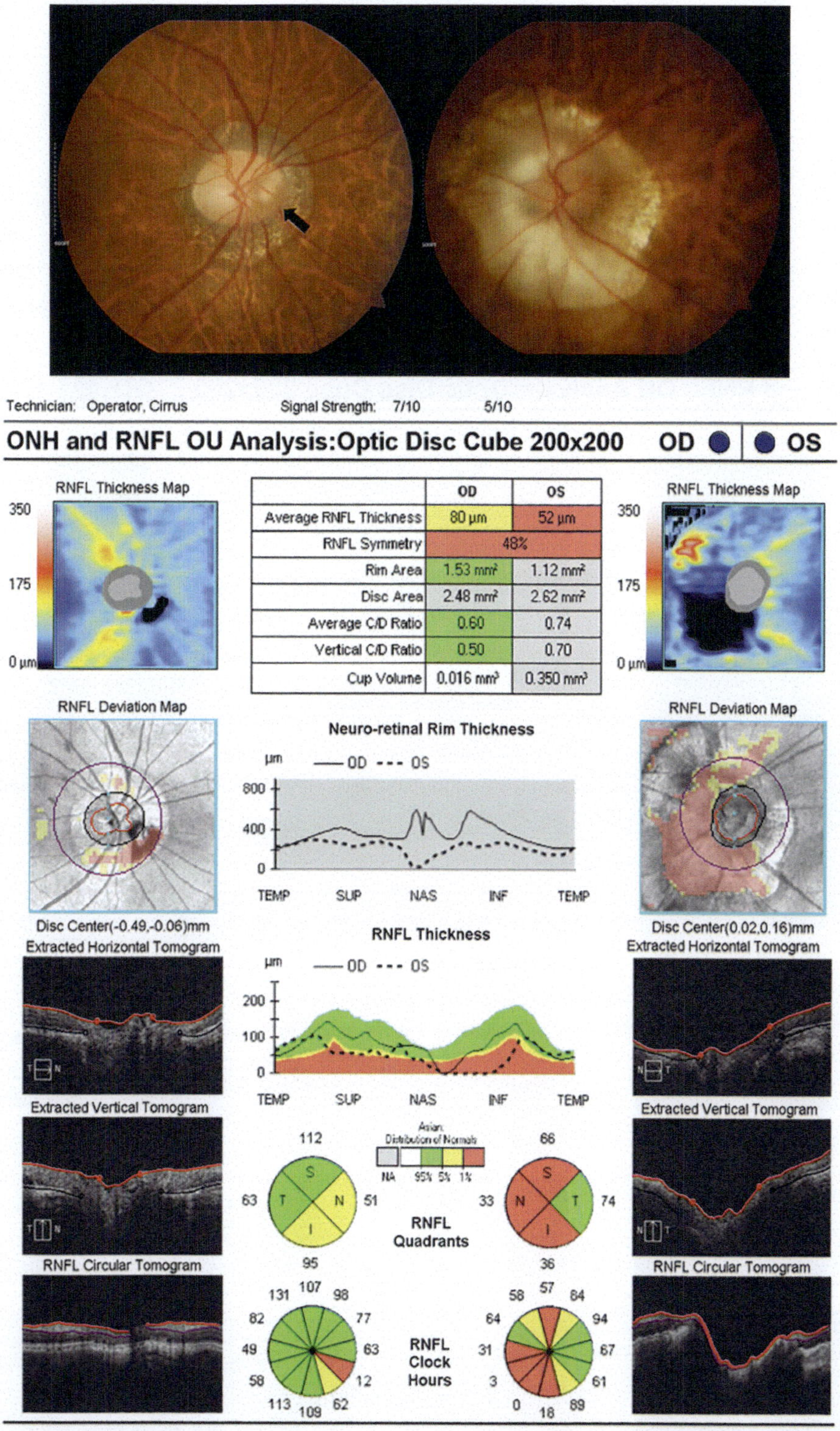

Fig. 4 Peripapillary staphyloma apparent in the left eye. The values on the TSNIT profile are zero in the region with segmentation error. The position of the Weiss ring in the right eye coincides with the RNFL calculation circle in the inferior quadrant in the right eye (black arrow). In cases where the Weiss ring blocks part of the calculation circle, it can affect the TSNIT graph and all of the pie charts

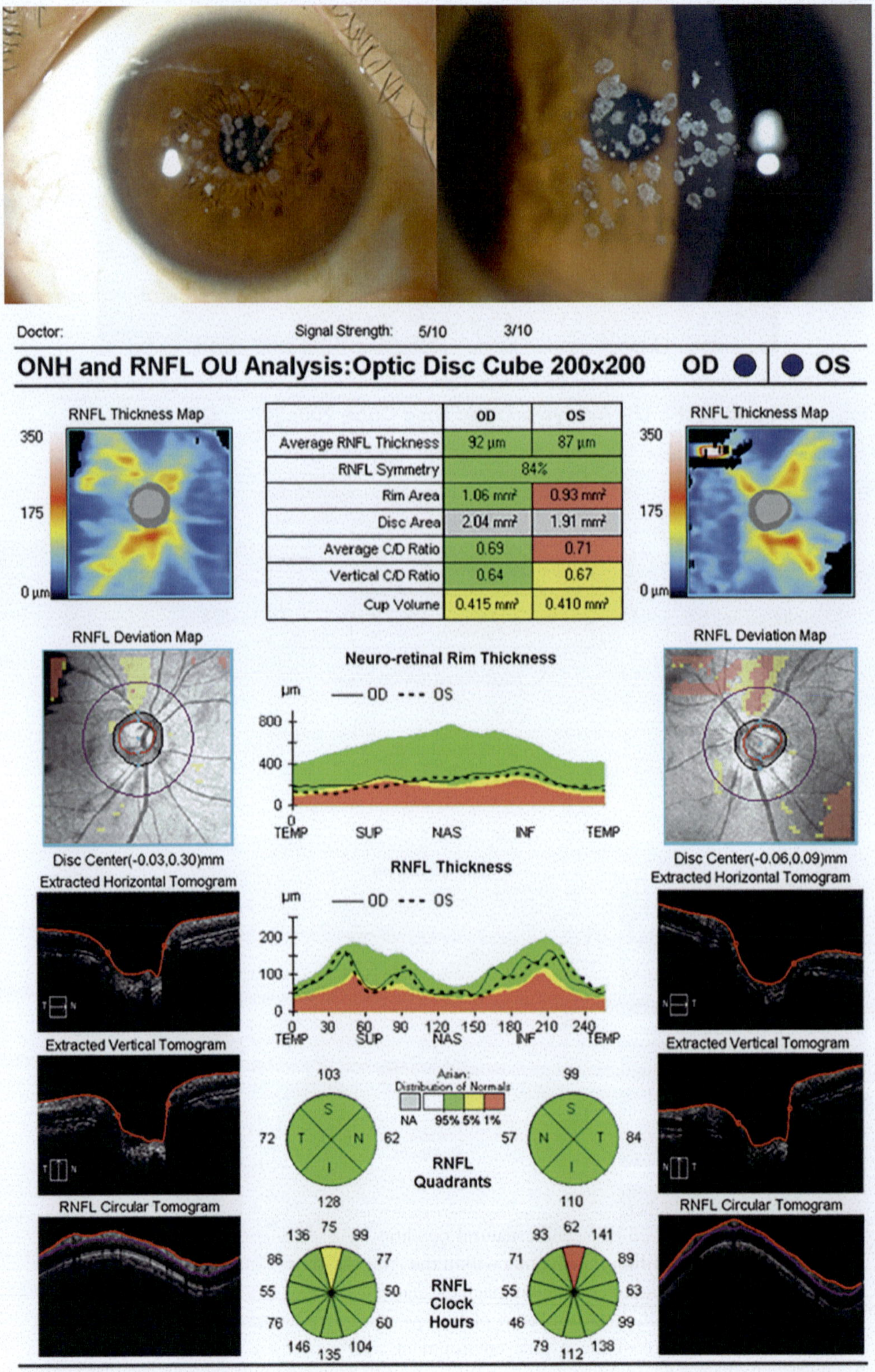

Fig. 5 OCT scan with low signal strength and multiple artifacts for both eyes diagnosed with Avellino corneal dystrophy. Note that the signal strength is 5 on the right and 3 on the left. The interpreter needs to recognize this kind of artifact on the RNFL thickness map as an area of scanning failure or block

3.4.1 Dry Eye and Cataract

Glaucoma, dry eye, and cataract frequently coexist, due to their prevalence in aging populations (Congdon et al. 2004; Weinreb et al. 2014). In addition, ocular surface diseases such as dry eye syndrome are common in patients using topical ocular hypotensive drugs (Anwar et al. 2013). OCT studies have shown that these diminish the scan quality index and decrease RNFL thickness measures (Stein et al. 2006; Mwanza et al. 2011; Bambo et al. 2014). Patients are commonly instructed not to blink during camera alignment and scan acquisition; however, this may cause tear film evaporation and breakup, particularly in patients with preexisting ocular surface disorders. Patients should be encouraged to blink a few times immediately before scan capture to ensure uniform tear film distribution and to preserve adequate scan quality. This may also improve patient comfort, thus decreasing the likelihood of blink or motion artifacts during scan acquisition.

Cataracts are one of the most common causes of low-quality scans (Fig. 6). To obtain acceptable image quality, fine adjustments of the camera alignment may be attempted to purposely redirect the light beam through the areas of least opacity. Unfortunately, the detrimental effects of cataracts on OCT scan quality are difficult to overcome, unless cataract surgery is performed (Mwanza et al. 2011; Savini et al. 2006). Multifocal lenses may affect the quality of the OCT scan, leading to wavy horizontal artifacts (Inoue et al. 2009). How these artifacts affect RNFL measurements remains to be seen, but nonetheless, it is an important factor to consider as increasing numbers of patients receive multifocal lens implants.

3.4.2 Weiss Ring

Floating vitreous opacities, most commonly such as Weiss rings, can manifest and disappear on different scans as their position changes with eye movements. As the Weiss ring moves in front of the retina, it blocks the OCT signal in different areas of the optic nerve head or retina on different scans (Fig. 4). It can cause red disease artifacts, even when not overlying the calculation circle. Additionally, it may cause green disease artifacts located over the optic nerve.

3.5 Vitreoretinal Interface Problems

A prominent vitreoretinal interface opacity can cause errors in the segmentation of RNFL thickness. OCT algorithms attempt to identify the internal limiting membrane as the upper boundary of the RNFL. Occasionally a prominent vitreous opacity will be incorrectly identified as the internal limiting membrane, which will result in an artifactually thickened RNFL measurement.

3.5.1 Peripapillary Vitreoretinal Traction

Vitreoretinal traction can result in an artificially high increase of RNFL thickness and may lead thereby to green disease artifact. This situation can occur when posterior vitreous detachment is developing or be due to posterior hyaloid thickening. Segmentation errors may also occur as the results of the presented average RNFL thickness values being much higher than expected (Figs. 7 and 8). Unless details of the vitreous interface with the internal limiting membrane are visible, a potential area of artifact could easily be overlooked. If the vitreous completely separates from the retina, RNFL thickness may decrease significantly and reveal the actual extent of RNFL loss. Clinicians should be careful not to interpret the reduction of RNFL thickness upon release of vitreoretinal traction as structural glaucoma progression.

3.5.2 Epiretinal Membrane

Epiretinal membrane can also cause artificially high RNFL thickness measurements and result in green disease (Asrani et al. 2014). The software algorithm identifies the upper boundary of the epiretinal membrane as that of the upper edge of the RNFL or as the internal limiting membrane of the retina, leading to erroneous measurements (Figs. 8 and 9). It is easily visible with SD-OCT machines that show the details of the vitreous-

a

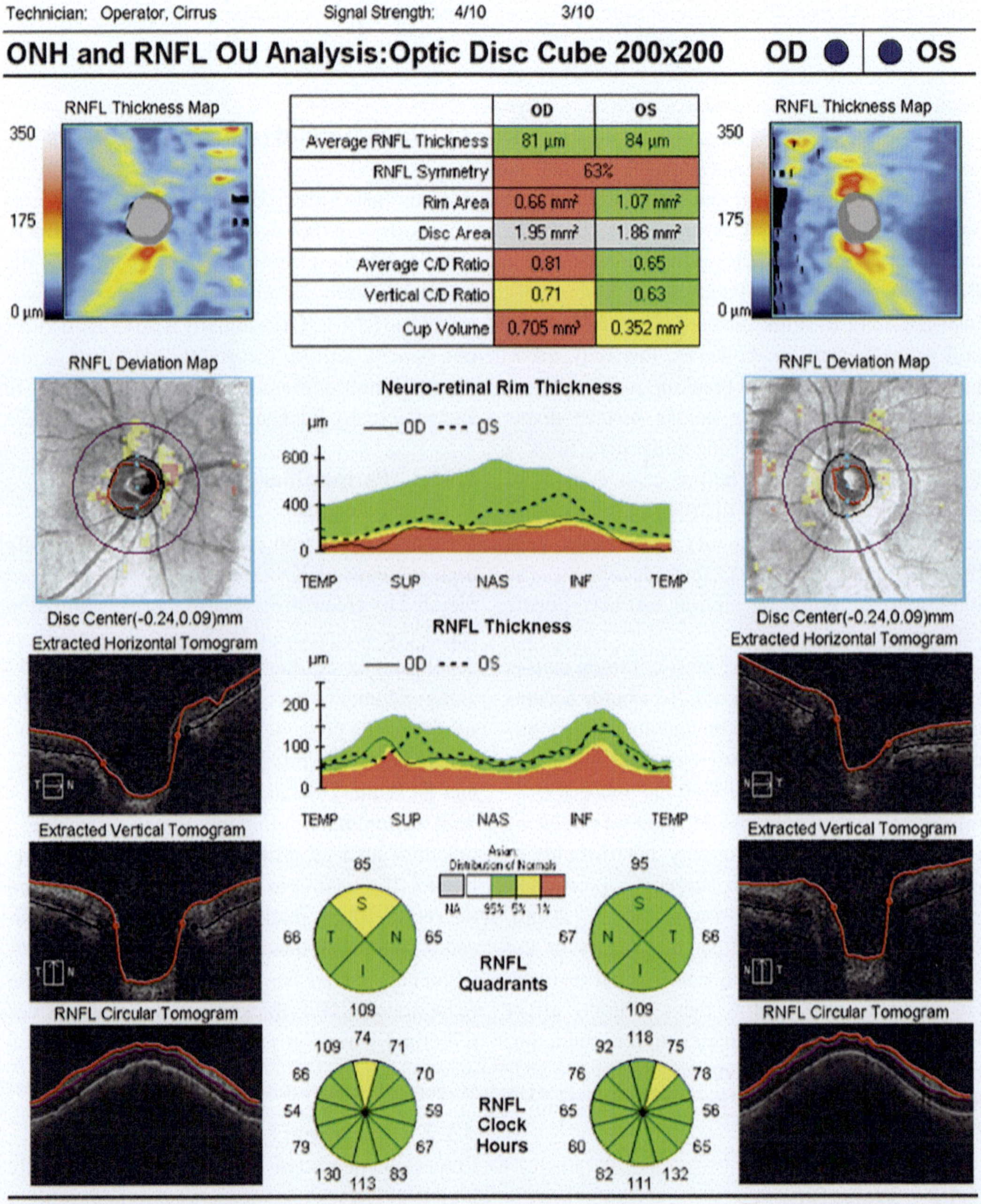

Fig. 6 (**a**) Very poor-quality Cirrus HD-OCT scan in a patient with bilateral cataract. Note the low signal strength values of 4 on the right eye and 3 on the left eye. The patient's cataract prevented a good-quality scan, and the RNFL thickness map shows areas that were not scanned (black areas on the RNFL thickness map). The TSNIT profile, quadrant and clock-hour graphs also show mild thinning caused by poor image quality. (**b**) Cirrus HD-OCT of the same patient after bilateral cataract surgery. Now the signal strength is 7 in both eyes, and the RNFL thickness maps are free of artifacts. The TSNIT profile, quadrant and clock-hour graphs show less damage after cataract removal

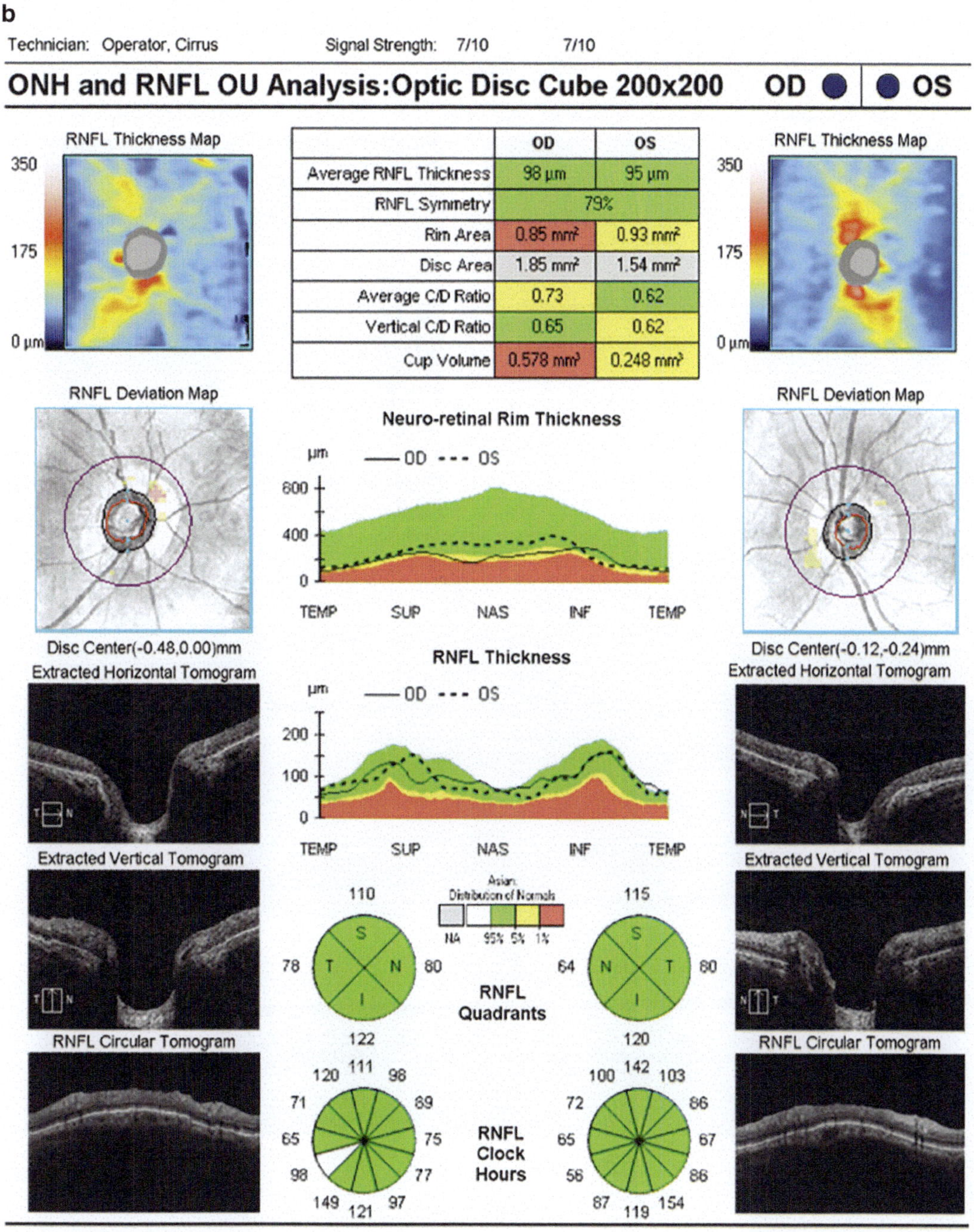

Fig. 6 (continued)

internal limiting membrane interface. The presence of an epiretinal membrane in a macular thickness scan should alert the physician to the possibility of an artifact on the RNFL scan.

3.5.3 Peripapillary Retinoschisis

Peripapillary retinoschisis is characterized by splitting of the peripapillary RNFL. It has been described in patients with different types of

a

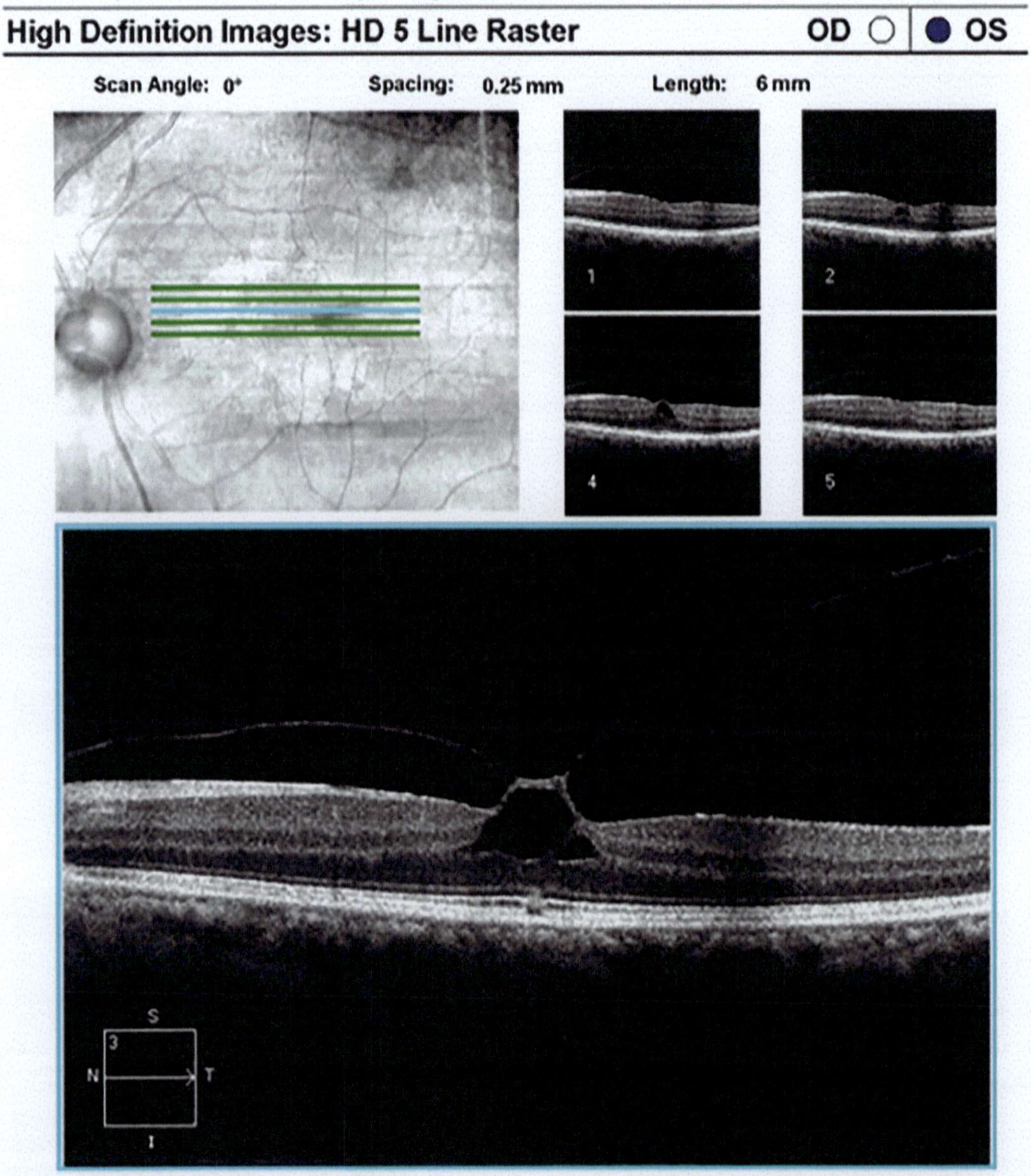

Fig. 7 (**a**) Cirrus HD-OCT demonstrating vitreoretinal traction in the left eye. (**b**) Areas of vitreous RNFL adhesions lead to tractions and artificial thickening of RNFL on the RNFL thickness map (red arrows)

b

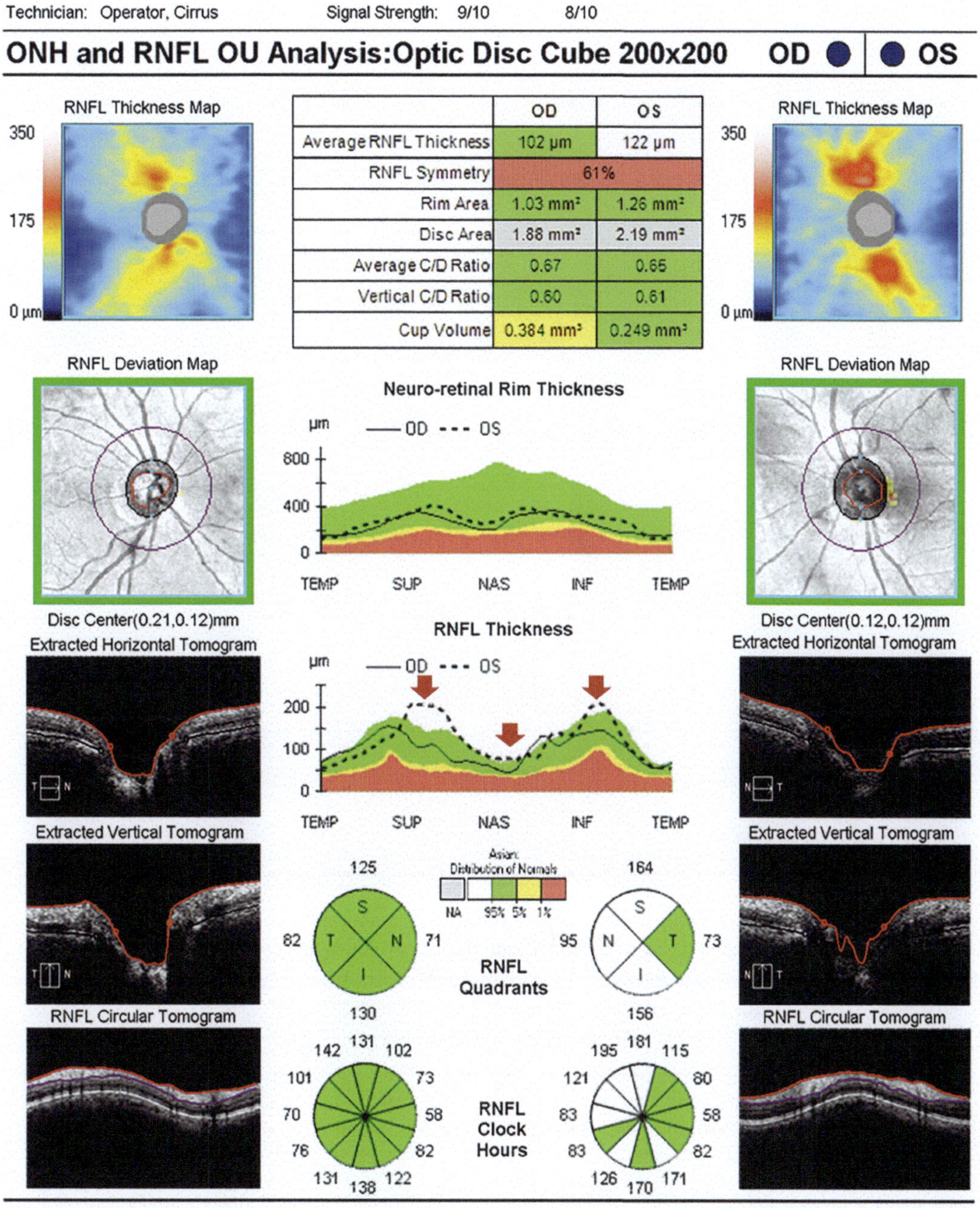

Fig. 7 (continued)

glaucoma, including primary open-angle glaucoma, angle-closure glaucoma, and pseudoexfoliation glaucoma (Zhao and Li 2011; Hollander et al. 2005; Kahook et al. 2007; Örnek et al. 2013). Temporary increase in RNFL thickness measurements is found in eyes with peripapillary retinoschisis, and after resolution of the retinoschisis, RNFL thickness may decrease remarkably (Hwang et al. 2014; Bayraktar et al. 2016) (Fig. 10). If a clinician simply looks at the mea-

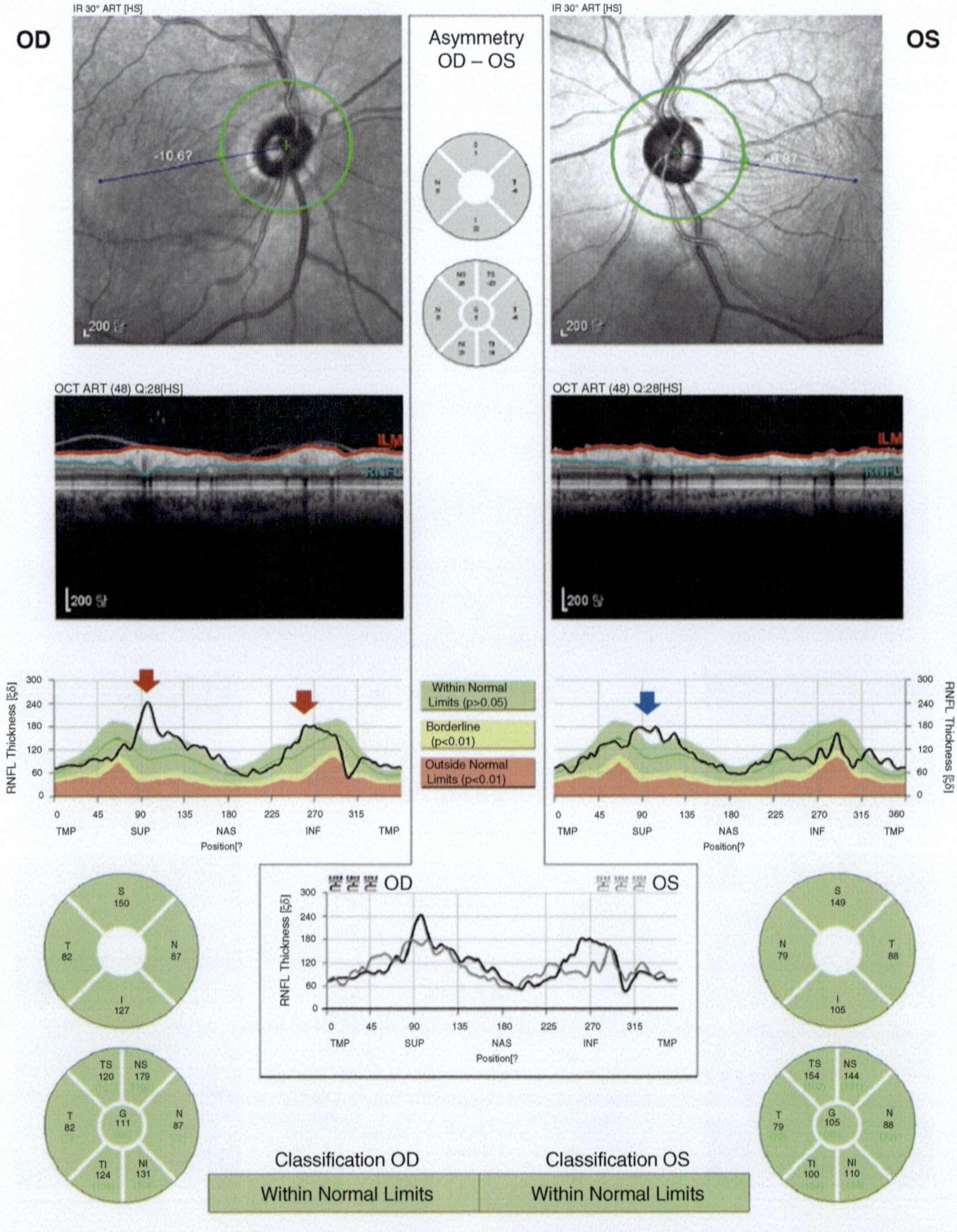

Fig. 8 Spectralis OCT demonstrating vitreoretinal traction in the right eye and epiretinal membrane in the left eye. In the right eye, the areas of vitreous RNFL adhesions lead to tractions and artificial thickening of the RNFL (red arrows). In the left eye, the software algorithm has misidentified the boundary of the epiretinal membrane as the upper edge of the RNFL, leading to an erroneously elevated RNFL measure in that region (blue arrow)

surement data without noticing the retinoschisis, such a decrease may be considered to be a rapid progression of glaucoma. Clinicians should examine thickness maps as well as horizontal B-scans in order to detect retinoschisis, so as not to overestimate RNFL thickness or misinterpret the resolution of retinoschisis as rapid structural progression.

3.5.4 Edema of Retina

Edema of the retina can have a large effect on the signal strength of the layers under it and, thus too, on the accuracy of segmentation by OCT. Green disease may appear in the form of thinning in certain sectors in eyes with very high RNFL thickness values. In diabetic macular edema, RNFL thickness measurements may be high due to the retinal edema, despite the fact that the presence of glaucomatous damage and green classification in these sectors may obscure the glaucomatous damage (Fig. 11). Also, edema caused by uveitis or age-related macular degeneration may mask glaucomatous RNFL thinning, thus leading to green disease (Moore et al. 2015). In peripapillary retinoschisis, there is a temporary increase in RNFL thickness, the values returning to normal after its resolution (Bayraktar et al. 2016; Hwang et al. 2011).

3.6 Optic Nerve Head Pathologies

In addition to the aforementioned diseases, optic nerve head pathologies can make segmentation inaccurate in the RNFL thickness plot and optic nerve head. Failed segmentation can often be identified as an area of absolute loss in the Cirrus RNFL deviation map that does not follow the normal arcuate pathway of the RNFL. Errors in segmentation can also be seen by examining the TSNIT RNFL thickness plot, which is available on most commercially available OCT displays (Fig. 12). Also, the segmentation algorithm may report a disc area

a

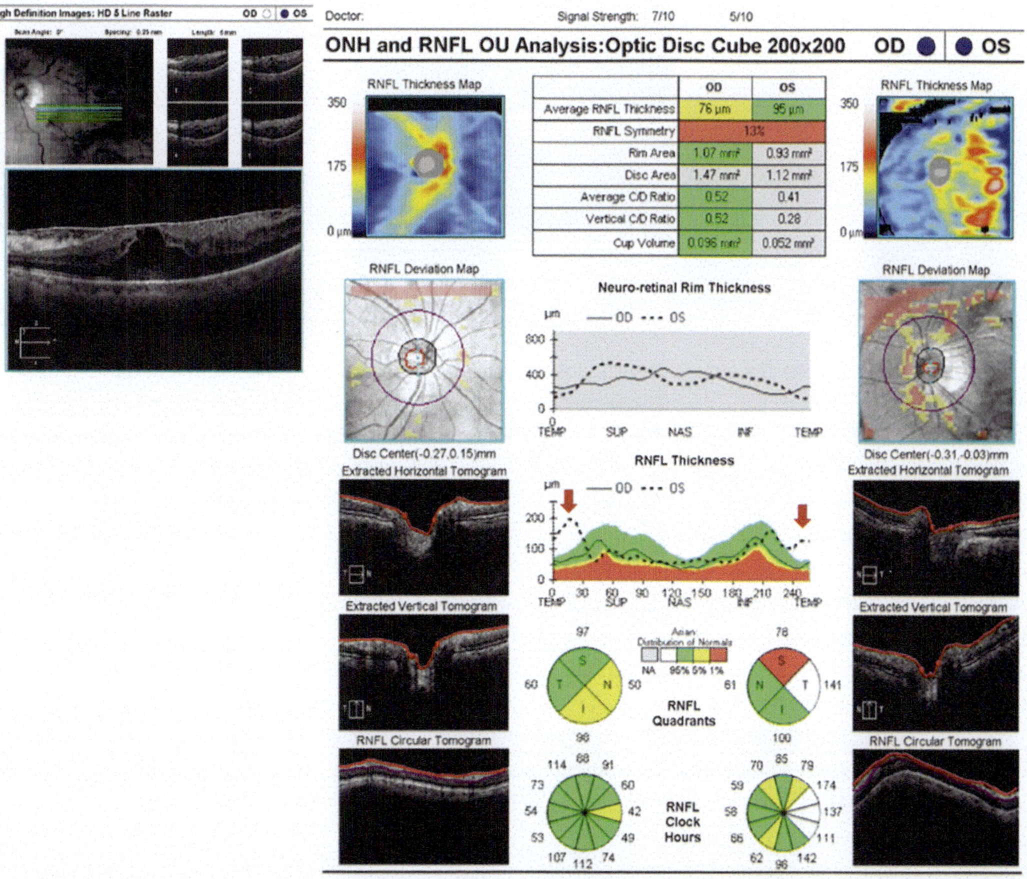

Fig. 9 (**a**) Cirrus HD-OCT demonstrating epiretinal membrane in the left eye. Multiple segmentation errors are present and the thickness of the RNFL in the temporal quadrant is increased. This was most likely caused by the traction forces on the retina. (**b**) Cirrus HD-OCT of the same patient after epiretinal membrane removal surgery. The RNFL thickness of the temporal quadrant is within normal range

b

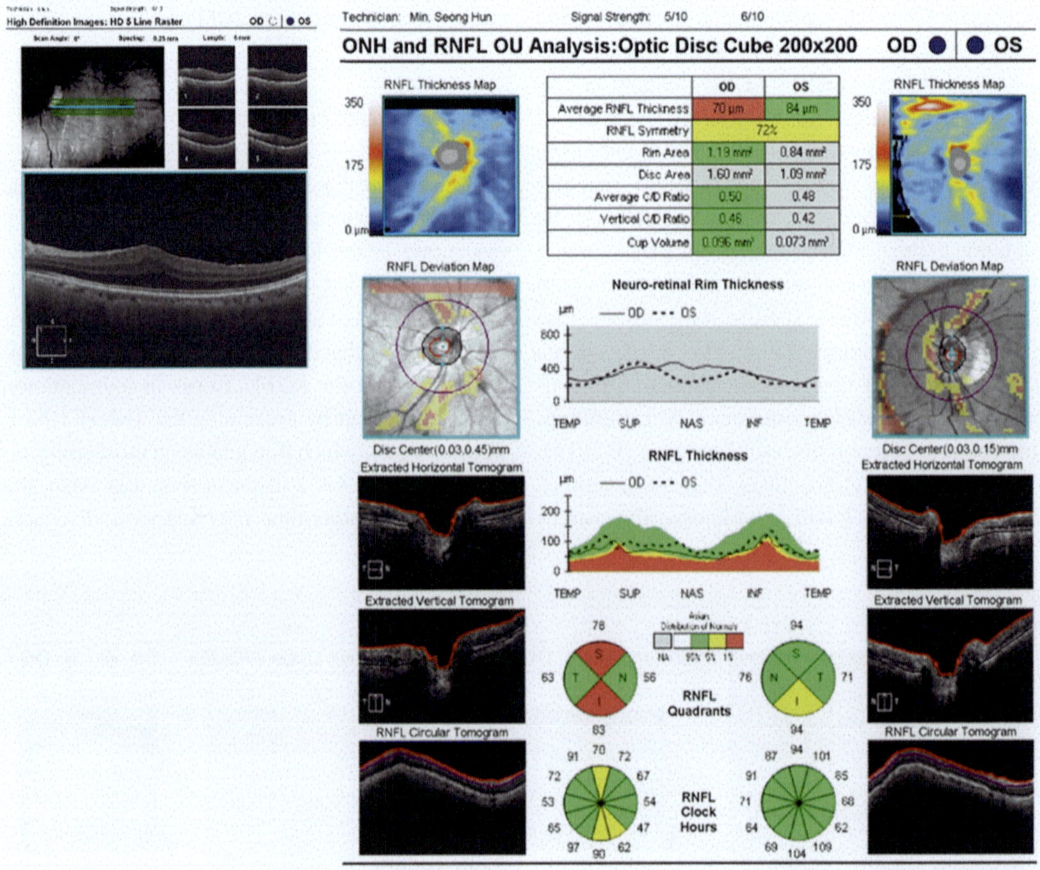

Fig. 9 (continued)

larger than its true size because the termination point of the Bruch's membrane and its termination at the neural canal opening are inaccurately located more proximally (Chen and Kardon 2016). In the case of an oversized optic nerve head, the peripapillary RNFL scanning ring will pass close to the disc margin, leading to inaccurate results (Bayer and Akman 2020). Errors in the determination of the border of the neural canal (disc area) will adversely affect the determination of the location and area of the rim as well as the cup-to-disc ratio.

In optic nerve head drusen, the cup area or volume is very small or at a value near zero despite a normal disc size. Also, neuroretinal rim thickness above the normal values is conspicuous. The presence of a myelinated nerve fiber layer can also lead to an increase in RNFL thickness that can lead in turn to overestimation of the number of axons in the corresponding location. Thickly myelinated nerve fibers can hide glaucomatous RNFL loss and may cause inaccurate segmentation and green disease. Again, in such cases, the peripapillary scan should be repeated with a larger ring diameter, or alternatively, macular and optic nerve head analyses should be performed.

In eyes with optic nerve head pathologies, it can be very difficult to isolate the glaucomatous damage by structural or functional tests. Progression analysis can be beneficial if there is suspicion or diagnosis of glaucoma; however, it should be noted that optic nerve head pathologies such as optic disc drusen itself may also cause progressive RNFL and visual field losses in a manner similar to glaucoma (Savino et al. 1979; Roh et al. 1998).

3.7 Pupil Size

Small pupil size may potentially reduce the amount and quality of the signal detected by

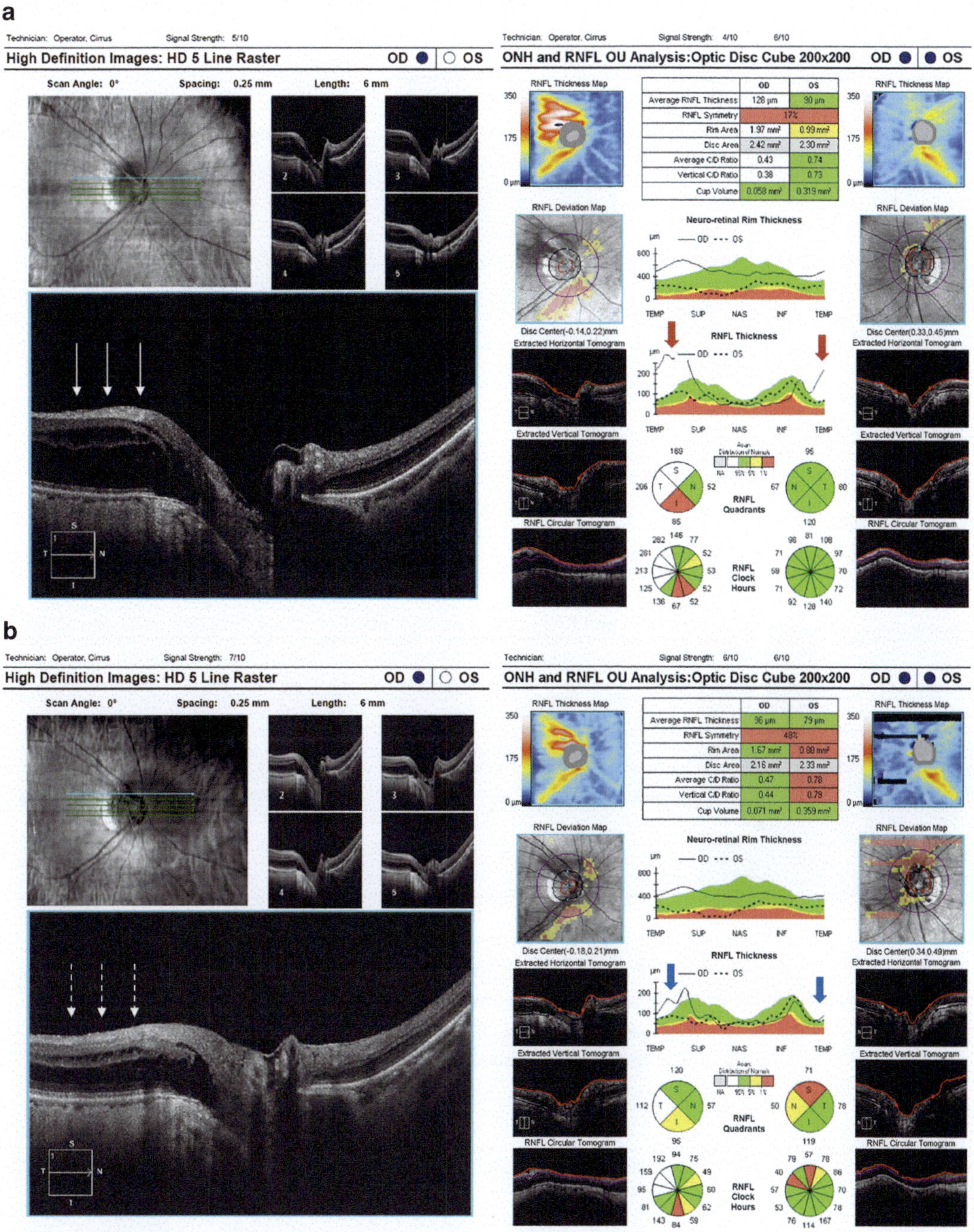

Fig. 10 (**a**) Peripapillary retinoschisis observed in the right eye (white arrows). The RNFL thickness curve is well above the expected values in the location corresponding to the region of retinoschisis. (**b**) Two years later, the extension of retinoschisis has become smaller (white dotted arrows). A remarkable decrease in the RNFL thickness in the superior and temporal areas also can be seen (blue arrows). (**c**) Guided progression analysis map showing progressive RNFL loss that can be misinterpreted as structural progression of glaucoma

c

Guided Progression Analysis: (GPA ™)

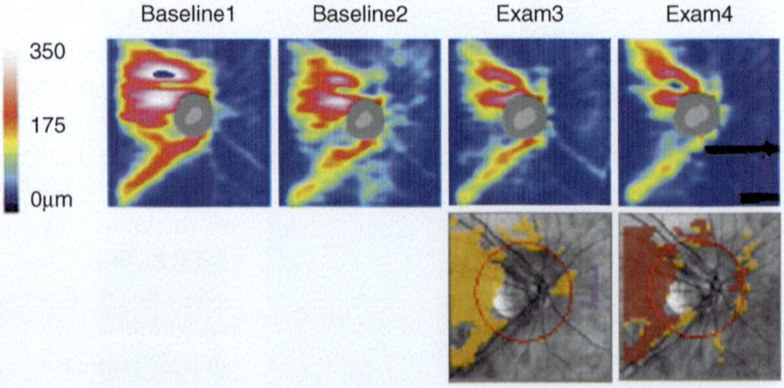

Fig. 10 (continued)

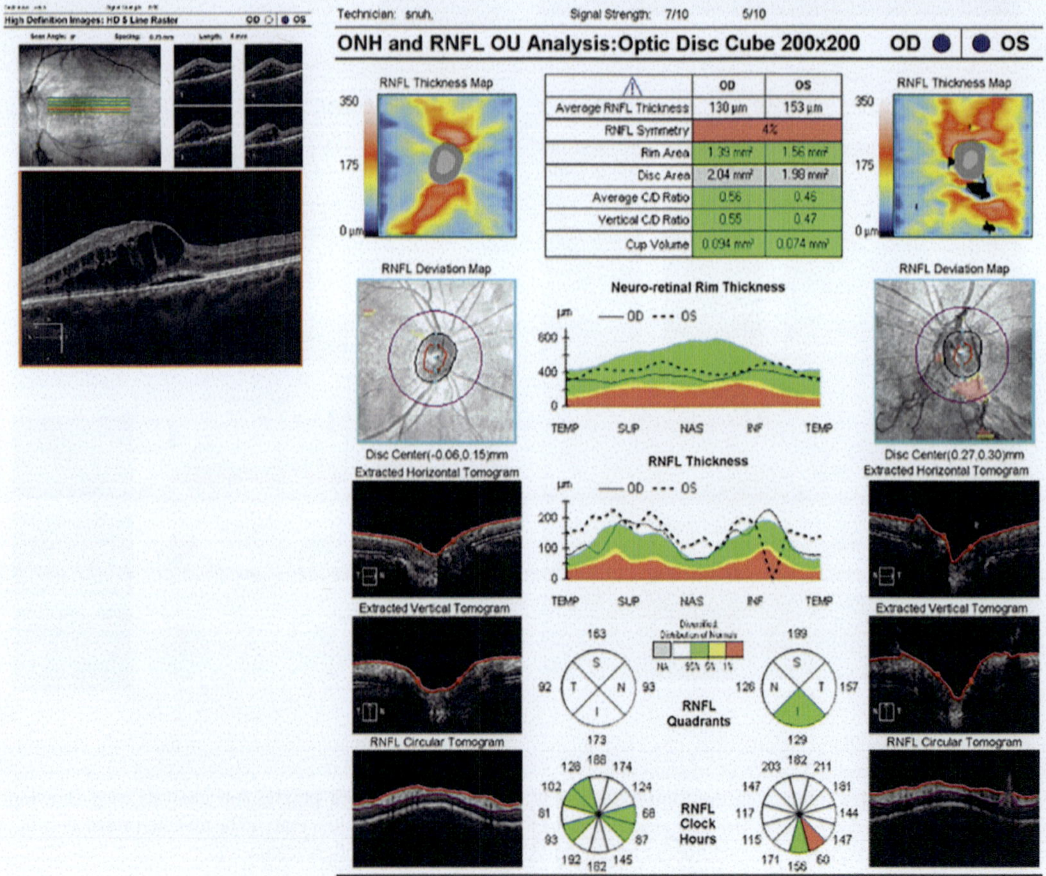

Fig. 11 Cirrus HD-OCT showing a patient with diabetic retinopathy and macular edema. In the TSNIT profile, the thickness curve is seen to be above normal limits. The optic nerve head parameters are within normal range, possibly due to the adhesions between the vitreous and the optic disc. In the inferotemporal area with peripapillary vitreoretinal traction, note the segmentation error resulting in the RNFL thickness of zero

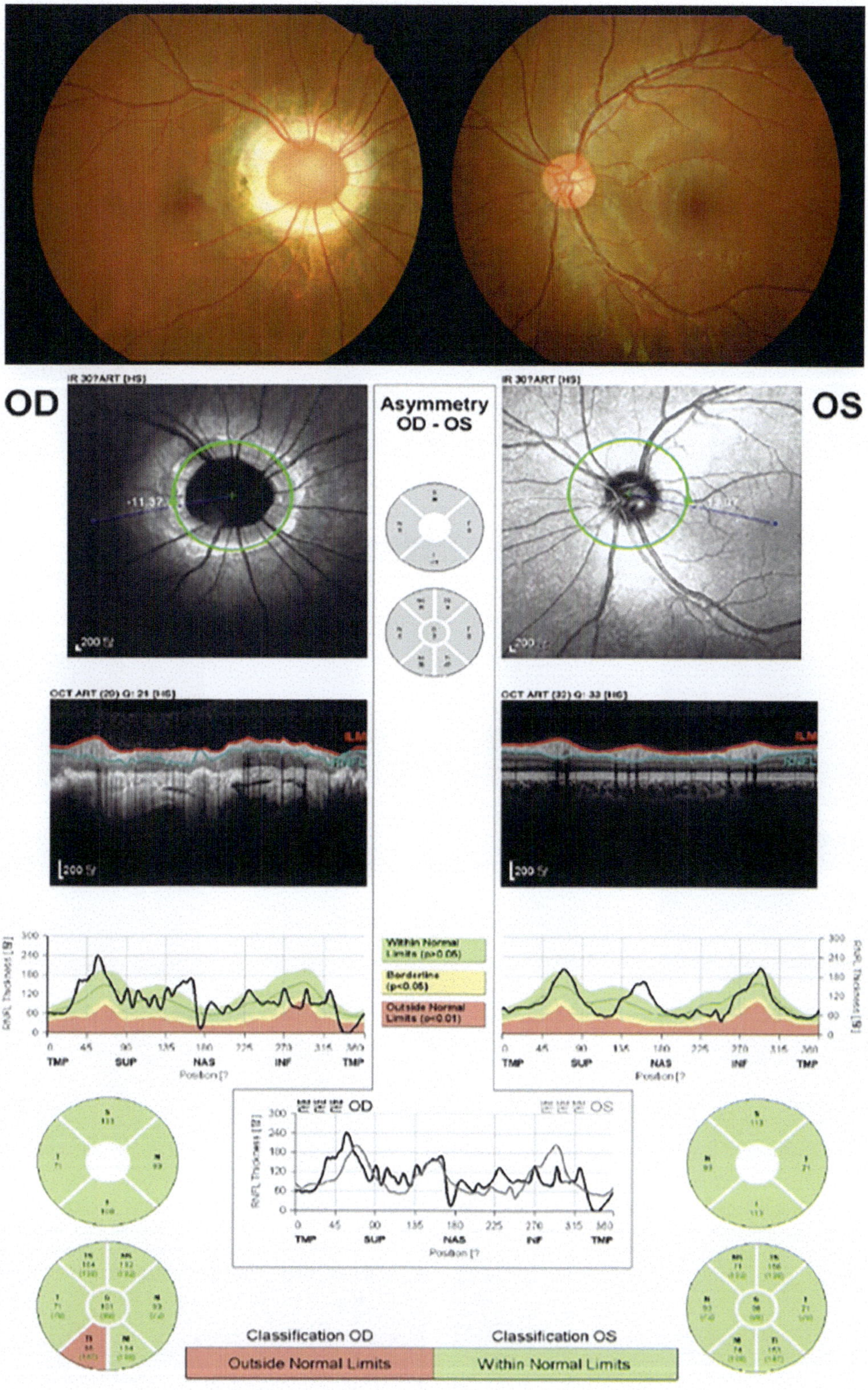

Fig. 12 Morning glory syndrome in the right eye causing segmentation artifact. On the TSNIT profile, it is seen that RNFL thickness has a value near 0 in the nasal quadrant and 0 in the temporal quadrant

a

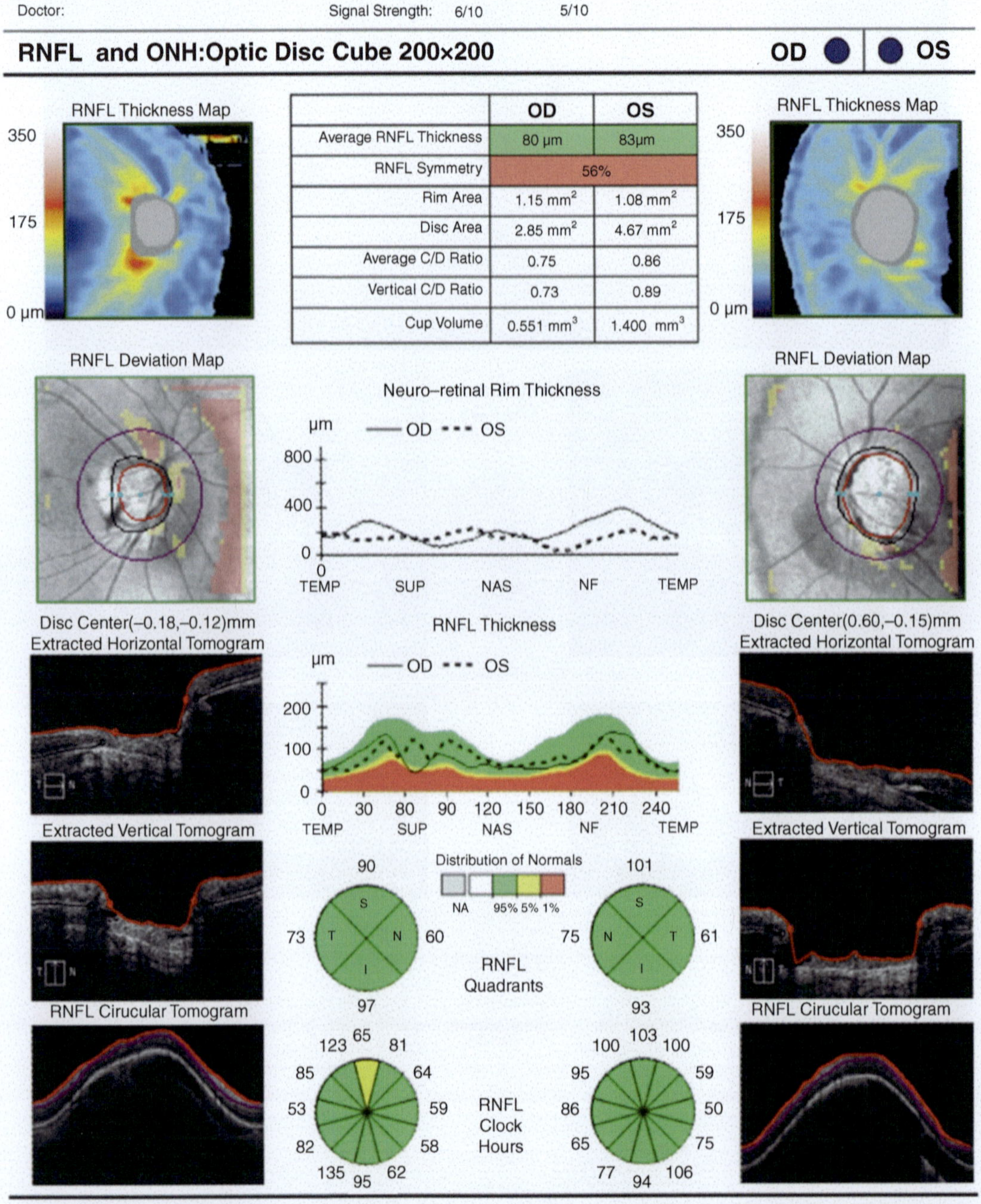

Fig. 13 (**a**) Borderline-quality Cirrus HD-OCT scan with signal strength of 6 in the right eye and 5 in the left eye of a small-pupil patient. Small pupil may have reduced the amount and quality of the signal detected by the instrument. (**b**) Cataract formation in both eyes of the same small-pupil patient. The coexisting cataract diminished the scan quality (signal strength, both eyes: 3) and decreased the RNFL thickness measures

b

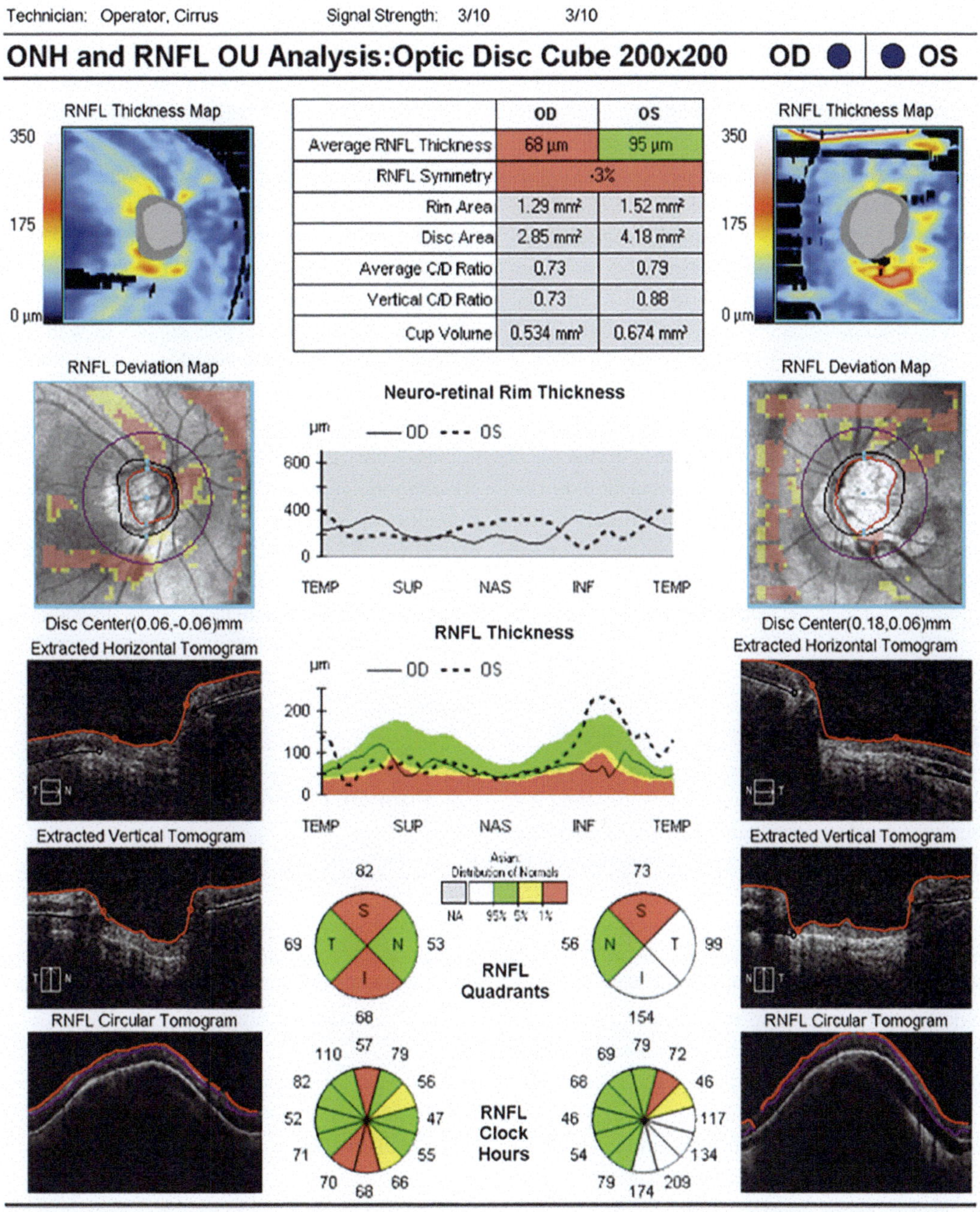

Fig. 13 (continued)

OCT (Fig. 13). Scans can be obtained in eyes with a pupil diameter greater than 2 mm. Recent studies have not found significant changes in RNFL thickness before and/or after dilation, which suggests that the effect of pupil size is insignificant (Massa et al. 2010; Savini et al. 2010). However, pharmacological dilation may be necessary in selected cases of small pupil size.

3.8 Motion Artifact

Motion artifact results from eye movements (e.g., horizontal saccades) during scan acquisition. Improvements in SD-OCT scanning speed and acquisition time have reduced the likelihood of motion artifact. However, for devices lacking an eye-tracking system or motion correction algorithms, eye movements remain a potential problem. Careful interpretation of results, including retinal vessels, optic disc shape, and clock-hour RNFL thickness, is warranted in scans with motion artifacts passing through the optic disc (Taibbi et al. 2014). Patients' steady fixation is required to avoid motion artifacts. It may be noticed during scanning that the disc or macula is not well centered. In such cases, a clear explanation of the scanning procedures and timely notification to the patient of imminent image acquisition may be helpful. Rescans should be attempted, and if necessary, an external fixation point can be used.

3.9 Blink Artifact

Although image acquisition time is less than 2 s, blinking may yet occur during this time frame. The effects of blink artifact on OCT depend on its position within the scan area (Fig. 14). In the absence of an eye-tracking system, the acquisition process continues even in the presence of blinking. This leads to transient loss of data, which is proportional to the duration of a single blink. Blink artifacts can be prevented by allowing the examinee to blink freely until the completion of the camera alignment process, followed by prompt notification of the imminent start of scan acquisition. In selected cases, artificial tears or other lubricants may be useful.

4 Instrument Factors

4.1 Poor Image Quality

A good-quality scan is essential for a reliable OCT result. All OCT devices use quality-control systems for assessing image quality. The "strength" of the light signal backscattered by the ocular structures, calculated as the signal-to-noise ratio, has been conventionally used as an objective measure of scan quality. Cirrus HD-OCT uses the "signal strength" parameter for this purpose and recommends a repeated scan if the signal strength is below 6. Spectralis OCT uses a quality score, or the "Q" coefficient, for the same purpose; values less than 20 require repetition of the test. Poor signal strength has been demonstrated as a major source of artifacts in previous studies as well and precludes the ability to detect change in the RNFL overtime (Vizzeri et al. 2009; Wu et al. 2007). Poor scanning quality can lead to inaccurate RNFL thickness measurements, specifically thinner-than-actual values (Rao et al. 2014; Huang et al. 2011; Russell et al. 2014). Several ocular-related factors may play a role in OCT scan quality, as outlined above (Stein et al. 2006; Mwanza et al. 2011; Bambo et al. 2014; Savini et al. 2010). In addition, operator-dependent factors, such as improper OCT lens cleaning or poor image centration, may affect results.

4.2 Poor OCT Device Performance

As an OCT device gets older and undergoes heavy use, the power of the superluminescent-light-emitting diode decays over time, the optics become dirty, and images opaque. The result is poor-quality scans in almost all patients, especially those with early cataracts or dry eyes.

4.3 Inaccurate Optic Disc Margin Delineation

Adequate optic disc assessment relies on the ability of the automated algorithm to identify the termination of the Bruch's membrane corresponding to the optic disc edge (Strouthidis et al. 2009a, b). Accurate delineation of the optic disc margin is incorporated in the optic disc center location. In eyes with peripapillary atrophy, the OCT signal reflectance alters due to retinal pigment epithelium disruption and choriocapillaris atrophy

a

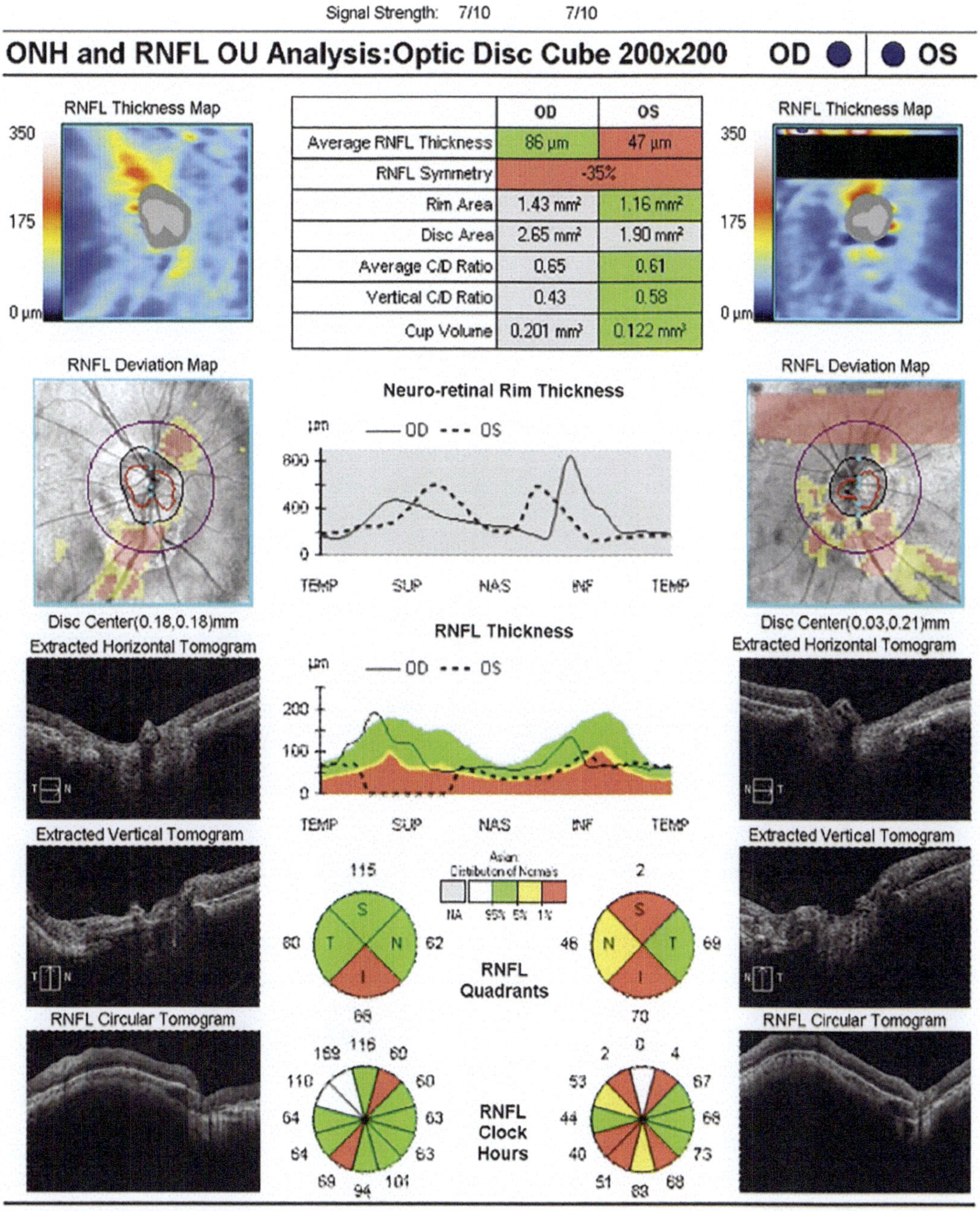

Fig. 14 (**a**) Blink artifact in the left eye. The blink produced a well-demarcated rectangular area of missing data and red superpixels spanning the entire width of the RNFL thickness map. (**b**) Rescan of the same patient. The RNFL thickness of the superior quadrant in the right eye as measured was within the normal range

b

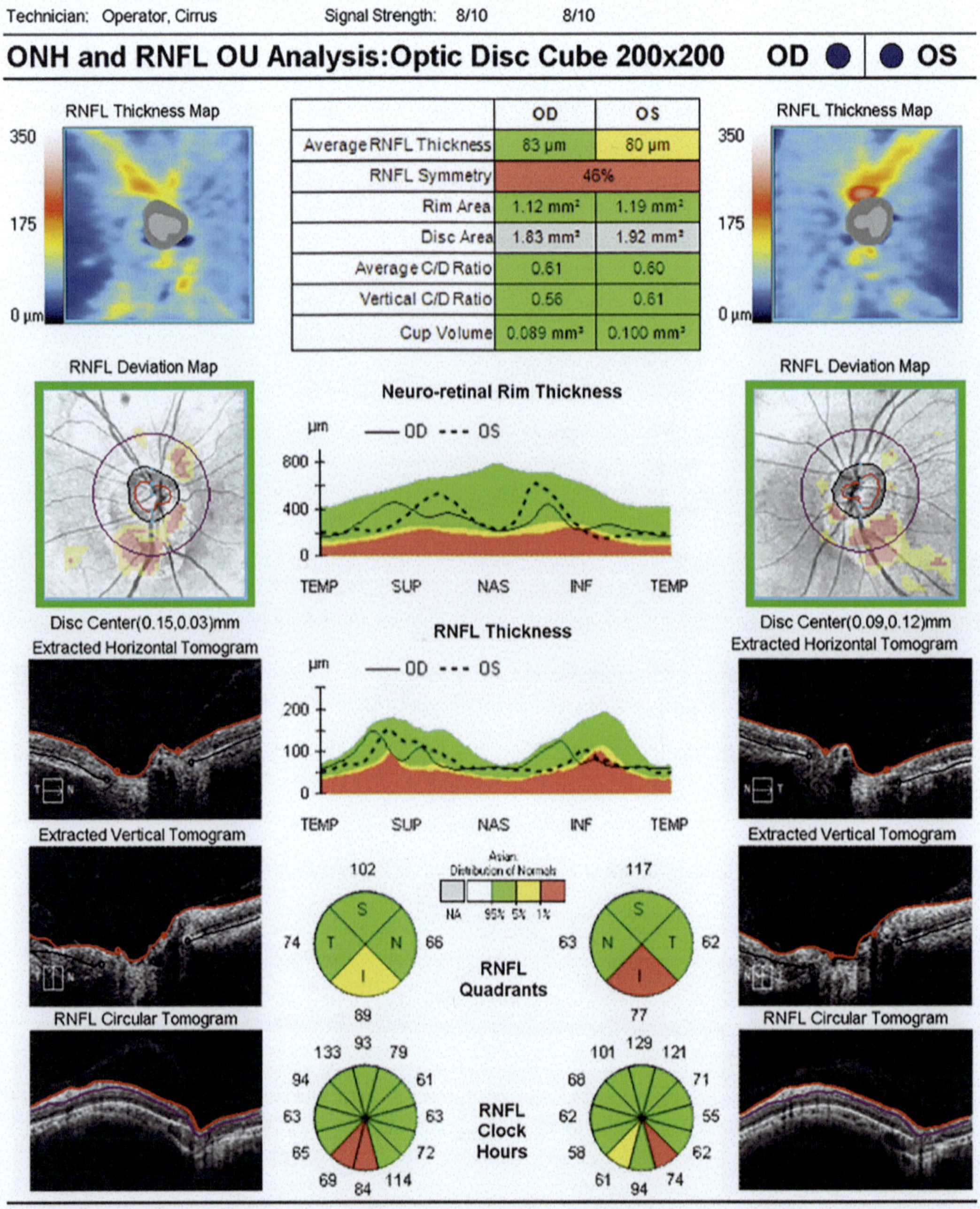

Fig. 14 (continued)

(Manjunath et al. 2011), coupled with Bruch's membrane changes (Curcio et al. 2000). This possibly affects the identification of the optic disc margin (Fig. 15). Blinking or optic disc cup truncation may also lead to unreliable optic disc parameters. Therefore, for each scan, careful inspection of the en-face image and the tomograms intersecting the optic disc is necessary. Moreover, rescans should be attempted in order to obtain accurate optic disc margin outlining.

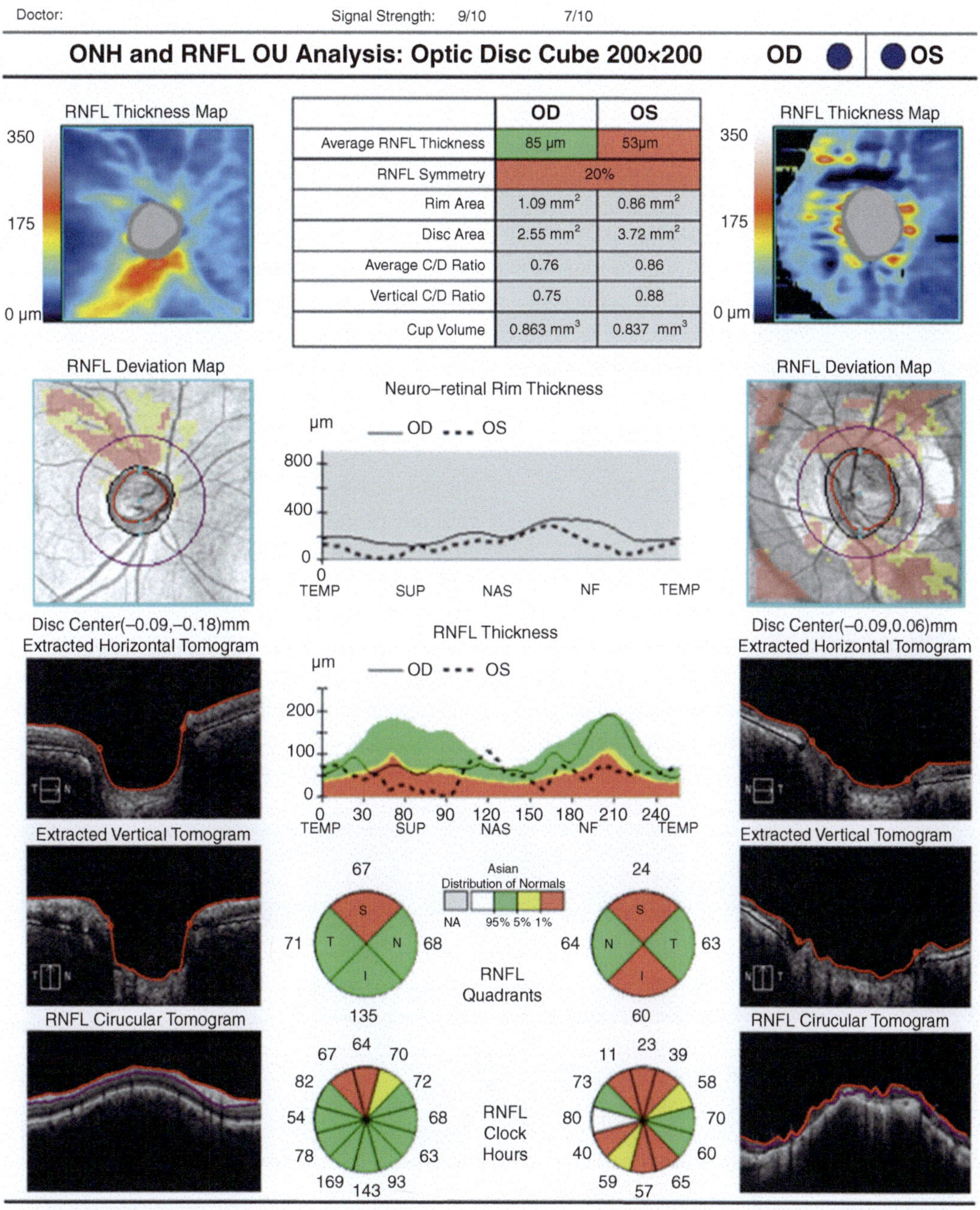

Fig. 15 Inaccurate optic disc margin delineation and segmentation artifact in Cirrus HD-OCT imaging of RNFL in a patient with large peripapillary atrophy in the left eye. The inaccurate delineation of the disc resulted in the artifacts of RNFL thickness. The RNFL thickness was measured as zero with large areas of abnormal thickness flagged as red areas

4.4 Segmentation Errors

All OCT devices have segmentation algorithms or layer-seeking algorithms to enable analysis and measure a target retinal layer. Segmentation errors occur when the software is unable to determine the layers correctly. Several mechanisms may be responsible for inaccurate RNFL segmentation, such as OCT signal attenuation with decreased reflectance of the RNFL caused by media opacities. The OCT signal may be interrupted by the effects of blinking or floaters, causing localized failure to identify the RNFL boundaries and decreased RNFL thickness measures. Moreover, truncation of the inner retinal layers may determine algorithm failure or obvious RNFL segmentation errors. Finally, motion artifacts intersecting the scan circle may incur inaccurate RNFL segmentation. In such cases, the RNFL or other retinal layer being assessed is measured as thicker or, more commonly, thinner than it actually is. RNFL thickness could be measured as zero and flagged as a red area (Fig. 16). Very low measurement of RNFL thickness, usually thinner than 30 μm, is due mostly to segmentation or imaging error (Chan and Miller 2007; Groth et al. 2013).

5 Operator Factors

5.1 Registration Error of Age

Thickness measurements obtained from an OCT device are compared against age-matched controls in order to identify significant thinning or thickening. There is a natural attrition of the RNFL with aging (Budenz et al. 2007; Parikh et al. 2007). One study reported that the overall mean RNFL thickness on OCT decreases by 0.365 mm for every year increase in age (Celebi and Mirza 2013). Therefore, not accounting for age effects can significantly affect estimates of disease progression (Leung et al. 2013). Entering the incorrect date of birth could cause abnormalities in the probability plots of thickness measurements that could lead to erroneous interpretation.

5.2 OCT Lens Opacities

Opacities of the OCT lens may occur from fingerprints or the patient's accidental contact with the lens. They can decrease image quality and directly affect RNFL thickness measures. On the final printout, they typically maintain an identical shape and occupy the same position on the en-face image over repeated testing. Periodic lens cleaning coupled with careful handling of the device by test operators and patients is necessary to prevent the occurrence of such artifacts.

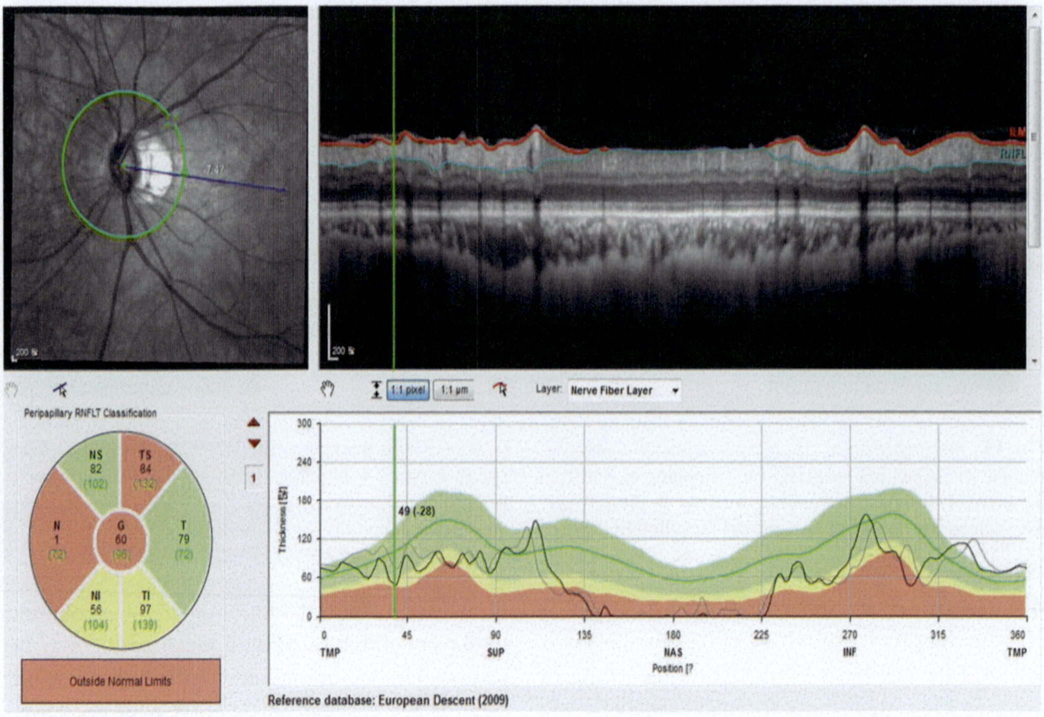

Fig. 16 Segmentation artifact in Spectralis OCT imaging of RNFL in a patient with myopic tilted disc. An incorrectly segmented posterior RNFL led to an RNFL thickness measurement of zero at the nasal quadrant

5.3 Incorrect Scan-Circle Placement

Incorrect RNFL scan-circle placement is easily identifiable on the final printout. Although most of these artifacts have been reported to be mild, moderate-to-severe displacement of the circle may result in erroneous RNFL values (Asrani et al. 2014; Cheung et al. 2008) (Fig. 17).

a

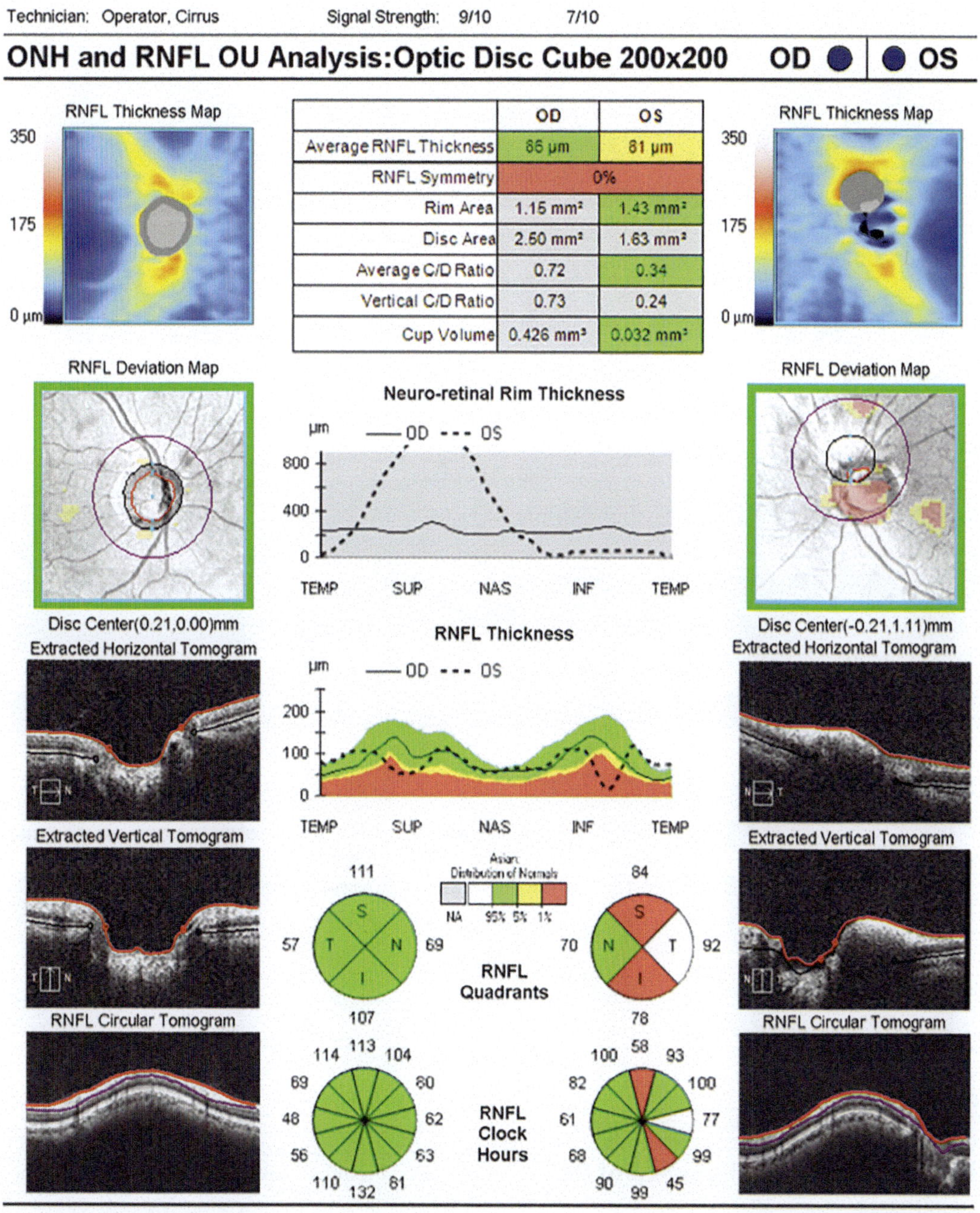

Fig. 17 (**a**) Incorrect RNFL circle resulting in artifacts of the RNFL thickness notwithstanding acceptable signal strength. (**b**) After replacing the RNFL circle, the RNFL thickness was within normal range

b

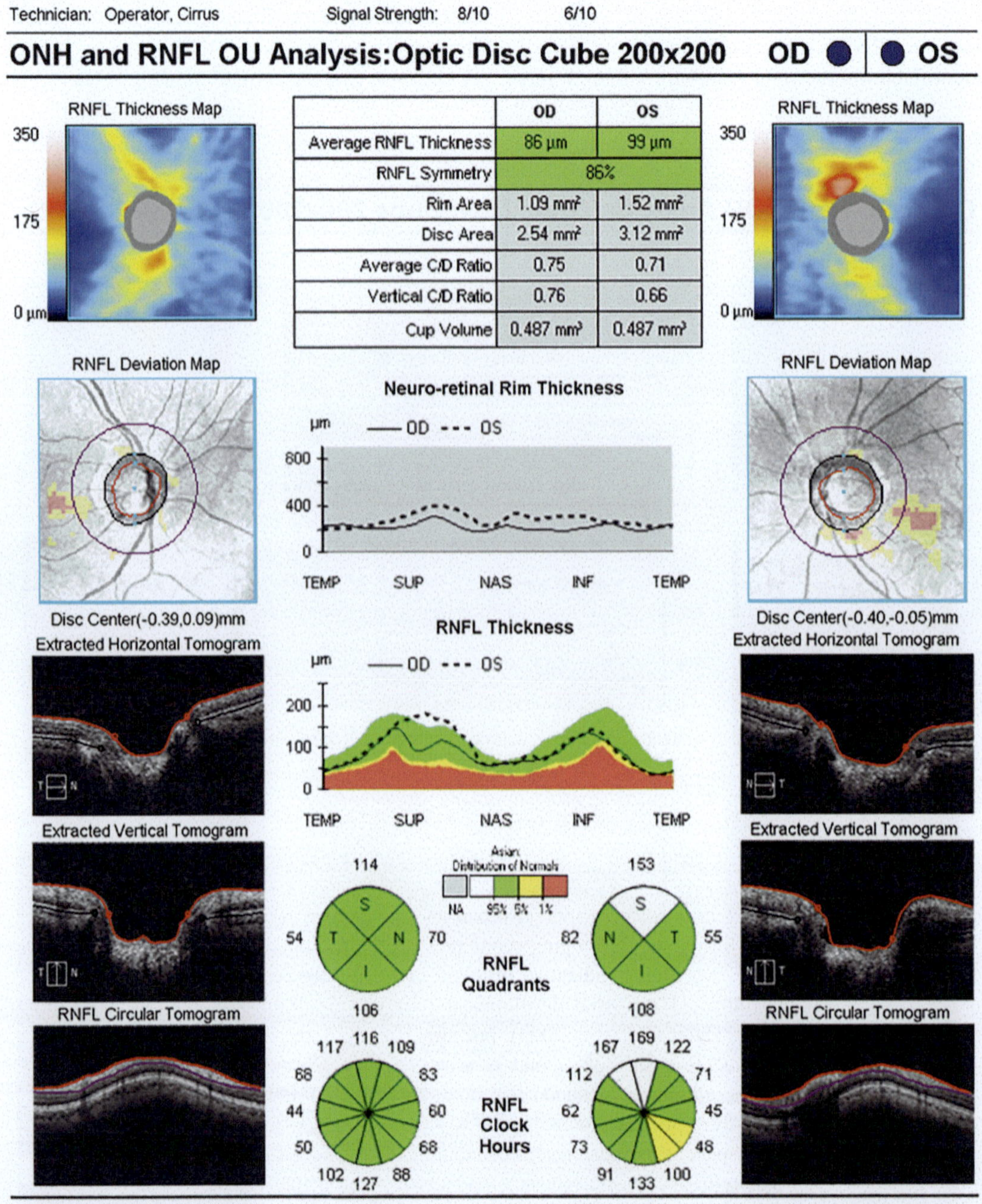

Fig. 17 (continued)

5.4 Incorrect Axial Alignment of OCT Image

Improper axial alignment of the scan in the z-axis occurs when the ocular structures are only partially included within the acquisition frame, resulting in image truncation (i.e., all edges of the image were not within the acquisition window). The areas of absolute loss on the RNFL thickness plot result in erroneous mean measure-

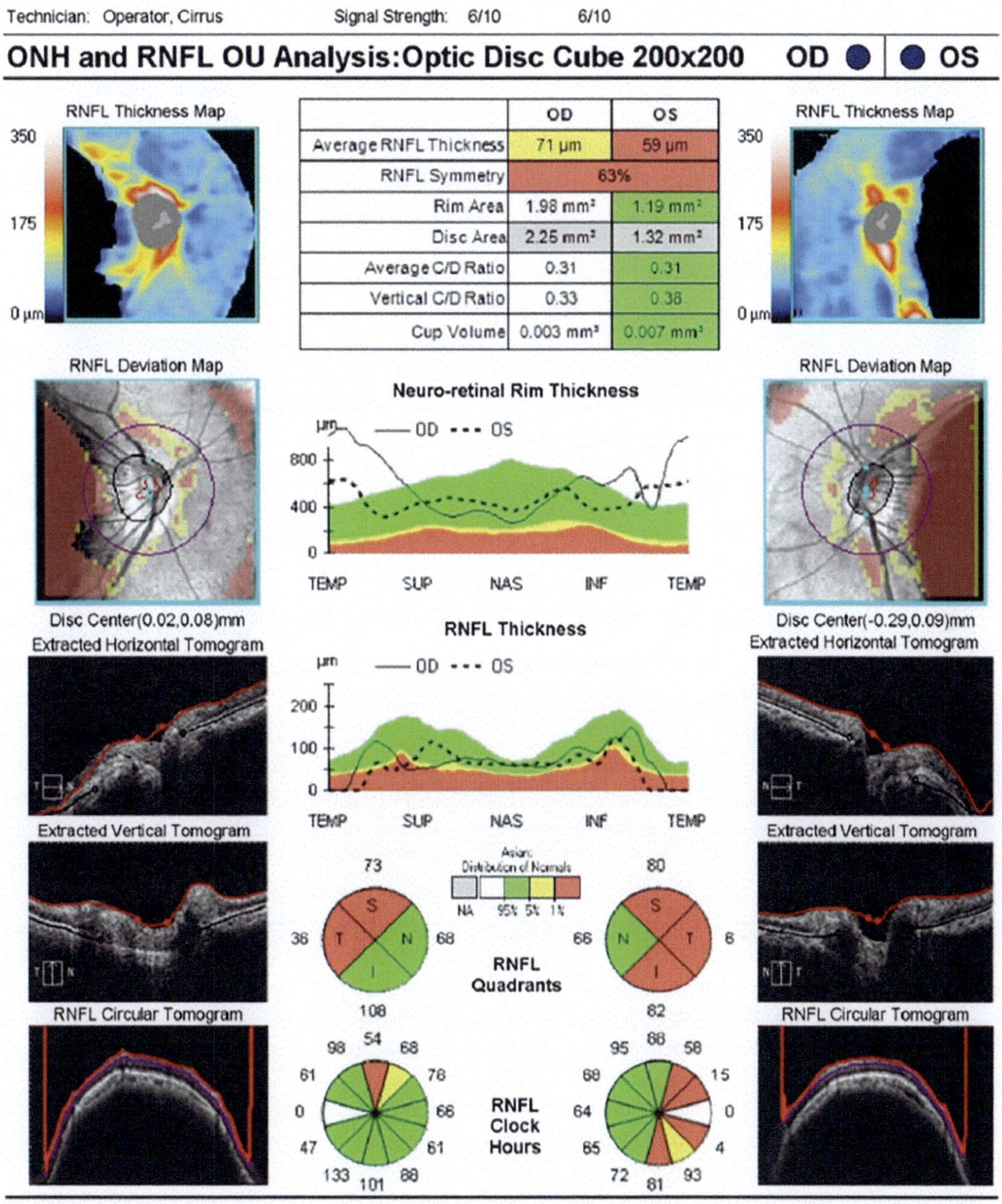

Fig. 18 Truncation of RNFL data due to decentering on z-axis. This resulted in regional errors in the derived RNFL thickness, which can be seen as irregular black areas of absolute thinning on the RNFL thickness map. Both eyes are predisposed to this z-axis truncation because of the presence of steep retinal curvature in myopic eyes

ments in the sector and in the global mean RNFL thickness values (Fig. 18). A clue to identifying such artifacts is the presence of RNFL values less than 30 μm or near zero. OCT image truncation commonly occurs in myopic eyes with a steep retinal curvature or in glaucomatous eyes with deep cupping, because the peripapillary RNFL may be difficult to capture on a single B-scan, due to the differences in height between the opposite sides of the circular RNFL scan. Other causes include improper distance between the eye and the device due to incorrect patient positioning and axial misalignment of the OCT scanning head.

6 OCT Artifacts in GCIPL Analysis

6.1 Macular GCIPL

Various studies have reported the prevalence of errors of RNFL and macular scans. Li and associates (2020) reported that artifacts were more common on peripapillary RNFL scans (43.7%) than on macular scans (30.0%), and Liu et al. (2015) reported a similar prevalence of RNFL artifacts (i.e., on 46.3% of scans). Asrani and associates (2014) reported that artifacts were more common on the macular scan (28.2%) than on the peripapillary RNFL scan (19.97%).

The commercially available segmentation algorithms are prone to segmentation failures of the GCIPL complex. Errors in segmentation occur in low-signal-strength scans, optic nerve edema, or in the cases of outer-retinal-layer structural abnormalities that affect segmentation of the inner retinal layers (Lee et al. 2010; Garvin et al. 2008). One sign of inaccurate inner-layer segmentation is the appearance of a non-pathologic shape, such as a corner of abnormal thinning, on the thickness and probability maps. Errors often appear as segments of blue (thinning) on the thickness map (Fig. 19). A GCIPL reading of less than 40 mm is also typically indicative of areas of segmentation error. On the B-scan, the algorithm's identification of the boundaries of the ganglion cell layer and inner plexiform layer often collapse together in the areas of artifact, thereby producing artifactual thinning.

Macular scan artifacts more commonly have been associated with dry eye or corneal opacities. The effect of corneal drying degrades many images including stereo disc photos (Stein et al. 2006). Encouraging the patient to blink may help improve the signal strength and reduce artifacts.

6.2 Interindividual Variation of Retinal Ganglion Cell Thickness Within Macula

In the macula thickness profile of normal eyes, the perifoveal location is the most variable site due to a wide variation in the thickness profile of the inner retina immediately surrounding the fovea. Therefore, an abnormal probability map in the perifoveal location should be spotlighted carefully and correlated with the clinical exam and functional tests. It is important to ensure that the fovea is correctly identified and centered by the OCT analysis. Otherwise, this may lead to artifactual thickening and thinning displayed as abnormal. However, true atrophy of the GCIPL may also cause perifoveal thinning and enlargement of the foveal depression, which renders difficult the differentiation of focal pathological thinning from normal variation in the perifoveal location (Chen and Kardon 2016).

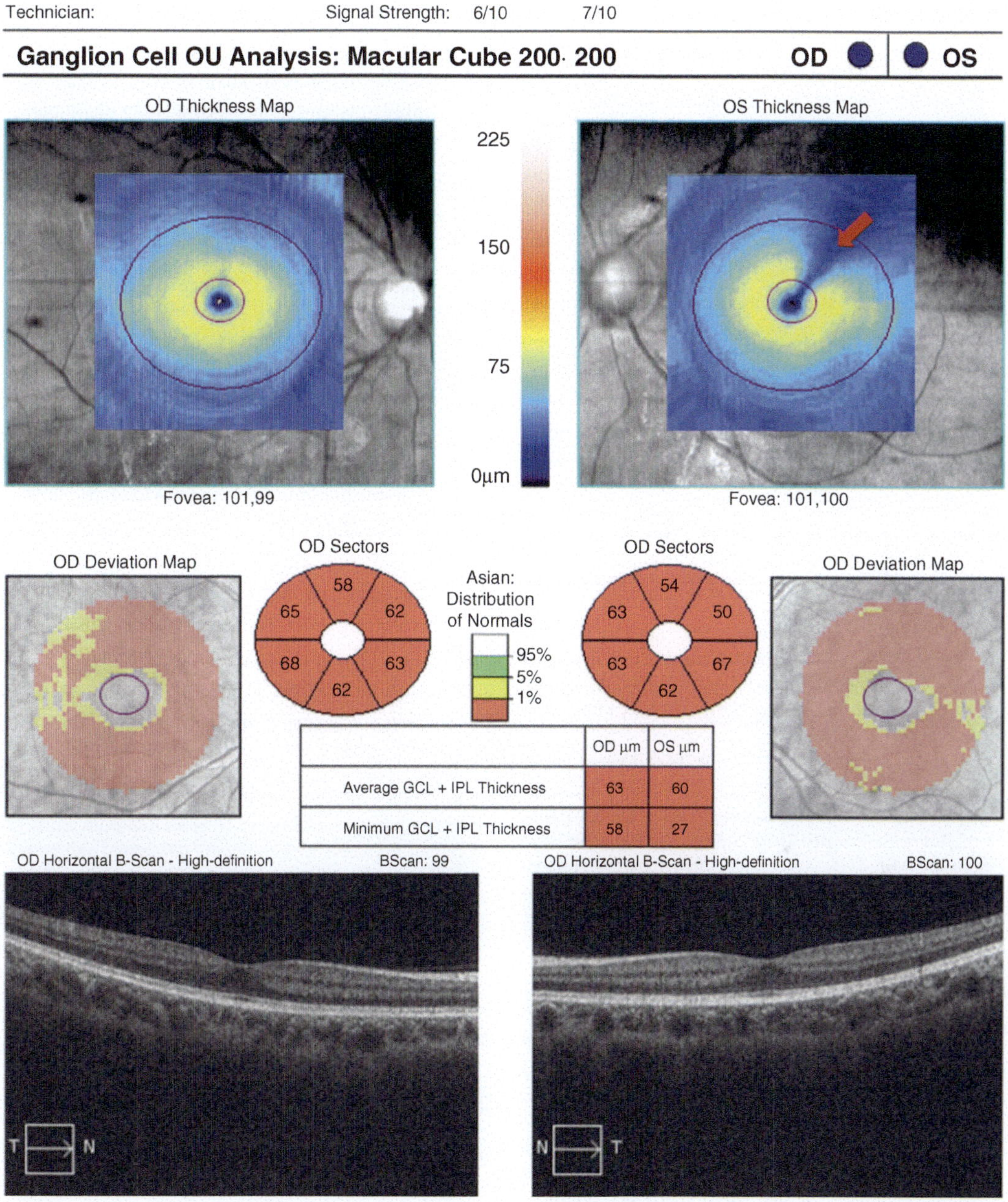

Fig. 19 Artificially decreased GCIPL complex thickness due to errors in segmentation. This can be seen as a segment of blue "thinning" on the thickness map (red arrow). The minimum thickness of GCIPL thickness is less than 40 mm in the left eye, which also is often an indication of segmentation error

References

Anwar Z, Wellik SR, Galor A. Glaucoma therapy and ocular surface disease: current literature and recommendations. Curr Opin Ophthalmol. 2013;24(2):136–43. https://doi.org/10.1097/ICU.0b013e32835c8aba.

Asrani S, Essaid L, Alder BD, Santiago-Turla C. Artifacts in spectral-domain optical coherence tomography measurements in glaucoma. JAMA Ophthalmol. 2014;132(4):396–402. https://doi.org/10.1001/jamaophthalmol.2013.7974.

Bambo MP, Garcia-Martin E, Otin S, et al. Influence of cataract surgery on repeatability and measurements of spectral domain optical coherence tomography. Br J Ophthalmol. 2014;98(1):52. https://doi.org/10.1136/bjophthalmol-2013-303752.

Bayer A, Akman A. Artifacts and anatomic variations in optical coherence tomography. Turk J Ophthalmol. 2020;50(2):99–106. https://doi.org/10.4274/tjo.galenos.2019.78000.

Bayraktar S, Cebeci Z, Kabaalioglu M, Ciloglu S, Kir N, Izgi B. Peripapillary retinoschisis in glaucoma patients. J Ophthalmol. 2016;2016:1612720. https://doi.org/10.1155/2016/1612720.

Bennett AG, Rudnicka AR, Edgar DF. Improvements on Littmann's method of determining the size of retinal features by fundus photography. Graefes Arch Clin Exp Ophthalmol. 1994;232(6):361–7. https://doi.org/10.1007/BF00175988.

Budenz DL, Anderson DR, Varma R, et al. Determinants of normal retinal nerve fiber layer thickness measured by Stratus OCT. Ophthalmology. 2007;114(6):1046–52. https://doi.org/10.1016/j.ophtha.2006.08.046.

Celebi AR, Mirza GE. Age-related change in retinal nerve fiber layer thickness measured with spectral domain optical coherence tomography. Invest Ophthalmol Vis Sci. 2013;54(13):8095–103. https://doi.org/10.1167/iovs.13-12634.

Chan CK, Miller NR. Peripapillary nerve fiber layer thickness measured by optical coherence tomography in patients with no light perception from long-standing nonglaucomatous optic neuropathies. J Neuro-ophthalmol. 2007;27(3):176–9. https://doi.org/10.1097/WNO.0b013e31814b1ac4.

Chen JJ, Kardon RH. Avoiding Clinical misinterpretation and artifacts of optical coherence tomography analysis of the optic nerve, retinal nerve fiber layer, and ganglion cell layer. J Neuro-ophthalmol. 2016;36(4):417–38. https://doi.org/10.1097/wno.0000000000000422.

Cheung CY, Leung CK, Lin D, Pang CP, Lam DS. Relationship between retinal nerve fiber layer measurement and signal strength in optical coherence tomography. Ophthalmology. 2008;115(8):1347–51, 51.e1–2. https://doi.org/10.1016/j.ophtha.2007.11.027.

Chong GT, Lee RK. Glaucoma versus red disease: imaging and glaucoma diagnosis. Curr Opin Ophthalmol. 2012;23(2):79–88. https://doi.org/10.1097/ICU.0b013e32834ff431.

Colen TP, Lemij HG. Prevalence of split nerve fiber layer bundles in healthy eyes imaged with scanning laser polarimetry. Ophthalmology. 2001;108(1):151–6. https://doi.org/10.1016/S0161-6420(00)00516-9.

Congdon N, Vingerling JR, Klein BE, et al. Prevalence of cataract and pseudophakia/aphakia among adults in the United States. Arch Ophthalmol (Chicago, Ill: 1960). 2004;122(4):487–94. https://doi.org/10.1001/archopht.122.4.487.

Curcio CA, Saunders PL, Younger PW, Malek G. Peripapillary chorioretinal atrophy: Bruch's membrane changes and photoreceptor loss. Ophthalmology. 2000;107(2):334–43. https://doi.org/10.1016/s0161-6420(99)00037-8.

Dong ZM, Wollstein G, Schuman JS. Clinical utility of optical coherence tomography in glaucoma. Invest Ophthalmol Vis Sci. 2016;57(9):Oct556–67. https://doi.org/10.1167/iovs.16-19933.

Gabriele ML, Wollstein G, Ishikawa H, et al. Optical coherence tomography: history, current status, and laboratory work. J Invest Ophthalmol Visual Sci. 2011;52(5):2425–36. https://doi.org/10.1167/iovs.10-6312.

Garvin MK, Abramoff MD, Kardon R, Russell SR, Wu X, Sonka M. Intraretinal layer segmentation of macular optical coherence tomography images using optimal 3-D graph search. IEEE Trans Med Imaging. 2008;27(10):1495–505. https://doi.org/10.1109/tmi.2008.923966.

Giani A, Cigada M, Choudhry N, et al. Reproducibility of retinal thickness measurements on normal and pathologic eyes by different optical coherence tomography instruments. Am J Ophthalmol. 2010;150(6):815–24. https://doi.org/10.1016/j.ajo.2010.06.025.

Groth SL, Harrison A, Grajewski AL, Lee MS. Retinal nerve fiber layer thickness using spectral-domain optical coherence tomography in patients with no light perception secondary to optic atrophy. J Neuro-ophthalmol. 2013;33(1):37–9. https://doi.org/10.1097/WNO.0b013e318272c7cd.

Han IC, Jaffe GJ. Evaluation of artifacts associated with macular spectral-domain optical coherence tomography. Ophthalmology. 2010;117(6):1177–89.e4. https://doi.org/10.1016/j.ophtha.2009.10.029.

Hollander DA, Barricks ME, Duncan JL, Irvine AR. Macular schisis detachment associated with angle-closure glaucoma. Arch Ophthalmol (Chicago, Ill: 1960). 2005;123(2):270–2. https://doi.org/10.1001/archopht.123.2.270.

Hong SW, Ahn MD, Kang SH, Im SK. Analysis of peripapillary retinal nerve fiber distribution in normal young adults. J Invest Ophthalmol Vis Sci. 2010;51(7):3515–23. https://doi.org/10.1167/iovs.09-4888.

Hood DC, Salant JA, Arthur SN, Ritch R, Liebmann JM. The location of the inferior and superior temporal blood vessels and interindividual variability of the retinal nerve fiber layer thickness. J Glaucoma. 2010;19(3):158–66. https://doi.org/10.1097/IJG.0b013e3181af31ec.

Huang J, Liu X, Wu Z, Sadda S. Image quality affects macular and retinal nerve fiber layer thickness measurements on fourier-domain optical coherence tomography. Ophthal Surg Lasers Imag. 2011;42(3):216–21. https://doi.org/10.3928/15428877-20110324-01.

Hwang YH, Lee JY, Kim YY. The effect of head tilt on the measurements of retinal nerve fibre layer and macular thickness by spectral-domain optical coherence tomography. Br J Ophthalmol. 2011;95(11):1547–51. https://doi.org/10.1136/bjo.2010.194118.

Hwang YH, Yoo C, Kim YY. Characteristics of peripapillary retinal nerve fiber layer thickness in eyes with myopic optic disc tilt and rotation. J Glaucoma. 2012;21(6):394–400. https://doi.org/10.1097/IJG.0b013e3182182567.

Hwang YH, Kim YY, Kim HK, Sohn YH. Effect of peripapillary retinoschisis on retinal nerve fibre layer thickness measurement in glaucomatous eyes. Br J Ophthalmol. 2014;98(5):669–74. https://doi.org/10.1136/bjophthalmol-2013-303931.

Inoue M, Bissen-Miyajima H, Yoshino M, Suzuki T. Wavy horizontal artifacts on optical coherence tomography line-scanning images caused by diffractive multifocal intraocular lenses. J Cataract Refract Surg. 2009;35(7):1239–43. https://doi.org/10.1016/j.jcrs.2009.04.016.

Jonas JB, Nguyen XN, Gusek GC, Naumann GO. Parapapillary chorioretinal atrophy in normal and glaucoma eyes. I. Morphometric data. Invest Ophthalmol Vis Sci. 1989;30(5):908–18.

Kahook MY, Noecker RJ, Ishikawa H, et al. Peripapillary schisis in glaucoma patients with narrow angles and increased intraocular pressure. Am J Ophthalmol. 2007;143(4):697–9. https://doi.org/10.1016/j.ajo.2006.10.054.

Kaliner E, Cohen MJ, Miron H, Kogan M, Blumenthal EZ. Retinal nerve fiber layer split bundles are true anatomic variants. Ophthalmology. 2007;114(12):2259–64. https://doi.org/10.1016/j.ophtha.2007.01.028.

Kang SH, Hong SW, Im SK, Lee SH, Ahn MD. Effect of myopia on the thickness of the retinal nerve fiber layer measured by cirrus HD optical coherence tomography. J Invest Ophthalmol Vis Sci. 2010;51(8):4075–83. https://doi.org/10.1167/iovs.09-4737.

Kim SY, Park H-YL, Park CK. The effects of peripapillary atrophy on the diagnostic ability of stratus and cirrus OCT in the analysis of optic nerve head parameters and disc size. J Invest Ophthalmol Vis Sci. 2012;53(8):4475–84. https://doi.org/10.1167/iovs.12-9682.

Lee K, Niemeijer M, Garvin MK, Kwon YH, Sonka M, Abramoff MD. Segmentation of the optic disc in 3-D OCT scans of the optic nerve head. IEEE Trans Med Imaging. 2010;29(1):159–68. https://doi.org/10.1109/TMI.2009.2031324.

Leung CK, Mohamed S, Leung KS, et al. Retinal nerve fiber layer measurements in myopia: an optical coherence tomography study. Invest Ophthalmol Vis Sci. 2006;47(12):5171–6. https://doi.org/10.1167/iovs.06-0545.

Leung CK, Cheng AC, Chong KK, et al. Optic disc measurements in myopia with optical coherence tomography and confocal scanning laser ophthalmoscopy. Invest Ophthalmol Vis Sci. 2007;48(7):3178–83. https://doi.org/10.1167/iovs.06-1315.

Leung CKS, Ye C, Weinreb RN, Yu M, Lai G, Lam DS. Impact of age-related change of retinal nerve fiber layer and macular thicknesses on evaluation of glaucoma progression. Ophthalmology. 2013;120(12):2485–92. https://doi.org/10.1016/j.ophtha.2013.07.021.

Li A, Thompson AC, Asrani S. Impact of Artifacts from optical coherence tomography retinal nerve fiber layer and macula scans on detection of glaucoma progression. Am J Ophthalmol. 2020;221:235–45. https://doi.org/10.1016/j.ajo.2020.08.018.

Liu Y, Simavli H, Que CJ, et al. Patient characteristics associated with artifacts in Spectralis optical coherence tomography imaging of the retinal nerve fiber layer in glaucoma. Am J Ophthalmol. 2015;159(3):565–76.e2. https://doi.org/10.1016/j.ajo.2014.12.006.

Manjunath V, Shah H, Fujimoto JG, Duker JS. Analysis of peripapillary atrophy using spectral domain optical coherence tomography. Ophthalmology. 2011;118(3):531–6. https://doi.org/10.1016/j.ophtha.2010.07.013.

Massa GC, Vidotti VG, Cremasco F, Lupinacci APC, Costa VP. Influence of pupil dilation on retinal nerve fibre layer measurements with spectral domain OCT. Eye. 2010;24(9):1498–502. https://doi.org/10.1038/eye.2010.72.

Moore DB, Jaffe GJ, Asrani S. Retinal nerve fiber layer thickness measurements: uveitis, a major confounding factor. Ophthalmology. 2015;122(3):511–7. https://doi.org/10.1016/j.ophtha.2014.09.008.

Mwanza JC, Bhorade AM, Sekhon N, et al. Effect of cataract and its removal on signal strength and peripapillary retinal nerve fiber layer optical coherence tomography measurements. J Glaucoma. 2011;20(1):37–43. https://doi.org/10.1097/IJG.0b013e3181ccb93b.

Mwanza JC, Budenz DL, Warren JL, et al. Retinal nerve fibre layer thickness floor and corresponding functional loss in glaucoma. Br J Ophthalmol. 2015;99(6):732–7. https://doi.org/10.1136/bjophthalmol-2014-305745.

Örnek N, Büyüktortop N, Örnek K. Peripapillary and macular retinoschisis in a patient with pseudoexfoliation glaucoma. BMJ Case Reports.

2013;2013:bcr2013009469. https://doi.org/10.1136/bcr-2013-009469.

Parikh RS, Parikh SR, Sekhar GC, Prabakaran S, Babu JG, Thomas R. Normal age-related decay of retinal nerve fiber layer thickness. Ophthalmology. 2007;114(5):921–6. https://doi.org/10.1016/j.ophtha.2007.01.023.

Qiu KL, Zhang MZ, Leung CK, et al. Diagnostic classification of retinal nerve fiber layer measurement in myopic eyes: a comparison between time-domain and spectral-domain optical coherence tomography. Am J Ophthalmol. 2011;152(4):646–53.e2. https://doi.org/10.1016/j.ajo.2011.04.002.

Rao HL, Addepalli UK, Yadav RK, Senthil S, Choudhari NS, Garudadri CS. Effect of Scan Quality on Diagnostic Accuracy of Spectral-Domain Optical Coherence Tomography in Glaucoma. Am J Ophthalmol. 2014;157(3):719–27.e1. https://doi.org/10.1016/j.ajo.2013.12.012.

Roh S, Noecker RJ, Schuman JS, Hedges TR 3rd, Weiter JJ, Mattox C. Effect of optic nerve head drusen on nerve fiber layer thickness. Ophthalmology. 1998;105(5):878–85. https://doi.org/10.1016/S0161-6420(98)95031-X.

Russell DJ, Fallah S, Loer CJ, Riffenburgh RH. A comprehensive model for correcting RNFL readings of varying signal strengths in cirrus optical coherence tomography. J Invest Ophthalmol Vis Sci. 2014;55(11):7297–302. https://doi.org/10.1167/iovs.14-14993.

Savini G, Zanini M, Barboni P. Influence of pupil size and cataract on retinal nerve fiber layer thickness measurements by Stratus OCT. J Glaucoma. 2006;15(4):336–40. https://doi.org/10.1097/01.ijg.0000212244.64584.c2.

Savini G, Carbonelli M, Parisi V, Barboni P. Effect of pupil dilation on retinal nerve fibre layer thickness measurements and their repeatability with Cirrus HD-OCT. Eye (London, England). 2010;24(9):1503–8. https://doi.org/10.1038/eye.2010.66.

Savini G, Barboni P, Parisi V, Carbonelli M. The influence of axial length on retinal nerve fibre layer thickness and optic-disc size measurements by spectral-domain OCT. Br J Ophthalmol. 2012;96(1):57–61. https://doi.org/10.1136/bjo.2010.196782.

Savino PJ, Glaser JS, Rosenberg MA. A clinical analysis of pseudopapilledema. II. Visual field defects. Arch Ophthalmol (Chicago, Ill: 1960). 1979;97(1):71–5. https://doi.org/10.1001/archopht.1979.01020010011002.

Sayed MS, Margolis M, Lee RK. Green disease in optical coherence tomography diagnosis of glaucoma. Curr Opin Ophthalmol. 2017;28(2):139–53.

Stein DM, Wollstein G, Ishikawa H, Hertzmark E, Noecker RJ, Schuman JS. Effect of corneal drying on optical coherence tomography. Ophthalmology. 2006;113(6):985–91. https://doi.org/10.1016/j.ophtha.2006.02.018.

Stein JD, Talwar N, Laverne AM, Nan B, Lichter PR. Trends in use of ancillary glaucoma tests for patients with open-angle glaucoma from 2001 to 2009. Ophthalmology. 2012;119(4):748–58. https://doi.org/10.1016/j.ophtha.2011.09.045.

Strouthidis NG, Yang H, Downs JC, Burgoyne CF. Comparison of clinical and three-dimensional histomorphometric optic disc margin anatomy. J Invest Ophthalmol Vis Sci. 2009a;50(5):2165–74. https://doi.org/10.1167/iovs.08-2786.

Strouthidis NG, Yang H, Fortune B, Downs JC, Burgoyne CF. Detection of optic nerve head neural canal opening within histomorphometric and spectral domain optical coherence tomography data sets. J Invest Ophthalmol Vis Sci. 2009b;50(1):214–23. https://doi.org/10.1167/iovs.08-2302.

Sull AC, Vuong LN, Price LL, et al. Comparison of spectral/Fourier domain optical coherence tomography instruments for assessment of normal macular thickness. Retina (Philadelphia, Pa). 2010;30(2):235–45. https://doi.org/10.1097/IAE.0b013e3181bd2c3b.

Taibbi G, Peterson GC, Syed MF, Vizzeri G. Effect of motion artifacts and scan circle displacements on cirrus HD-OCT retinal nerve fiber layer thickness measurements. J Invest Ophthalmol Vis Sci. 2014;55(4):2251–8. https://doi.org/10.1167/iovs.13-13276.

Vizzeri G, Bowd C, Medeiros FA, Weinreb RN, Zangwill LM. Effect of signal strength and improper alignment on the variability of stratus optical coherence tomography retinal nerve fiber layer thickness measurements. Am J Ophthalmol. 2009;148(2):249–55.e1. https://doi.org/10.1016/j.ajo.2009.03.002.

Wang G, Qiu KL, Lu XH, et al. The effect of myopia on retinal nerve fibre layer measurement: a comparative study of spectral-domain optical coherence tomography and scanning laser polarimetry. Br J Ophthalmol. 2011;95(2):255–60. https://doi.org/10.1136/bjo.2009.176768.

Weinreb RN, Aung T, Medeiros FA. The pathophysiology and treatment of glaucoma: a review. JAMA. 2014;311(18):1901–11. https://doi.org/10.1001/jama.2014.3192.

Wu Z, Vazeen M, Varma R, et al. Factors associated with variability in retinal nerve fiber layer thickness measurements obtained by optical coherence tomography. Ophthalmology. 2007;114(8):1505–12. https://doi.org/10.1016/j.ophtha.2006.10.061.

Yamashita T, Asaoka R, Tanaka M, et al. Relationship between position of peak retinal nerve fiber layer thickness and retinal arteries on sectoral retinal nerve fiber layer thickness. J Invest Ophthalmol Vis Sci. 2013;54(8):5481–8. https://doi.org/10.1167/iovs.12-11008.

Yamashita T, Kii Y, Tanaka M, et al. Relationship between supernormal sectors of retinal nerve fibre layer and axial length in normal eyes. Acta Ophthalmol. 2014;92(6):e481–7. https://doi.org/10.1111/aos.12382.

Yoo YC, Lee CM, Park JH. Changes in peripapillary retinal nerve fiber layer distribution by axial length. Optom Vis Sci. 2012;89(1):4–11. https://doi.org/10.1097/OPX.0b013e3182358008.

Zhao M, Li X. Macular retinoschisis associated with normal tension glaucoma. Graefe's Arch Clin Exp Ophthalmol. 2011;249(8):1255–8. https://doi.org/10.1007/s00417-011-1668-y.

The manufacturer's authorised representative in the EU is Springer Nature Customer Service Centre GmbH, Europaplatz 3, 69115 Heidelberg, Germany. If you have any concerns regarding our products, please contact ProductSafety@springernature.com

Printed and bound by CPI Group (UK) Ltd, Croydon, CR0 4YY
27/07/2026
02177354-0002